Clinical Diagnosis and Treatment of Chronic Pain

Clinical Diagnosis and Treatment of Chronic Pain

Guest Editors

Ferran Cuenca-Martínez
Luis Suso-Martí

MDPI

Basel • Beijing • Wuhan • Barcelona • Belgrade • Novi Sad • Cluj • Manchester

Guest Editors
Ferran Cuenca-Martínez
Department of Physiotherapy
University of Valencia
Valencia
Spain

Luis Suso-Martí
Department of Physiotherapy
University of Valencia
Valencia
Spain

Editorial Office
MDPI AG
Grosspeteranlage 5
4052 Basel, Switzerland

This is a reprint of the Special Issue, published open access by the journal *Diagnostics* (ISSN 2075-4418), freely accessible at: https://www.mdpi.com/journal/diagnostics/special_issues/U7HQ20R3F3.

For citation purposes, cite each article independently as indicated on the article page online and as indicated below:

Lastname, A.A.; Lastname, B.B. Article Title. *Journal Name* **Year**, *Volume Number*, Page Range.

ISBN 978-3-7258-6302-0 (Hbk)
ISBN 978-3-7258-6303-7 (PDF)
https://doi.org/10.3390/books978-3-7258-6303-7

Contents

About the Editors

Ferran Cuenca-Martínez

Ferran Cuenca-Martínez, researcher at the Faculty of Physiotherapy at the University of Valencia. He is interested in the study of pain and strategies of movement representation. For him, the most important aspect is not scientific productivity but surrounding himself with nice people and working happily.

Luis Suso-Martí

Luis Suso-Martí, researcher at the Faculty of Physiotherapy at the University of Valencia. He has a wide range of research interests, which makes him highly versatile. He has published more than 100 articles in international peer reviewed journals.

diagnostics

MDPI

Article

Oral Glucocorticoid Use and Long-Term Mortality in Patients with Chronic Musculoskeletal Non-Cancer Pain: A Cross-Sectional Cohort Study

Hey-Ran Choi [1,†], In-Ae Song [2,3,†] and Tak Kyu Oh [2,3,*]

1 Department of Anesthesiology and Pain Medicine, Inje University Seoul Paik Hospital, Seoul 04551, Republic of Korea; viovio04@naver.com
2 Department of Anesthesiology and Pain Medicine, Seoul National University Bundang Hospital, Seongnam 13620, Republic of Korea; songoficu@outlook.kr
3 Department of Anesthesiology and Pain Medicine, College of Medicine, Seoul National University, Seoul 01811, Republic of Korea
* Correspondence: airohtak@hotmail.com
† These authors contributed equally to the article and share first authorship.

Abstract: This study aimed to examine the associated factors of oral glucocorticoid (GC) use in patients with chronic non-cancer pain (CNCP) associated with musculoskeletal diseases (MSDs) in South Korea. Moreover, we examined whether oral GC use was associated with long-term mortality in patients with CNCP. This population-based cohort study used data from the national registration database in South Korea. Using a stratified random sampling technique, we extracted the data from 2.5% of adult patients diagnosed with MSDs in 2010. Patients with CNCP-associated MSDs who were prescribed oral GC regularly for ≥30 days were defined as GC users, while the other patients were considered to be non-GC users. A total of 1,804,019 patients with CNCP were included in the final analysis, and 9038 (0.5%) patients were GC users, while 1,794,981 (95.5%) patients were non-GC users. Some factors (old age, comorbid status, pain medication use, and MSD) were associated with GC use among patients with CNCP. Moreover, in the multivariable time-dependent Cox regression model, GC users showed a 1.45-fold higher 10-year all-cause mortality (hazard ratio: 1.45, 95% confidence interval: 1.36–1.54; $p < 0.001$) than non-GC users. In South Korea, the 10-year all-cause mortality risk increased in the patients with CNCP using GC.

Keywords: pain; glucocorticoids; steroids; arthritis; rheumatoid; osteoarthritis; gout

1. Introduction

Chronic non-cancer pain (CNCP) is chronic pain that is not associated with cancer [1], and its global prevalence was reported to be one adult in five in 2010 [2]. CNCP is associated with increased substance abuse, emergency department utilization, and inpatient hospitalization [3], exerting a substantial social and economic burden on affected individuals and societies [4].

Glucocorticoids (GCs) are steroid hormones and are commonly prescribed among patients with chronic medical illnesses for 1.2% in the United States [5] and 1.0% in the United Kingdom [6], respectively. Both immunosuppressive and anti-inflammatory effects are the main mechanisms of GCs [7], which inhibit the production of the two main inflammatory products such as prostaglandins and leukotrienes [8]. Therefore, oral GCs have been prescribed to patients with various chronic medical conditions because of their immunosuppressive and anti-inflammatory effects [9–12]. Moreover, oral GC can be prescribed as an adjuvant analgesic to patients who experience severe pain [13]. Therefore, patients diagnosed with musculoskeletal diseases (MSDs) with CNCP may be prescribed oral GC as an adjuvant analgesic. Oral GC use reportedly causes various side effects, such as dysfunction of major organ systems including gastrointestinal, cardiovascular, endocrine, and neuropsychiatric dysfunction [14]. Moreover, increased long-term mortality was observed in oral GC use in the general adult population in previous studies [15,16]. However, the association between long-term mortality and oral GC use in patients with MSDs and CNCP has not been elucidated.

Thus, we aimed to examine whether oral GC use was associated with long-term mortality. We hypothesized that oral GC use was associated with increased long-term mortality in patients with CNCP.

2. Materials and Methods

2.1. Study Design and Ethical Statement

We assert that all procedures contributing to this work comply with the ethical standards of the relevant national and institutional committees on human experimentation and the Helsinki Declaration of 1975, as revised in 2008. All human patient procedures were approved by the Institutional Review Board (IRB) of the Seoul National University Bundang Hospital (IRB approval number: X-2105-685-901). The Ethics Committee of (IRB of Seoul National University Bundang Hospital: X-2105-685-901) waived the requirement for informed consent because of the study's retrospective nature.

2.2. Data Source

The National Health Insurance Service (NHIS) database was used as a data source. The NHIS database includes information regarding all disease diagnoses and prescriptions for any drug or procedure because it is the sole public health insurance system in South Korea. The International Classification of Diseases and Related Health Issues 10th Revision (ICD-10) was used to register disease diagnoses in the NHIS database. The study protocol was approved by the NHIS Ethics Committee (NHIS approval number: NHIS-2021-1-615).

2.3. Study Population

The ICD-10 codes in Supplementary Material S1 were used to define all the patients with CNCP. MSDs associated with CNCP include rheumatoid arthritis (RA), osteoarthritis (OA), low back pain, neck pain, and other MSDs. Adult patients with CNCP-associated MSDs were included in this study.

2.4. GC Exposure

The prescription data of oral GC were initially collected from 1 January 2010, to 31 December 2019, and followed up to 31 December 2019. Patients with CNCP who were prescribed oral GC (prednisolone, methylprednisolone, or dexamethasone) for ≥30 days were defined as GC users. Individuals not prescribed any GC or prescribed GC for <30 days were classified as non-GC users. Exposure was defined as a prescription ≥30 days of oral GC based on the year, and the prescription date was used to determine this. For example, patients with a prescription of ≥30 days of oral GC on 1 January 2011, were considered as GC users in 2011, while those with a prescription of ≥30 days of oral GC on 31 December 2012, were considered as GC users in 2012. Although, if an oral GC user discontinued GC for more than 30 days within the same year, the patient was considered as a GC user for that year because the patient was exposed to GC for ≥30 days during that year.

Since only prescription history was used to define a GC user, it was included in the study even if a patient was prescribed for 30 days on 31 December 2010, and died before 30 January 2010.

In South Korea, when a physician prescribes a certain drug, such as GC, the relevant primary diagnosis has to be registered in the NHIS database for the patient to receive financial coverage for treatment costs. This study included the oral GC prescription data with registered ICD-10 codes of MSDs as the primary diagnosis. Therefore, oral GC prescribed in this study might be associated with CNCP-associated MSDs.

2.5. Covariates

Data on age and sex were extracted as demographic information. Information on employment status, household income level, and place of residence was collected to determine the socioeconomic status of patients with CNCP because socioeconomic status could affect pharmacological treatment in patients with CNCP [17]. Information on household income level was included in the NHIS database to determine the insurance premiums of the South Korean population. However, individuals who are too poor to pay their insurance premiums or have difficulty supporting themselves financially are assigned to the Medical Aid Program, a government program developed to cover almost all medical expenses to help reduce the burden of medical costs on individuals. Except for the patients in the Medical Aid Program, all patients were divided into four groups using the quartile ratio. Residences of all patients were classified into two groups: urban areas (Seoul and six other metropolitan cities [Incheon, Daejeon, Gwangju, Daegu, Ulsan, and Busan]) and rural areas (all other areas). Data on the Charlson comorbidity index (CCI) and details of any underlying disabilities were collected to determine the physical comorbidity status of the patients because chronic pain conditions associated MSDs could co-occur with various physical comorbidities [18]. The CCI was calculated using the registered ICD-10 codes, as shown in Supplementary Material S3. As patients with CNCP are prescribed pain medication such as opioids, gabapentin or pregabalin, paracetamol, and nonsteroidal anti-inflammatory drugs (NSAIDs), information regarding pain medication ($\geq$30 days) was also collected because history of other pain medication reflects pain severity of patients with CNCP.

2.6. Statistical Analyses

The clinicopathological characteristics between GC users and non-GC users are presented as numbers with percentages for categorical variables and mean values with standard deviation (SD) for continuous variables. *T*-tests and Chi-square tests were used to compare continuous and categorical variables among clinicopathological characteristics between GC users and non-GC users. We constructed a multivariable Cox regression model for GC use among patients with CNCP in 2010. All covariates were included in the model for multivariable adjustment, and results are presented as odds ratios (OR) with 95% confidence intervals (CI). The Hosmer–Lemeshow test was used to confirm that goodness of fit in the multivariable model was appropriate.

As exposure to GC varied between the GC and non-GC users in 2010 throughout the evaluation period (2011–2019), as shown in Supplementary Material S4, exposure to GC prescription was considered to be a time-dependent variable. All the other covariates were included in the time-dependent Cox regression model for multivariable adjustment, based on data in 2010 as time-fixed covariates. All-cause death from 1 January 2011 to 31 December 2019, was set as the event in the multivariable time-dependent Cox model.

In addition, we constructed 17 multivariable time-dependent Cox regression models for the 10-year disease-specific mortality. In these 17 models, all covariates were included for multivariable adjustment. As a sensitivity analysis, we made a multivariable time-dependent Cox regression model for 10-year all-cause mortality considering a lag-time period. In this sensitivity analysis, the evaluation period of 10-year all-cause mortality was 2012–2019, after excluding deaths in 2011, considering 2011 as a lag-time period. A variance inflation factor <2.0 was used to confirm no multicollinearity between variables in all models. The Cox regression results are presented as hazard ratios (HRs) with 95% CIs. All statistical analyses were performed using IBM SPSS (version 25.0; IBM SPSS Statistics for Windows, version 25.0, Armonk, NY, USA), and statistical significance was set at $p < 0.05$.

3. Results

3.1. Study Population

Initially, all patients were screened using the ICD-10 codes of MSDs from 2010 to 2019. The data of 800,000,000 cases of medical resource utilization with diagnoses of MSDs were extracted from the NHIS database. Owing to the large sample size, data from 2.5%

of cases with adult patients (aged ≥20 years) were extracted using a stratified random sampling technique, considering age and sex as exclusive strata for sampling. The study population was drawn from each stratum, with sizes proportional to the strata of the overall 800,000,000 cases. Finally, 19,645,161 cases were sampled using a stratified random sampling method using SAS version 9.4 (SAS Institute, Cary, NC, USA) 17. Among these, 874,171 patients diagnosed with cancer as a comorbidity were excluded to focus on those diagnosed with CNCP. Next, 756 patients who underwent surgery during the study period were excluded because acute pain after surgery could be a source of bias in determining patients with CNCP. Therefore, 18,770,234 adult patients were screened. Among them, 1,808,043 patients with CNCP in 2010 were selected. Finally, after excluding 4024 patients with CNCP who died in 2010, 1,804,019 patients with CNCP were included as shown in Figure 1.

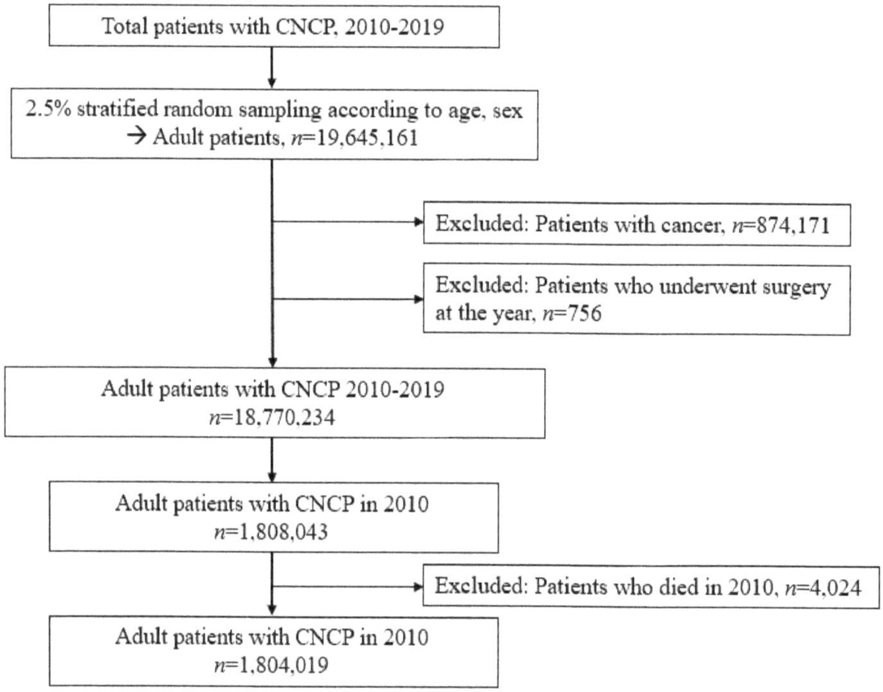

Figure 1. Patient selection flow chart.

3.2. GC Users in Cohort 2010

Table 1 shows the results of the comparison of clinicopathological characteristics between GC users and non-GC users in patients with CNCP in 2010. A total of 9038 (0.5%) patients were GC users, while 1,794,981 (95.5%) patients were non-GC users. The mean ages of the GC user and non-GC users were 57.9 ± 15.9 (mean age ± SD) and 45.9 ± 16.0 years, respectively ($p < 0.001$). Table 2 shows the results of the multivariable logistic regression model for GC use in the 2010 cohort with CNCP. Old age (OR: 1.02, 95% CI: 1.02–1.02; $p < 0.001$), living in a rural area (OR: 1.05, 95% CI: 1.01–1.09; $p = 0.037$), increased CCI (OR: 1.17, 95% CI: 1.16–1.19; $p < 0.001$), opioid use (OR: 5.40, 95% CI: 4.64–6.29; $p < 0.001$), gabapentin or pregabalin use (OR: 1.82, 95% CI: 1.63–2.04; $p < 0.001$), and NSAID use (OR: 3.49, 95% CI: 2.80–4.35; $p < 0.001$) were associated with higher odds of GC use among patients with CNCP. In addition, among MSDs, underlying RA (OR: 6.82, 95% CI: 6.45–7.21; $p < 0.001$), OA (OR: 1.19, 95% CI: 1.13–1.26; $p < 0.001$), and gout (OR: 1.77, 95% CI: 1.63–1.94; $p < 0.001$) were associated with higher odds of GC use among patients with CNCP.

Table 1. Comparison of clinicopathological characteristics between GC users and non-GC users in patients with CNCP in 2010.

Variable	GC Users n = 9038	Non-GC Users n = 1,794,981	p-Value
Age, year	57.9 (15.9)	45.9 (16.0)	<0.001
Sex, male	3396 (37.6)	872,619 (48.6)	<0.001
Having a job	4435 (49.1)	954,005 (53.1)	<0.001
Household income			<0.001
Medical aid	745 (8.2)	55,543 (3.1)	
Q1 (lowest)	1573 (17.4)	332,888 (18.5)	
Q2	1383 (15.3)	356,852 (19.9)	
Q3	2083 (23.0)	446,160 (24.9)	
Q4 (highest)	2951 (32.7)	546,506 (30.4)	
Unknown	303 (3.4)	57,032 (3.2)	
Residence			<0.001
Urban area	3839 (42.5)	834,290 (46.5)	
Rural area	5199 (57.5)	960,691 (53.5)	
CCI	0.8 (1.2)	2.3 (1.9)	<0.001
Pain medication			
Opioid use	733 (8.1)	7587 (0.4)	<0.001
Gabapentin or pregabalin	414 (4.6)	8896 (0.5)	<0.001
Paracetamol	531 (5.9)	6792 (0.4)	<0.001
NSAIDs	102 (1.1)	1686 (0.1)	<0.001
Underlying MSDs			
RA	2793 (30.9)	31,757 (1.8)	<0.001
OA	4247 (47.0)	287,524 (16.0)	<0.001
LBP	4362 (48.3)	422,588 (23.5)	<0.001
Neck pain	1302 (14.4)	132,105 (7.4)	<0.001
Gout	672 (7.4)	22,356 (1.2)	<0.001
Other MSD	6326 (70.0)	449,647 (25.1)	<0.001

GC, glucocorticoid; CNCP, chronic non-cancer pain; CCI, Charlson comorbidity index; NSAIDs, non-steroidal anti-inflammatory drugs; MSD, musculoskeletal disease; RA, rheumatoid arthritis; OA, osteoarthritis; and LBP, low back pain.

Table 2. Multivariable logistic regression model for GC use in the 2010 cohort with CNCP.

Variable	OR (95% CI)	p-Value
Age, year	1.02 (1.02, 1.02)	<0.001
Sex, male (vs. female)	0.99 (0.95, 1.04)	0.668
Having a job	1.01 (0.96, 1.05)	0.771
Household income		
Medical aid	1	
Q1 (lowest)	0.85 (0.77, 0.94)	0.001
Q2	0.78 (0.70, 0.86)	<0.001
Q3	0.86 (0.78, 0.94)	0.001
Q4 (highest)	0.85 (0.78, 0.93)	<0.001
Unknown	0.89 (0.77, 1.02)	0.085
Residence		
Urban area	1	
Rural area	1.05 (1.01, 1.09)	0.037
CCI, point	1.17 (1.16, 1.19)	<0.001
Pain medication		
Opioid use	5.40 (4.64, 6.29)	<0.001
Gabapentin or pregabalin	1.82 (1.63, 2.04)	<0.001
Paracetamol	0.80 (0.66, 0.94)	0.007
NSAIDs	3.49 (2.80, 4.35)	<0.001

Table 2. *Cont.*

Variable	OR (95% CI)	*p*-Value
Underlying MSDs		
RA	6.82 (6.45, 7.21)	<0.001
OA	1.19 (1.13, 1.26)	<0.001
LBP	0.96 (0.91, 1.01)	0.080
Neck pain	0.92 (0.86, 0.98)	0.008
Gout	1.77 (1.63, 1.94)	<0.001
Other MSD	2.67 (2.53, 1.94)	<0.001

GC, glucocorticoid; CNCP, chronic non-cancer pain; OR, odds ratio; CI, confidence interval; CCI, Charlson comorbidity index; NSAIDs, non-steroidal anti-inflammatory drugs; MSD, musculoskeletal disease; RA, rheumatoid arthritis; OA, osteoarthritis; and LBP, low back pain.

3.3. Survival Analyses

Table 3 shows the results of the multivariable time-dependent Cox regression model for 10-year all-cause mortality among cohorts with CNCP in 2010. GC users showed a 1.69-fold higher 10-year all-cause mortality (HR: 1.45, 95% CI: 1.36–1.54; $p < 0.001$) than non-GC users. All other HRs with 95% CIs in the multivariable time-dependent Cox regression model were presented in Supplementary Material S5. In a sensitivity analysis considering the lag-time period, GC users showed a 1.39-fold higher 10-year all-cause mortality (HR: 1.39, 95% CI: 1.35–1.43; $p < 0.001$) than non-GC users. Table 4 shows the results of the survival analyses of the 10-year disease-specific mortality. The GC users showed a higher 10-year mortality than non-GC users due to infection (HR: 2.00, 95% CI: 1.64–2.57; $p < 0.001$); cancer (HR: 1.18, 95% CI: 1.05–1.30; $p = 0.005$); blood disease (HR: 3.25, 95% CI: 1.90–5.02; $p < 0.001$); circulatory disease (HR: 1.30, 95% CI: 1.20–1.45; $p < 0.001$); respiratory disease (HR: 3.00, 95% CI: 2.75–3.30; $p < 0.001$); digestive disease (HR: 1.28, 95% CI: 1.05–1.51; $p = 0.032$); skin disease (HR: 3.40, 95% CI: 1.85–6.00; $p < 0.001$); MSD (HR: 8.50, 95% CI: 6.25–10.25; $p < 0.001$); genitourinary disease (HR: 1.58, 95% CI: 1.25–1.95; $p < 0.001$); abnormal clinical and laboratory findings (HR: 1.30, 95% CI: 1.13–1.50; $p = 0.001$); and injury, poisoning and certain other consequences of external causes (HR: 1.22, 95% CI: 1.05–1.41; $p = 0.010$).

Table 3. Multivariable time-dependent Cox regression model for 10-year all-cause mortality among cohort with CNCP in 2010.

Variable	HR (95% CI)	*p*-Value
Multivariable model		
GC user (vs. non-GC users)	1.45 (1.36, 1.54)	<0.001
Sensitivity analysis considering lag-time period		
GC user (vs. non-GC users)	1.39 (1.35, 1.43)	<0.001

GC, glucocorticoid; CNCP, chronic non-cancer pain; HR, hazard ratio; and CI, confidence interval.

Table 4. Survival analyses of the 10-year disease-specific mortality using time-dependent Cox regression model.

Mortality	Event (*n*, %)	HR (95% CI)	*p*-Value
Infectious mortality			
Non-GC user	3091/1,794,981 (0.2)	1	
GC user	81/9038 (0.9)	2.00 (1.64, 2.57)	<0.001
Cancer mortality			
Non-GC user	28,271/1,794,981 (1.6)	1	
GC user	307/9038 (3.4)	1.18 (1.05, 1.30)	0.005
Blood disease mortality			
Non-GC user	281/1,794,981 (0.0)	1	
GC user	11/9038 (0.1)	3.25 (1.90, 5.02)	<0.001

Table 4. *Cont.*

Mortality	Event (*n*, %)	HR (95% CI)	*p*-Value
Endocrine disease mortality			
Non-GC user	4527/1,794,981 (0.3)	1	
GC user	89/9038 (1.0)	1.20 (0.90, 1.42)	0.072
Mental disease mortality			
Non-GC user	2029/1,794,981 (0.1)	1	
GC user	16/9038 (0.2)	0.78 (0.45, 1.25)	0.215
Nervous disease mortality			
Non-GC user	4547/1,794,981 (0.3)	1	
GC user	62/9038 (0.7)	1.21 (0.85, 1.42)	0.320
Circulatory disease mortality			
Non-GC user	24,965/1,794,981 (1.4)	1	
GC user	412/9038 (4.6)	1.30 (1.20, 1.45)	<0.001
Respiratory disease mortality			
Non-GC user	11,881/1,794,981 (0.7)	1	
GC user	450/9038 (5.0)	3.00 (2.75, 3.30)	<0.001
Digestive disease mortality			
Non-GC user	4645/1,794,981 (0.3)	1	
GC user	69/9038 (0.8)	1.28 (1.05, 1.51)	0.032
Skin disease mortality			
Non-GC user	230/1,794,981 (0.0)	1	
GC user	10/9038 (0.1)	3.40 (1.85, 6.00)	<0.001
Musculoskeletal disease mortality			
Non-GC user	607/1,794,981 (0.0)	1	
GC user	73/9038 (0.8)	8.50 (6.25, 10.25)	<0.001
Genitourinary disease mortality			
Non-GC user	2876/1,794,981 (0.2)	1	
GC user	74/9038 (0.8)	1.58 (1.25, 1.95)	<0.001
Mortality due to event during pregnancy, childbirth, and the puerperium			
Non-GC user	15/1,794,981 (0.0)	1	
GC user	0/9038 (0.0)	0.00 (0.00-)	0.995
Congenital disease mortality			
Non-GC user	48/1,794,981 (0.0)	1	
GC user	2/9038 (0.0)	3.48 (0.85, 15.85)	0.102
Mortality associated symptoms, signs, and abnormal clinical and laboratory findings			
Non-GC user	10,300/1,794,981 (0.6)	1	
GC user	149/9038 (1.6)	1.30 (1.13, 1.50)	0.001
Mortality due to injury, poisoning, and certain other consequences of external causes			
Non-GC user	10,848/1,794,981 (0.6)	1	
GC user	118/9038 (1.3)	1.22 (1.05, 1.41)	0.010
Mortality due to factors influencing health status and contact with health services			
Non-GC user	41/1,794,981 (0.0)	1	
GC user	0/9038 (0.0)	0.00 (0.00-)	0.970

GC, glucocorticoid; HR, hazard ratio; and CI.

3.4. Proportion of GC Use in Patients with CNCP from 2010 to 2019

Figure 2 shows the proportion of GC users among patients with CNCP from 2010 to 2019. In 2010, the proportion of GC users was 0.5% (9194/1,808,043), gradually increasing to 0.8% (14,566/1,892,913) in 2019. The overall proportion of GC users among patients with CNCP was 0.6% (119,834/18,770,234) during 2010–2019.

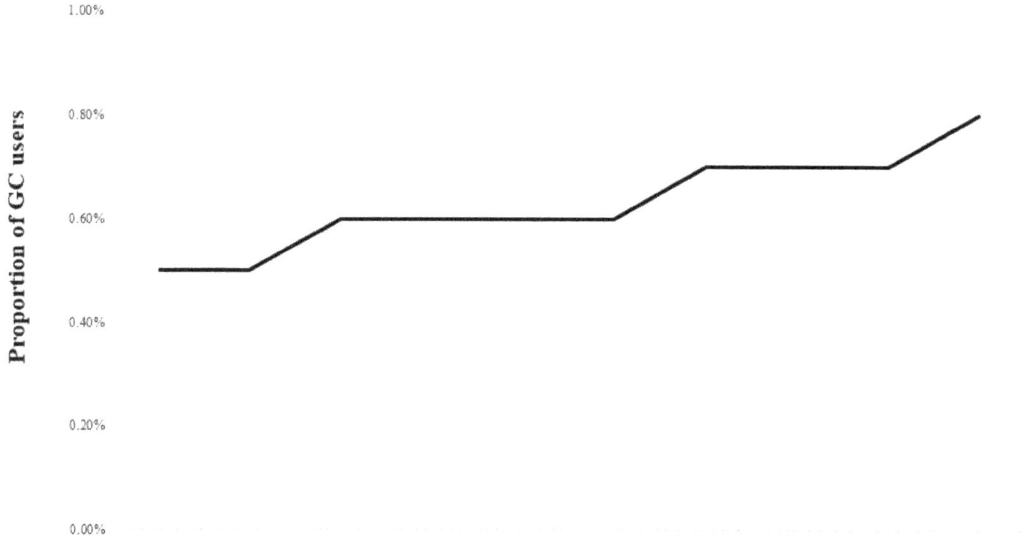

Year	2010	2011	2012	2013	2014	2015	2016	2017	2018	2019
GC user, *n*	9,194	10,049	10,760	11,195	11,666	12,331	12,724	13,296	14,053	14,566
GC user, %	0.50%	0.50%	0.60%	0.60%	0.60%	0.60%	0.70%	0.70%	0.70%	0.80%
Total, *n*	1,808,043	1,835,044	1,855,017	1,869,978	1,887,462	1,901,335	1,907,627	1,908,562	1,904,253	1,892,913

Figure 2. Proportion of glucocorticoid (GC) users in patients with chronic non-cancer pain (CNCP) from 2010 to 2019.

4. Discussion

This population-based cohort study showed that certain factors (old age, comorbid status, pain medication, and MSD) were identified as potential risk factors for GC use among patients with CNCP. Moreover, GC use was associated with an increased 10-year all-cause mortality among patients with CNCP. Our results suggest that GC use may be a potential risk factor for poor long-term survival among patients with CNCP. The proportion of GC use also increased from 2010 to 2019 in South Korea.

Some analgesics, such as opioids, gabapentin, pregabalin, and NSAIDs, were associated with GC use among patients with CNCP. A previous cohort study reported that NSAIDs and opioid use were associated with GC use among patients with RA [19]. Moreover, GCs are commonly prescribed with opioids and NSAIDs for patients with rheumatic diseases, such as RA, ankylosing spondylitis, and psoriatic arthritis [20], which has been reported to be associated with increased NSAIDs and opioid use with GC among these patients. GC is an adjuvant analgesic often prescribed with other analgesics, such as NSAIDs and opioids [13,21]. Patients with MSDs and CNCP might be prescribed other analgesics, such as NSAIDs and opioids, first, and GC might be prescribed as a secondary adjuvant analgesic for patients with severe CNCP. In addition to RA, underlying OA and gout were associated with increased GC use among patients with CNCP. GC is prescribed to alleviate inflammation, pain, and other symptoms in patients with OA and gout [22]. However, the benefit of GC administration in patients with gout remains controversial [23] and requires further research.

GC users have lower average CCI points than non-users (as depicted in Table 1), while higher CCI was associated with higher odds of GC use among patients with CNCP (as depicted in Table 2). The results in Table 2 are more important because all covariates were included in that multivariable model. There are two points that might explain these results. First, patients with severe pain are more likely to have other underlying medical conditions [18]. Second, patients with chronic pain are likely to visit medical institutions more frequently than those without pain, so there is a possibility that other diseases can be diagnosed more easily [24].

The relationship between GC exposure and increased mortality has been examined in patients with asthma and RA [25,26]. In South Korea, the number of GC users in the adult population has grown and is associated with an elevated risk of long-term mortality [16]. Long-term GC administration is known to cause serious adverse effects such as immunosuppression, which increases the risk of infection [27] and impairs immunotherapy outcomes [28,29]. In this study, the risk of 10-year infectious mortality was 2.08-fold higher in GC users than in non-GC users among patients with CNCP.

Interestingly, the 10-year mortality risk due to MSDs was highest at 7.04 HR in GC users compared to non-GC users among patients with CNCP. In this study, most MSD-related deaths were due to age-related osteoporosis with current pathological fractures (M80). As long-term GC exposure is known to cause osteoporotic fractures [30], GC users among patients with CNCP had a higher mortality risk due to osteoporotic fractures than non-GC users. Moreover, the 10-year mortality risk due to respiratory diseases was higher (HR: 3.14) in GC users than non-GC users among patients with CNCP. Most respiratory disease-related deaths occur because of pneumonia (J18) and chronic obstructive pulmonary disease with acute lower respiratory tract infection (J44). An increased risk of infection is a well-documented major side effect of long-term GC exposure owing to its immunosuppressive effect [31]. Moreover, a previous cohort study reported that lower respiratory tract infection was the most common complication in patients who received systemic GC [32], consistent with the present study's findings.

There were several limitations in this study. As we extracted only 2.5% of patients as sampled using a stratified random sampling technique, there might be differences between the sampled patients with CNCP and total patients with CNCP in South Korea. Second, we could not evaluate and adjust the severity of MSD. For example, the duration and severity of pain in each MSD might influence the use of GC and lead to increased long-term mortality in GC users. Third, some important information, such as body mass index and lifestyle factors, were not used as covariates in this study because the NHIS database did not contain it. Fourth, as we used GC prescription data for determining its users, the actual compliance of GC among GC users was not evaluated in this study. Fifth, as we used registered ICD-10 codes of MSDs to define our study population, it was not definite that our population with MSDs had CNCP. Therefore, the results should be carefully interpreted. Lastly, there might be the possibility of confounding by indication. GC users might have more severe diseases, such as medical conditions, leading to poor long-term survival outcomes. Moreover, GC could also be a surrogate of high MSD activities, which themselves already contribute to poor outcomes. Therefore, the results should be interpreted carefully.

5. Conclusions

In conclusion, certain factors, such as old age, comorbid status, pain medicines (opioid, gabapentin or pregabalin, NSAIDs) use, and MSD (RA, OA, and gout) were potential risk factors for GC use among patients with CNCP. In addition, the 10-year all-cause mortality risk increased among the patients with CNCP using GC. Our results suggest that patients with CNCP who were prescribed GC were at high risk of poor long-term survival outcomes.

Supplementary Materials: The following supporting information can be downloaded at: https://www.mdpi.com/article/10.3390/diagnostics13152521/s1, Supplementary Material S1. ICD-10 codes, Supplementary Material S2. ICD-code for disease-specific mortality, Supplementary Material S3. The ICD-10 codes used by comorbidity to compute the Charlson comorbidity index, Supplementary Material S4. GC exposure during 2011–2019, Supplementary Material S5. Multivariable time-dependent Cox regression model for all-cause mortality during 2012–2019 among cohort with CNCP in 2010.

Author Contributions: T.K.O. and H.-R.C. contributed to the study design, analyzed the data, and drafted the first manuscript. I.-A.S. contributed to the data acquisition, analyzed the data, and drafted the revised version of manuscript. All authors have read and agreed to the published version of the manuscript.

Funding: This research received no external funding.

Institutional Review Board Statement: All human patient procedures were approved by the Institutional Review Board (IRB) of the Seoul National University Bundang Hospital (IRB approval number: X-2105-685-901, approval date: 29 April 2021).

Informed Consent Statement: The requirement for informed consent was waived by the Ethics Committee of (IRB of Seoul National University Bundang Hospital: X-2105-685-901) because of the retrospective nature of the study.

Data Availability Statement: All data are available upon reasonable request from the corresponding author.

Conflicts of Interest: The authors declare no conflict of interest.

References

1. Fishman, S.M. *Bonica's Management of Pain*; LWW: Philadelphia, PA, USA, 2012.
2. Vos, T.; Flaxman, A.D.; Naghavi, M.; Lozano, R.; Michaud, C.; Ezzati, M.; Shibuya, K.; Salomon, J.A.; Abdalla, S.; Aboyans, V.; et al. Years lived with disability (YLDs) for 1160 sequelae of 289 diseases and injuries 1990–2010: A systematic analysis for the Global Burden of Disease Study 2010. *Lancet* **2012**, *380*, 2163–2196. [CrossRef] [PubMed]
3. John, W.S.; Wu, L.-T. Chronic non-cancer pain among adults with substance use disorders: Prevalence, characteristics, and association with opioid overdose and healthcare utilization. *Drug Alcohol Depend.* **2020**, *209*, 107902. [CrossRef]
4. Turk, D.C.; Wilson, H.D.; Cahana, A. Treatment of chronic non-cancer pain. *Lancet* **2011**, *377*, 2226–2235. [CrossRef]
5. Overman, R.A.; Yeh, J.-Y.; Deal, C.L. Prevalence of oral glucocorticoid usage in the United States: A general population perspective. *Arthritis Care Res.* **2012**, *65*, 294–298. [CrossRef] [PubMed]
6. Van Staa, T.P.; Leufkens, H.G.M.; Abenhaim, L.; Begaud, B.; Zhang, B.; Cooper, C. Use of oral corticosteroids in the United Kingdom. *QJM Int. J. Med.* **2000**, *93*, 105–111. [CrossRef]
7. Boumpas, D.T.; Chrousos, G.P.; Wilder, R.L.; Cupps, T.R.; Balow, J.E. Glucocorticoid Therapy for Immune-Mediated Diseases: Basic and Clinical Correlates. *Ann. Intern. Med.* **1993**, *119*, 1198–1208. [CrossRef] [PubMed]
8. Goppelt-Struebe, M.; Wolter, D.; Resch, K. Glucocorticoids inhibit prostaglandin synthesis not only at the level of phospholipase A2 but also at the level of cyclo-oxygenase/PGE isomerase. *Br. J. Pharmacol.* **1989**, *98*, 1287–1295. [CrossRef] [PubMed]
9. Keatings, V.M.; Jatakanon, A.; Worsdell, Y.M.; Barnes, P.J. Effects of inhaled and oral glucocorticoids on inflammatory indices in asthma and COPD. *Am. J. Respir. Crit. Care Med.* **1997**, *155*, 542–548. [CrossRef]
10. Tait, A.S.; Butts, C.L.; Sternberg, E.M. The role of glucocorticoids and progestins in inflammatory, autoimmune, and infectious disease. *J. Leukoc. Biol.* **2008**, *84*, 924–931. [CrossRef]
11. Berthelot, J.-M. Comments about the article by Mouterde et al. entitled "Indications of glucocorticoids in early arthritis and rheumatoid arthritis: Recommendations for clinical practice based on data from the literature and expert opinions". Joint Bone Spine 2010;77:597-603. Low-dose prednisone and biologics: Allies rather than competitors? *Jt. Bone Spine* **2011**, *79*, 103–104. [CrossRef]
12. Dimeloe, S.; Nanzer, A.; Ryanna, K.; Hawrylowicz, C. Regulatory T cells, inflammation and the allergic response—The role of glucocorticoids and Vitamin D. *J. Steroid Biochem. Mol. Biol.* **2010**, *120*, 86–95. [CrossRef] [PubMed]
13. Watanabe, S.; Bruera, E. Corticosteroids as adjuvant analgesics. *J. Pain Symptom Manag.* **1994**, *9*, 442–445. [CrossRef] [PubMed]
14. Oray, M.; Abu Samra, K.; Ebrahimiadib, N.; Meese, H.; Foster, C.S. Long-term side effects of glucocorticoids. *Expert Opin. Drug Saf.* **2016**, *15*, 457–465. [CrossRef] [PubMed]
15. Einarsdottir, M.J.; Ekman, P.; Molin, M.; Trimpou, P.; Olsson, D.S.; Johannsson, G.; Ragnarsson, O. High Mortality Rate in Oral Glucocorticoid Users: A Population-Based Matched Cohort Study. *Front. Endocrinol.* **2022**, *13*, 918356. [CrossRef]
16. Oh, T.K.; Song, I.-A. Trends in long-term glucocorticoid use and risk of 5-year mortality: A historical cohort study in South Korea. *Endocrine* **2020**, *69*, 634–641. [CrossRef] [PubMed]
17. Atkins, N.; Mukhida, K. The relationship between patients' income and education and their access to pharmacological chronic pain management: A scoping review. *Can. J. Pain* **2022**, *6*, 142–170. [CrossRef]
18. Davis, J.A.; Robinson, R.L.; Le, T.K.; Xie, J. Incidence and impact of pain conditions and comorbid illnesses. *J. Pain Res.* **2011**, *4*, 331–345. [CrossRef]
19. Black, R.J.; Lester, S.; Buchbinder, R.; Barrett, C.; Lassere, M.; March, L.; Whittle, S.; Hill, C.L. Factors associated with oral glucocorticoid use in patients with rheumatoid arthritis: A drug use study from a prospective national biologics registry. *Thromb. Haemost.* **2017**, *19*, 253. [CrossRef]
20. Hunter, T.; Nguyen, C.; Birt, J.; Smith, J.; Shan, M.; Tan, H.; Lisse, J.; Isenberg, K. Pain Medication and Corticosteroid Use in Ankylosing Spondylitis, Psoriatic Arthritis, and Rheumatoid Arthritis in the United States: A Retrospective Observational Study. *Rheumatol. Ther.* **2021**, *8*, 1371–1382. [CrossRef]

21. Vyvey, M. Steroids as pain relief adjuvants. *Can. Fam. Physician* **2010**, *56*, 1295–1297.
22. Savvidou, O.; Milonaki, M.; Goumenos, S.; Flevas, D.; Papagelopoulos, P.; Moutsatsou, P. Glucocorticoid signaling and osteoarthritis. *Mol. Cell Endocrinol.* **2018**, *480*, 153–166. [CrossRef]
23. Liu, X.; Sun, D.; Ma, X.; Li, C.; Ying, J.; Yan, Y. Benefit-risk of corticosteroids in acute gout patients: An updated meta-analysis and economic evaluation. *Steroids* **2017**, *128*, 89–94. [CrossRef] [PubMed]
24. Foley, H.E.; Knight, J.C.; Ploughman, M.; Asghari, S.; Audas, R. Association of chronic pain with comorbidities and health care utilization: A retrospective cohort study using health administrative data. *Pain* **2021**, *162*, 2737–2749. [CrossRef] [PubMed]
25. del Rincón, I.; Battafarano, D.F.; Restrepo, J.F.; Erikson, J.M.; Escalante, A. Glucocorticoid Dose Thresholds Associated with All-Cause and Cardiovascular Mortality in Rheumatoid Arthritis. *Arthritis Rheumatol.* **2014**, *66*, 264–272. [CrossRef] [PubMed]
26. Lee, H.; Ryu, J.; Nam, E.; Chung, S.J.; Yeo, Y.; Park, D.W.; Park, T.S.; Moon, J.-Y.; Kim, T.-H.; Sohn, J.W.; et al. Increased mortality in patients with corticosteroid-dependent asthma: A nationwide population-based study. *Eur. Respir. J.* **2019**, *54*, 1900804. [CrossRef]
27. Klein, N.C.; Go, C.H.-U.; Cunha, B.A. Infections associated with steroid use. *Infect. Dis. Clin. N. Am.* **2001**, *15*, 423–432. [CrossRef]
28. Wolfe, F.; Caplan, L.; Michaud, K. Treatment for rheumatoid arthritis and the risk of hospitalization for pneumonia: Associations with prednisone, disease-modifying antirheumatic drugs, and anti–tumor necrosis factor therapy. *Arthritis Rheum.* **2006**, *54*, 628–634. [CrossRef]
29. Flint, T.R.; Janowitz, T.; Connell, C.M.; Roberts, E.W.; Denton, A.E.; Coll, A.P.; Jodrell, D.I.; Fearon, D.T. Tumor Induced IL-6 Reprograms Host Metabolism to Suppress Anti-tumor Immunity. *Cell Metab.* **2016**, *24*, 672–684. [CrossRef]
30. Buckley, L.; Humphrey, M.B. Glucocorticoid-Induced Osteoporosis. *New Engl. J. Med.* **2018**, *379*, 2547–2556. [CrossRef]
31. Brassard, P.; Bitton, A.; Suissa, A.; Sinyavskaya, L.; Patenaude, V.; Suissa, S. Oral Corticosteroids and the Risk of Serious Infections in Patients with Elderly-Onset Inflammatory Bowel Diseases. *Am. J. Gastroenterol.* **2014**, *109*, 1795–1802. [CrossRef]
32. Fardet, L.; Petersen, I.; Nazareth, I. Common Infections in Patients Prescribed Systemic Glucocorticoids in Primary Care: A Population-Based Cohort Study. *PLoS Med.* **2016**, *13*, e1002024. [CrossRef] [PubMed]

diagnostics

MDPI

Article

Pressure Pain Thresholds and Central Sensitization in Relation to Psychosocial Predictors of Chronicity in Low Back Pain

Anke Steinmetz [1,*], Franziska Hacke [2] and Karl-Stefan Delank [3]

1 Physical and Rehabilitation Medicine, Department of Trauma, Reconstructive Surgery and Rehabilitation Medicine, University Medicine Greifswald, 17475 Greifswald, Germany
2 Department of Geriatrics, Martin-Luther-University Halle-Wittenberg, 06120 Halle/Saale, Germany
3 Department of Orthopedic and Trauma Surgery, Martin-Luther-University Halle-Wittenberg, 06120 Halle/Saale, Germany
* Correspondence: anke.steinmetz@med.uni-greifswald.de; Tel.: +49-3834-86-6695

Abstract: (1) Background: Peripheral, as well as central, sensitization have been described in chronic low back pain (cLBP). The purpose of this study is to investigate the influence of psychosocial factors on the development of central sensitization. (2) Methods: This prospective study investigated local and peripheral pressure pain thresholds and their dependence on psychosocial risk factors in patients with cLBP receiving inpatient multimodal pain therapy. Psychosocial factors were assessed using the Örebro Musculoskeletal Pain Screening Questionnaire (ÖMPSQ). (3) Results: A total of 90 patients were included in the study, 61 (75.4% women, 24.6% men) of whom had significant psychosocial risk factors. The control group consisted of 29 patients (62.1% women, 37.9% men). At baseline, patients with psychosocial risk factors showed significantly lower local and peripheral pressure pain thresholds, suggesting central sensitization, compared to the control group. Sleep quality, measured by the Pittsburgh Sleep Quality Index (PSQI), was also correlated with altered PPTs. After multimodal therapy, all participants reported increased local pain thresholds compared to at admission, independent of psychosocial chronification factors. (4) Conclusions: Psychosocial chronicity factors measured using the ÖMPSQ have a significant influence on pain sensitization in cLBP. A 14-day multimodal pain therapy increased local, but not peripheral, pressure pain thresholds.

Keywords: pressure pain thresholds; central sensitization; Örebro Musculoskeletal Pain Screening Questionnaire (ÖMPSQ); yellow flags; cLBP; sleep disorders; Pittsburgh Sleep Quality Index (PSQI)

1. Introduction

Chronic musculoskeletal pain is associated with reduced pressure pain thresholds [1–6]. In chronic pain, this phenomenon occurs not only locally, but also on peripheral locations far from the primary pain region. As such, in the context of central sensitization, pain thresholds decline at a distance from the original pain region [1,4,6]. In contrast, generalized hyperalgesia is not observed in patients with new-onset or acute pain syndromes [1,7,8].

However, it is not only chronic pain patients who experience a lowering of pain thresholds. Psychological disorders can also have an influence on pain sensitivity. Patients with major depression showed significantly reduced pressure pain thresholds compared to healthy control subjects [9,10]. With regard to therapeutic options for improving hyperalgesia, mainly individual treatment methods (e.g., training on the bicycle ergometer, segmental stabilization exercises) have been investigated for their potential in changing lowered pressure pain thresholds. Various studies have showed desensitization directly after completing a therapy session [7,11,12]. Only Cho et al. investigated an exercise program over several weeks and was also able to demonstrate an increase in pressure pain thresholds [13]. However, it is not yet known how a complex inpatient therapy program affects central and peripheral sensitization in contrast to individual outpatient therapies.

Especially in the case of degenerative spinal pathologies, conservative or combined treatment approaches with minimally invasive therapies have been discussed and investigated in recent years [14]. Precise diagnostics in chronic back pain must of course collect and evaluate clinical and radiological findings in order to be able to interpret the function and morphological changes, as well as psychosocial factors [15]. Because chronic pain, especially back pain, often occurs in combination with psychological disorders, it is frequently difficult to differentiate the cause of the hyperalgesia. Meints et al. demonstrated that pain sensitization was associated with greater catastrophizing [16]. The question arises whether chronic back pain patients with typical psychosocial factors and predictors for chronification also have lowered pressure pain thresholds compared to solely back pain patients.

Difficulties falling asleep, frequent awakenings, reduced sleep time and reduced sleep quality are factors that patients with chronic low back pain suffer from significantly more often than healthy people [17–20]. Despite the use of pain medication, the estimated prevalence of sleep disturbance is 58.7% [21]. A total of 42% of patients with chronic low back pain sleep less than six hours per night, and about one fifth of them even report less than four hours of sleep [22]. The risk of developing sleep problems increases up to 3.8 fold after a week of experiencing back pain [20]. Alsaadi et al. were able to demonstrate a bidirectional relationship between pain and sleep problems. The day after poor sleep showed increased pain intensity and, conversely, after days of severe pain, sleep quality decreased [23].

Patients affected by both back pain and sleep disturbances also frequently develop depressive episodes and anxiety disorders. Conversely, back pain patients with depressive episodes and anxiety disorders are additionally more often diagnosed with sleep disorders [24].

Furthermore, reduced sleep quality is also highly relevant in chronic pain patients. Although statistically significant correlations between chronic lumbar back pain and sleep disturbances have already been demonstrated [17–20], and chronic pain is already associated with reduced pressure pain thresholds [1,3,6], little is known about how far sleep affects pressure pain thresholds in chronic low back pain. Only for patients with rheumatoid arthritis has an association of sleep disturbances with lowered pressure pain thresholds been detected [25].

The influence of sleep on central sensitization mechanisms has gained particular attention since the recently introduced pain mechanism of nociplastic pain developed by the IASP [IASP website (https://www.iasp-pain.org/resources/terminology/?ItemNumber=1698, accessed on 15 January 2023]). Sleep disorders are listed here as one of the associated comorbidities of nociplastic pain [26].

The aim of this study was to investigate to what extent psychosocial factors, indicating a risk of developing chronic pain, influence central nociceptive sensitization processes among patients with chronic lumbar back pain. The primary question was whether patients with chronic low back pain and psychosocial risk factors exhibited generalized hyperalgesia in the context of central pain processing with reduced remote pain thresholds, in addition to a reduction in local pressure pain thresholds. Furthermore, the effect of 14-day multimodal pain therapy on local and peripheral pressure pain thresholds should be investigated, with particular focus on the potential dependence or association with the psychosocial risk factors. To our knowledge, this aspect has not yet been addressed in the literature. Secondly, the impact of sleep disturbances on peripheral and central pain sensitization in patients with cLBP should be investigated in detail to understand to what extent differences in both the quality and quantity of sleep are evident.

It is of particular interest whether inpatient multimodal pain therapy is able to eliminate local and central sensitization mechanisms and lead to general desensitization.

2. Materials and Methods

2.1. Study Design

A cross-sectional design with a prospective follow-up was used to investigate local and peripheral pressure pain thresholds. Patients with psychosocial risk factors (case group) were compared with patients without psychosocial risk factors (control group). The case group consisted of patients with chronic lumbar pain syndromes and a high risk of chronicity, defined by the cut-off of 100 points (or more) in the Örebro Musculoskeletal Pain Screening Questionnaire (ÖMPSQ) [27]. The control group consisted of patients with chronic lumbar pain syndromes and an ÖMPSQ score lower than 100, with a therefore assumed lower risk of chronicity [27].

The investigator of the pressure pain thresholds was blinded to group membership to avoid measurement bias. The research project was reviewed and approved by the Ethics Committee of the Medical Faculty of the University (ethics committee no. 2014-81), in accordance with the declaration of Helsinki of 1975 (in the current, revised version). Written informed consent was obtained from all patients. The study was retrospectively registered at the German Register of Clinical Trials (DRKS00028286).

2.2. Participants

Participants were recruited from patients treated in a conservative orthopedic ward at a University Hospital. Patients suitable for the study were comprehensively informed about the procedure and objectives of the study on the day of admission and included in the study after giving their written consent. A total of 114 patients were recruited from 21 July 2014 to 29 February 2016. Inclusion criteria included the presence of chronic lumbar back pain for at least a twelve-weeks duration, aged over 18 years, and sufficient knowledge of the German language. Exclusion criteria were previous spinal surgery, known traumas, infections or tumors of the spine. Female patients were not allowed to be pregnant or breastfeeding.

The case number calculation (assuming a mean effect size of $d = 0.5$, as well as $\alpha = 0.05$ and $\beta = 0.80$) indicated a group size of 41 patients each in order to obtain sufficient power. This number of cases could not be achieved in the control group despite several extensions of the implementation period, as the patient collective mainly comprised patients with a high risk of chronicity. This resulted in an unevenly distributed sample size of 61 case patients and 29 control patients.

2.3. Pressure Pain Thresholds

Pressure pain thresholds were determined using the FORCE ONE FDIX DIGITAL FORCE GAGE digital pressure algometer from Wagner Instruments (Riverside, CT, USA). The algometer was set to measure at a rate of 100 readings per second and always displayed the highest pressure measured. The round attachment surface had a diameter of 1.12 cm. Newton (N) was set as the unit of measurement on the device. Later, it was converted to kilopascals (kPa) to enable comparability with other studies.

On the day of admission, the patients were comprehensively informed about the study. Subsequently, after consenting to participate, the first measurement of the pressure pain thresholds took place (T0). The pain thresholds were determined locally over the lumbar spine and peripherally on the extremities. Local measurements were carried out in the least painful resting position for the patient, for example, in the standing or prone position in the area of the facet joints of the fourth lumbar vertebra. The pressure pain thresholds of the extremities were determined in the sitting position. For the lower extremity, measurements were taken centrally over the tibialis anterior muscle and for the upper extremity, measurements were taken over the deltoid muscle about 5 cm caudal to the acromion.

All measurements were performed bilaterally and repeated three times, and they were not measured again at exactly the same point to avoid influencing the pain threshold by the previous measurements. The time interval between measurements over the same muscle was approximately 10 s [7,28]. After 14 days of multimodal therapy, mechanical pain thresholds were measured again on the eve of discharge (T1) to investigate the influence of inpatient pain therapy on pressure pain thresholds.

2.4. Örebro Musculoskeletal Pain Screening Questionnaire (ÖMPSQ)

The ÖMPSQ was developed to determine the individual risk of developing chronic/ persistent musculoskeletal pain and contains questions addressing psychosocial factors, which have also been described as "yellow flags", contributing to the chronification process.

In the present study, this instrument was used to assess the presence of "yellow flags" in patients with chronic back pain. The cut-off set by Linton at 90 and 105 points (from 212 points maximum) is now outdated in the literature. According to a study by Linton and Boersma, with a score of 100 points, the specificity (74%) roughly corresponds to the sensitivity (76%), which is why this value was chosen as the cut-off here [27]. With a score of at least 100, increased psychosocial risk factors contributing to the persistence of back pain problem was assumed.

2.5. German Pain Questionnaire

For this study, the following parameters of the German Pain Questionnaire (2006) were used and evaluated: von Korff Questionnaire (pain intensity, disability points, severity); Hospital Anxiety and Depression Scale (HADS); and general well-being.

The combination of pain intensity, disability points and severity, according to von Korff, describe the grade of pain severity (Grade I–IV).

Severity according to von Korff was described as follows: 0 = no pain; 1 = low pain intensity (<50) and low pain-related impairment (<3 disability points); 2 = high pain intensity (>50), low pain-related impairment (<3 disability points); 3 = high pain-related impairment, moderately limiting (3–4 disability points); and 4 = high pain-related impairment, severely limiting (5–6 disability points).

The Hospital Anxiety and Depression Scale (HADS) is a screening questionnaire for anxiety and depression. For both parameters, a value greater than seven is considered borderline and a value greater than ten is considered abnormal [29].

General well-being was determined using the Marburg Questionnaire on Habitual Well-being (MFHW). A score of less than ten points indicates low general well-being.

2.6. Pittsburgh Sleep Quality Index (PSQI)

The German version of the PSQI was used to assess the subjective sleep quality of the last four weeks before admission. The total score can assume values between 0 and 21. If the cut-off of five points was exceeded, a patient was defined as a poor sleeper [30]. In addition, the average sleep time (PSQI: question 4) was considered separately. The six-hour mark was chosen as the cut-off (analogous to Marty et al., Artner et al. [17,22]).

2.7. Multimodal Pain Therapy

During the inpatient stay, the patients received multimodal pain therapy. The therapy consisted of an individual combination of the following therapy methods: interventional pain therapy; optimization of oral pain medication; manual medicine; physiotherapy; sensomotoric training; medical training therapy; relaxation methods; psychoeducational training; and psychotherapy. As a rule, about 30 passive and active therapy sessions of 30 min each on average took place within 14 days.

2.8. Statistics

For the study design, a sample size calculation was carried out using the program nQuery. The data obtained were transferred to Excel (Microsoft) and collected. IBM SPSS Statistics 22.0 for Windows was then used for the statistical evaluation and the creation of tables and graphics. The statistical processing of the metric variables was initially carried out using descriptive statistics. Means, standard deviations and 95% confidence intervals were calculated and presented. The groups were tested for homogeneity with regard to gender, age and BMI using the Chi^2 test and the t-test. Furthermore, mean differences of the pressure pain thresholds were analyzed with the help of two-sided t-tests for paired and unpaired samples. Missing values were excluded list by list. The test for equality of variance of the groups presented was carried out in each case using Levene's test. In order to determine the pairwise correlation of the individual test characteristics with each other, bivariate correlations were carried out using Pearson's correlation coefficient. The significance level was set at $p < 0.05$ in the study design.

3. Results

3.1. Demographics

Of the 90 patients included, 61 patients had an elevated ÖMPSQ score of > 100 points and were included in the case group. The control group (ÖMPSQ score $\leq$ 100 points) comprised a total of 29 patients. The age of all included patients ranged between 26 and 90 years. The body mass index showed values above normal weight on average for both patient groups. A total of 41 of the patients examined had a BMI above 30 kg/m^2 and thus manifested obesity. Neither group showed significant differences of gender distribution, mean age or BMI (see Table 1).

Table 1. Demographics.

ÖMPSQ	>100 pts. (Case Group)	<100 pts. (Control Group)	*p*
N	61	29	N.A.
Sex Female (N/%) Male (N/%)	46 (75) 15 (25)	18 (62) 11 (38)	0.192
Age (yrs) Mean (SD)	65.1 (12.5)	63.8 (11.8)	0.638
BMI (kg/m^2) Mean (SD)	30 (5.5)	29.5 (5.3)	0.715

N: number; ÖMPSQ: Örebro Musculoskeletal Pain Screening Questionnaire.

3.2. Questionnaires

The case and control groups showed significant differences ($p < 0.05$) in the questionnaire scores regarding pain intensity, severity of chronification according to v. Korff, depression, anxiety and well-being (see Table 2).

With regard to the factors of anxiety and depressiveness, the mean values of the case group with 9.38 and 9.03 points, respectively, were in the borderline range of abnormality. Correspondingly, 41% and 36% of the patients in the case group showed abnormal values of over 10 points. In the control group, the average values of 6.66 and 6.38 were within the normal range. Only 17.2% and 13.8% of the patients in the control group had abnormal scores. While both patient groups were, on average, assigned a high-pain-related impairment of a moderately limiting character according to von Korff (severity level 3 according to von Korff), the subjective pain intensity with 72.23 (of 100) points was on average significantly higher in the case group compared to the control group (60.40 points) ($p = 0.003$).

Sleep quality was reduced on average in both groups. A total of 67 out of the 90 patients were found to be poor sleepers. The prevalence of sleep disorders in this cohort was thus 74.4%. In the case group, the percentage was even higher at 80.3% compared to the control group (62.1%). The PSQI score achieved, with an average of 10.38 points, was also significantly different from the control group's score of 7.64 points.

The general well-being was only limited in the case group. With an average of 7.86 points, the score fell below the ten-point limit, while patients in the control group were still within the normal range with an average of 13.52 points (see Table 2).

Table 2. Questionnaire scores in case and control group.

		N	M	SD	SEM	*p*
ÖMPSQ	Case	61	133.28	22.496	2.880	<0.001
	Control	29	87.59	16.240	3.016	
HADS-A	Case	61	9.03	4.626	0.592	0.009
	Control	29	6.38	3.802	0.706	
HADS-D	Case	61	9.38	4.140	0.530	0.004
	Control	29	6.66	3.810	0.708	
Pain intensity	Case	61	72.23	15.959	2.043	0.003
	Control	29	60.40	19.985	3.711	
Pain severity v. Korff	Case	61	3.75	0.977	0.125	0.009
	Control	29	3.03	1.239	0.230	
MFHW	Case	58	7.86	8.008	1.051	0.003
	Control	29	13.52	8.175	1.518	
PSQI	Case	60	10.38	4.748	0.613	0.009
	Control	28	7.64	3.783	0.715	
Sleeping time [h]	Case	60	5.80	1.619	0.209	0.206
	Control	28	6.30	1.940	0.367	

N: number; M: mean; SD: standard deviation; SEM: standard error of the mean; P: *p*-value; ÖMPSQ: Örebro Musculoskeletal Pain Screening Questionnaire; HADS-A: Hospital Anxiety and Depression Scale-Anxiety; HADS-D: Hospital Anxiety and Depression Scale-Depression; MFHW: Marburg Questionnaire on Habitual Well-being; PSQI: Pittsburgh Sleep Quality Index.

3.3. Pressure Pain Thresholds

Pressure pain thresholds of the back measured at T0 were significantly lower in the case group compared to the control group ($p = 0.047$). In this group, decreased PPTs were not only displayed over the facet joints, but also peripherally over the deltoid ($p = 0.044$) and tibialis ant. ($p = 0.046$) muscles, indicating central sensitization in the patients with psychosocial factors (see Table 3). In the control group, PPTs of the back and the deltoid muscle were nearly identical, while even higher pressures were allowed above the tibialis anterior muscle. Overall, higher pressures were tolerated over the tibialis anterior muscle than over the deltoid muscle. The pain thresholds measured locally on the back were lower than the peripheral thresholds in both groups (see Table 3).

Table 3. Pain pressure thresholds case/control group T0.

		N	MW	SD	SEM	*p*
PPT Facet joints [kPa]	Case	60	222.08	119.496	15.427	0.047
	Control	29	276.70	120.326	22.344	
PPT Deltoid muscle [kPa]	Case	60	230.66	96.704	12.484	0.044
	Control	29	278.52	116.429	21.620	
PPT Tibialis anterior muscle [kPa]	Case	60	270.70	106.779	13.785	0.046
	Control	29	318.87	102.353	19.006	

N: number; M: mean; SD: standard deviation; SEM: standard error of the mean; P: *p*-value; PPT: pain pressure threshold.

The inpatient treatment of the investigated back pain patients with multimodal pain therapy resulted in a significant improvement in the mechanical pain threshold above the spine both in the case group and in the control group (without increased psychosocial factors) at T1 (Table 4). In the case group, PPTs continued to be lowered peripherally and, in fact, were significantly reduced further, so that therapy did not lead to a decline in central sensitization. In the control group, peripheral PPTs showed no significant changes compared with T0.

Table 4. Influence of multimodal pain therapy on pressure pain thresholds.

			MW	SD	SEM	p
PPT Facet joints [kPa]	Case	T0	222.08	119.496	15.427	0.005
		T1	256.33	116.098	14.988	
	Control	T0	276.70	120.326	22.344	0.006
		T1	321.07	107.573	19.976	
PPT Deltoid muscle [kPa]	Case	T0	230.66	96.703	12.484	0.025
		T1	212.39	91.527	11.816	
	Control	T0	278.52	116.429	21.620	0.123
		T1	255.06	107.512	19.965	
PPT Tibialis anterior muscle [kPa]	Case	T0	270.70	106.779	13.785	<0.001
		T1	237.27	92.713	11.969	
	Control	T0	318.87	102.353	19.006	0.133
		T1	297.10	103.604	19.239	

M: mean; SD: standard deviation; SEM: standard error of the mean; P: *p*-value; PPT: pain pressure threshold.

3.4. Correlations of Demographic Factors, Questionnaire Scores and PPTs

Finally, bivariate correlations between the PPTs, questionnaire scores and demographic variables were considered (see Table 5). This showed that with higher age, less anxiety ($p = 0.015$) was reported. The local pressure pain thresholds on the back were also less sensitive ($p = 0.001$). Furthermore, gender also had an influence on pain sensitivity. Men had higher local ($p = 0.015$) and peripheral pressure pain thresholds than women ($p = 0.001$). The higher the score in the ÖMSPQ, the higher the individual scores for depression ($p < 0.001$), anxiety ($p = 0.001$), pain intensity ($p < 0.001$) and degree of impairment according to von Korff ($p < 0.001$). General well-being, on the other hand, decreased with an increase in ÖMPSQ score ($p < 0.001$). PSQI scores also correlated positively with scores for depression ($p = 0.007$), anxiety ($p < 0.001$) and pain intensity ($p = 0.021$). General well-being was again lower the higher the PSQI score increased ($p = 0.033$).

Table 5. Correlations of demographics, questionnaire scores and PPTs.

		Age	Gender ♂	BMI	HADS-D	HADS-A	PI	v. Korff	MFHW	PSQI
Age	r	1000	0.106	0.001	−0.035	−0.256 *	−0.191	−0.059	0.130	−0.150
	P		0.319	0.996	0.742	0.015	0.071	0.580	0.231	0.163
	n	90	90	84	90	90	90	90	87	88
Gender ♂	r	0.106	1000	0.071	0.164	0.111	−0.012	−0.013	0.080	−0.213
	P	0.319		0.521	0.123	0.298	0.908	0.905	0.464	0.046
	n	90	90	84	90	90	90	90	87	88
BMI	r	0.001	0.071	1000	0.112	−0.058	−0.070	0.043	0.024	−0.100
	P	0.996	0.521		0.311	0.599	0.526	0.695	0.832	0.364
	n	84	84	84	84	84	84	84	81	84
ÖMPSQ	r	0.109	0.035	0.137	0.556 **	0.413 **	0.437 **	0.419 **	0.445 **	0.241
	P	0.306	0.741	0.215	0.000	0.000	0.000	0.000	0.000	0.024
	n	90	90	84	90	90	90	90	87	88
PPT Facet Joints	r	0.380 **	0.255 *	−0.165	−0.161	−0.181	−0.265 *	−0.139	0.194	−0.413 **
	P	0.000	0.015	0.134	0.130	0.088	0.011	0.193	0.071	0.000
	n	90	90	84	90	90	90	90	87	88

Table 5. *Cont.*

		Age	Gender ♂	BMI	HADS-D	HADS-A	PI	v. Korff	MFHW	PSQI
PPT Deltoid muscle	r	0.031	0.395 **	−0.062	−0.099	−0.054	−0.063	−0.010	0.151	−0.417 **
	P	0.773	0.000	0.576	0.355	0.617	0.560	0.926	0.166	0.000
	n	89	89	83	89	89	89	89	86	87
PPT Tibialis anterior muscle	r	0.058	0.339 **	−0.309 **	−0.168	−0.116	−0.045	−0.017	0.089	−0.368 **
	P	0.584	0.001	0.004	0.114	0.275	0.673	0.877	0.415	0.000
	n	90	90	84	90	90	90	90	87	88

Gender ♂: male; BMI: body mass index; HADS-D: Hospital Anxiety and Depression Scale-Depression; HADS-A: Hospital Anxiety and Depression Scale-Anxiety; PI: pain intensity; v. Korff: grade of severity; MFHW: Marburg Questionnaire on Habitual Well-being; PSQI: Pittsburgh Sleep Quality Index, r: Pearson; P: *p*-value; n: number; ÖMPSQ: Örebro Musculoskeletal Pain Screening Questionnaire; PPT: pain pressure threshold. * Correlation is significant at level 0.05 (two-sided), ** Correlation is significant at level 0.01 (two-sided), both shaded gray. Metric correlations were represented by Pearson's correlation coefficient. The correlations of the metric variables with gender are represented by the coefficient Eta.

4. Discussion

At baseline (T0), patients in the case group showed significantly lower pressure pain thresholds both locally and peripherally. As such, central sensitization can be assumed compared to the control group. This suggests that psychosocial chronicity factors, assessed using the ÖMPSQ at T0, are associated with pain sensitization in chronic lumbar back pain. The more pronounced the "yellow flags" are, the lower the pressure pain thresholds become.

In the literature, the overall ÖMPSQ score has not yet been linked to pressure pain thresholds. However, evidence can be found for the association of individual psychological chronicity factors, such as depression or anxiety, with pressure pain thresholds. A higher questionnaire score in anxiety and/or depression is associated with lower pressure pain thresholds [2,5,9,10]. Interestingly, Lautenbacher et al. postulated completely opposite results. Patients with depression had significantly higher pressure pain thresholds [31]. Regarding the risk factors of pain intensity and severity of impairment, a review by Hübscher et al. can be considered, in which the level of pressure pain thresholds made it possible to distinguish between patients with and without pain, without being able to predict pain intensity or severity of impairment [32]. The present results only allow a group classification (high vs. low psychosocial factors), and not a direct correlation of pain thresholds to questionnaire scores. It is therefore neither possible to predict the exact risk of chronicity via pain thresholds nor to determine the pain thresholds via the questpptionnaire scores.

One of the main results was that pain sensitization does not only occur at the site of the pain focus, but that it rather leads to generalized hyperalgesia. Comparable results were also found in other studies. Patients with chronic back pain had significantly lower pressure pain thresholds (ppts) both locally and peripherally than healthy controls [1,4,6]. In addition, Meints et al. showed that regardless of increased pain sensitivity compared to healthy controls, within the cLBP group, greater catastrophizing was associated with both greater experimental pain sensitivity and clinical pain, with deep-tissue hyperalgesia mediating between the extent of catastrophizing and clinical pain [16]. That psychosocial factors, such as catastrophizing, contribute to central pain sensitization has been discussed in several studies [33,34], but to our knowledge no studies have been conducted using a psychosocial predictive score for the development of chronic pain syndrome, such as the ÖMPSQ, so far. Based on this, the present study underscores that cLBP patients with varying degrees of psychosocial factors differ with respect to the fact that central sensitization takes place. These findings are in line with recent findings by Aoyagi et al., showing that the 2011 FM survey (Fibromyalgia Criteria and Severity Scales) identifies a subgroup of cLBP patients who exhibit central sensitization in association with greater catastrophizing, anxiety and depressive symptoms [35].

When comparing the absolute measured values in the literature, large differences can be found. While the mean values of this study range between 222 kPa and 318 kPa, depending on the case or control group and pressure location, O'Neill et al. measured significantly higher values with an average of 450 kPa or even 680 kPa in patients with chronic lumbar back pain [1,28]. Starkweather et al., on the other hand, described rather lower values with an average of 180 kPa [8]. These discrepancies can be explained, for example, by the use of different pressure algometers with headpieces of different sizes. Furthermore, the composition of the patient collective could also explain the poor comparability. This study included patients who required 14 days of inpatient pain therapy, which implies high suffering levels and a long course of the disease.

A study by Corrêa et al., which also included healthy subjects, however, shows a similar pain threshold level in the results [6]. Unfortunately, the study does not provide any information on the size of the algometer headpiece used, so it is not possible to determine beyond doubt whether the results are really comparable. Nevertheless, this study provides the opportunity to compare the pain thresholds of the control group of the present study with the pain thresholds of completely healthy subjects. Patients with chronic lumbar back pain showed lumbar ppts of 253 kPa and ppts of 262 kPa over the tibialis anterior muscle [6], which roughly correspond to the pressure pain thresholds of the present study. Healthy subjects without back pain showed lumbar ppts of 343 kPa, which were significantly higher than those of the back pain patients in this study (222 kPa and 277 kPa). This suggests that in the present study, local sensitization took place in both the case and control groups, which was to be expected due to the chronification of the pain syndrome that had taken place. However, the mean values of the peripheral pain thresholds in the healthy subjects (322 kPa) of Corrêa hardly exceed our values of the patients with back pain without psychosocial risk factors (319 kPa) [6]. This supports our hypothesis that no central sensitization took place in the control group of our study.

After 14 days of multimodal inpatient treatment, all participants showed higher local pain thresholds than at admission (T0). This phenomenon was present in the case and control groups, independent of psychosocial chronification factors. Consequently, the therapy must have contributed to the desensitization of the previously hyperalgesic areas. An increase in pressure pain thresholds after various physical therapy procedures has been described in the literature [7,11,12]. In the present study, infiltration techniques, oral analgesics and psychological therapies may additionally have supported desensitization. There are very few studies on these widespread therapeutic approaches, especially on drug effects, in the context of pressure pain thresholds. For benzodiazepines, Vuilleumer et al. could not prove an antihyperalgesic effect. Peripherally, however, inpatient treatment led to further sensitization instead of a subsequent reduction in central sensitization [36]. Nevertheless, Vaegter et al. also demonstrated improvements in local ppts on the back and no changes in remote trapezius ppts during 12-week cognitive functional therapy (a physiotherapy-guided intervention with physical, lifestyle and psychological targets), indicating no change in central sensitization [37].

From the present results, it can be concluded that the local changes regarding sensitization are reduced by 14-day pain therapy. The central processes, represented by peripheral pain thresholds, however, do not seem to have decreased in this short period of time. On the contrary, peripheral sensitization even seemed to continue in the case group. Provided that pain threshold measurement is subject to good test–retest reliability [38,39], it remains to be considered which factors could be responsible for the decrease in peripheral pain thresholds. It might well be that proinflammatory mechanisms continue to be present peripherally and maintain sensitization, which has been resolved locally by the treatment. Perhaps the local pain relief also causes a kind of shift in perception. The back is no longer the center of attention, so peripheral pain stimuli are not superimposed and rather reach the consciousness. Further studies are obviously necessary in this regard.

The prevalence of sleep disturbances was 74.4% in the entire patient population. This value is consistent with the data from the literature for patients with chronic lumbar back pain [19,20,22]. The prevalence of sleep disturbance was even higher with an ÖMPSQ score above 100 (80,3%). Furthermore, in accordance with the literature, a positive correlation of the PSQI to the individual chronicity factors mapped by the HADS-D, HADS-A, pain intensity and negatively to the MFHW can be observed [24]. It can therefore be stated that chronic back pain patients with psychosocial chronicity factors sleep less well or that pain patients who sleep less well tend to have psychosocial factors. The exact relationship between the factors cannot be deduced from the present results.

Furthermore, this study showed that poor sleepers with a PSQI score of more than five points have significantly lower pressure pain thresholds over the facet joints and the deltoid muscle. How sleep quality affects the pressure pain thresholds of chronic back pain patients has not yet been discussed in studies, so no comparative values are available. Because the PSQI correlates with other risk factors, it is also possible that only these are represented here.

Another factor that supports the importance of sleep in this context is absolute sleep time. Subjectively, this was around six hours on average. In the literature, subjective sleep times range between six and eight hours on average, regardless of the presence of chronic back pain [18,19,23,40]. Artner et al. show in their study that 42% of back pain patients sleep less than six hours [22]. In the present patient collective, about 45% of the subjects slept less than six hours per night. Additionally, they showed significantly reduced pain thresholds in comparison. This phenomenon was observed both locally and peripherally. Patients who sleep less than six hours seem to be prone to generalized hyperalgesia. Age may have acted as a possible confounding factor in this evaluation. The patients with less sleep time were significantly younger. However, a study by Donat et al. shows that pressure pain thresholds do not differ significantly in different age groups [41]. At most, there is a slight decrease in values with an increase in age, but not an increase. The correlations drawn in this study also do not reveal any correlations between age and peripheral pressure pain threshold. Nevertheless, there is a lack of comparable study results that support the influence of sleep time on pressure pain thresholds. It becomes clear that greater attention should be paid to the topic of sleep in research and therapy as a whole.

Limitations

Over the observation period, a total of 114 patients were recruited and of these, 90 patients were finally included in the study. A total of 61 patients were assigned to the case group and 29 patients were assigned to the control group. The recruitment phase was extended from the originally planned eight months to nineteen months. In total, even more than the originally planned 82 participants were recruited, but there was still asymmetry with regard to group size, which could have reduced the planned power. The patient collective of the conservative orthopedic ward of a University Hospital mainly comprised patients with a high risk of chronification. The sample size is comparable to that of similarly structured studies on the topic of pressure pain thresholds [7,8,10,25]. Asymmetries in group size can also be observed here.

Above all, the exclusion of all patients who had undergone back surgery further reduced the number of patients who could be recruited. On the other hand, studies have not yet investigated the extent to which spinal surgery influences pressure pain thresholds. As such, distortion by this could not be ruled out. Another minimizing factor was the fact that a control examination was to be carried out in all patients after the 14-day pain therapy. Because 22 patients who were already recruited discontinued the treatment prematurely, there was a further reduction in the number of patients.

Another possible limiting factor to be discussed would be that patients with a pathological score in the HADS were not excluded. However, as no correlations between the HADS-A and HADS-D with pressure pain thresholds could be shown, it can be assumed that abnormal values in the HADS did not distort the results. Nevertheless, in future studies, the presence of depression or anxiety should definitely be excluded.

5. Conclusions

In this study, we were able to demonstrate for the first time that central sensitization in patients with chronic back pain is associated with the extent of psychosocial factors known as "yellow flags" measured with the ÖMPSQ, although we cannot conclude the exact relationship from the results. Furthermore, a 14-day multimodal pain therapy influences local pressure pain thresholds, which are significantly reduced in both (case and control) groups. Central sensitization, however, could not be influenced by the therapy; unexpectedly, it even increased. Further studies are warranted to understand these mechanisms and to develop therapy strategies for the reduction and reversal of central sensitization.

Author Contributions: Conceptualization, A.S. and K.-S.D.; methodology, A.S. and F.H.; validation, A.S., F.H. and K.-S.D.; formal analysis, F.H.; investigation, F.H.; resources, K.-S.D.; data curation, F.H.; writing—original draft preparation, A.S.; writing—review and editing, A.S.; visualization, F.H.; supervision, K.-S.D.; project administration, A.S. All authors have read and agreed to the published version of the manuscript.

Funding: This research received no external funding.

Institutional Review Board Statement: The study was conducted in accordance with the Declaration of Helsinki and approved by the Institutional Review Board (or Ethics Committee) of the Medical Faculty of the University of Halle/Saale (ethics committee no. 2014-81).

Informed Consent Statement: Informed consent was obtained from all subjects involved in the study.

Data Availability Statement: The data presented in this study are available on reasonable request from the corresponding author.

Acknowledgments: We thank Sean Wiebersch for his help in language editing.

Conflicts of Interest: The authors declare no conflict of interest.

References

1. O'Neill, S.; Kjaer, P.; Graven-Nielsen, T.; Manniche, C.; Arendt-Nielsen, L. Low pressure pain thresholds are associated with, but does not predispose for, low back pain. *Eur. Spine J.* **2011**, *20*, 2120–2125. [CrossRef]
2. Sjörs, A.; Larsson, B.; Persson, A.L.; Gerdle, B. An increased response to experimental muscle pain is related to psychological status in women with chronic non-traumatic neck-shoulder pain. *BMC Musculoskelet. Disord.* **2011**, *12*, 230. [CrossRef]
3. Imamura, M.; Chen, J.; Matsubayashi, S.R.; Targino, R.A.; Alfieri, F.M.; Bueno, D.K.; Hsing, W.T. Changes in pressure pain threshold in patients with chronic nonspecific low back pain. *Spine* **2013**, *38*, 2098–2107. [CrossRef]
4. Borstad, J.; Woeste, C. The role of sensitization in musculoskeletal shoulder pain. *Braz. J. Phys. Ther.* **2015**, *19*, 251–256. [CrossRef] [PubMed]
5. Bagnato, G.; de Andres, I.; Sorbara, S.; Verduci, E.; Corallo, G.; Ferrera, A.; Morgante, S.; Roberts, W.N., Jr.; Bagnato, G. Pain threshold and intensity in rheumatic patients: Correlations with the Hamilton Depression Rating scale. *Clin. Rheumatol.* **2015**, *34*, 555–561. [CrossRef]
6. Correa, J.B.; Pena Costa, L.O.; Bastos de Oliveira, N.T.; Sluka, K.A.; Liebano, R.E. Central sensitization and changes in conditioned pain modulation in people with chronic nonspecific low back pain: A case-control study. *Exp. Brain Res.* **2015**, *233*, 2391–2399. [CrossRef]
7. Meeus, M.; Roussel, N.A.; Truijen, S.; Nijs, J. Reduced pressure pain thresholds in response to exercise in chronic fatigue syndrome but not in chronic low back pain: An experimental study. *J. Rehabil. Med.* **2010**, *42*, 884–890. [CrossRef]
8. Starkweather, A.R.; Ramesh, D.; Lyon, D.E.; Siangphoe, U.; Deng, X.; Sturgill, J.; Heineman, A.; Elswick, R.K.; Dorsey, S.G.; Greenspan, J. Acute Low Back Pain: Differential Somatosensory Function and Gene Expression Compared With Healthy No-Pain Controls. *Clin. J. Pain* **2016**, *32*, 933–939. [CrossRef]
9. Euteneuer, F.; Schwarz, M.J.; Hennings, A.; Riemer, S.; Stapf, T.; Selberdinger, V.; Rief, W. Depression, cytokines and experimental pain: Evidence for sex-related association patterns. *J. Affect. Disord.* **2011**, *131*, 143–149. [CrossRef]
10. Hennings, A.; Schwarz, M.J.; Riemer, S.; Stapf, T.M.; Selberdinger, V.B.; Rief, W. The influence of physical activity on pain thresholds in patients with depression and multiple somatoform symptoms. *Clin. J. Pain* **2012**, *28*, 782–789. [CrossRef]
11. Kumar, S.P. Efficacy of segmental stabilization exercise for lumbar segmental instability in patients with mechanical low back pain: A randomized placebo controlled crossover study. *N. Am. J. Med. Sci.* **2011**, *3*, 456–461. [CrossRef]

12. Yu, X.; Wang, X.; Zhang, J.; Wang, Y. Changes in pressure pain thresholds and Basal electromyographic activity after instrument-assisted spinal manipulative therapy in asymptomatic participants: A randomized, controlled trial. *J. Manip. Physiol. Ther.* **2012**, *35*, 437–445. [CrossRef]
13. Cho, H.; Kim, E.-H.; Kim, J. Effects of the CORE Exercise Program on Pain and Active Range of Motion in Patients with Chronic Low Back Pain. *J. Phys. Ther. Sci.* **2014**, *26*, 1237–1240. [CrossRef]
14. Alexandre, A.; Corò, L.; Paradiso, R.; Dall'aglio, R.; Alexandre, A.M.; Fraschini, F.; Spaggiari, P.G. Treatment of symptomatic lumbar spinal degenerative pathologies by means of combined conservative biochemical treatments. *Acta Neurochir. Suppl.* **2011**, *108*, 127–135. [CrossRef] [PubMed]
15. Scarcia, L.; Pileggi, M.; Camilli, A.; Romi, A.; Bartolo, A.; Giubbolini, F.; Valente, I.; Garignano, G.; D'Argento, F.; Pedicelli, A.; et al. Degenerative Disc Disease of the Spine: From Anatomy to Pathophysiology and Radiological Appearance, with Morphological and Functional Considerations. *J. Pers. Med.* **2022**, *12*, 1810. [CrossRef] [PubMed]
16. Meints, S.M.; Mawla, I.; Napadow, V.; Kong, J.; Gerber, J.; Chan, S.-T.; Wasan, A.D.; Kaptchuk, T.J.; McDonnell, C.; Carriere, J.; et al. The relationship between catastrophizing and altered pain sensitivity in patients with chronic low-back pain. *Pain* **2019**, *160*, 833–843. [CrossRef]
17. Marty, M.; Rozenberg, S.; Duplan, B.; Thomas, P.; Duquesnoy, B.; Allaert, F.; Rhumatol, S.R.S.F. Quality of sleep in patients with chronic low back pain: A case-control study. *Eur. Spine J.* **2008**, *17*, 839–844. [CrossRef] [PubMed]
18. van de Water, A.T.M.; Eadie, J.; Hurley, D.A. Investigation of sleep disturbance in chronic low back pain: An age- and gender-matched case-control study over a 7-night period. *Man. Ther.* **2011**, *16*, 550–556. [CrossRef]
19. Bahouq, H.; Allali, F.; Rkain, H.; Hmamouchi, I.; Hajjaj-Hassouni, N. Prevalence and severity of insomnia in chronic low back pain patients. *Rheumatol. Int.* **2013**, *33*, 1277–1281. [CrossRef] [PubMed]
20. Axen, I. Pain-related Sleep Disturbance A Prospective Study With Repeated Measures. *Clin. J. Pain* **2016**, *32*, 254–259. [CrossRef]
21. Alsaadi, S.M.; McAuley, J.H.; Hush, J.M.; Maher, C.G. Prevalence of sleep disturbance in patients with low back pain. *Eur. Spine J.* **2011**, *20*, 737–743. [CrossRef]
22. Artner, J.; Cakir, B.; Spiekermann, J.-A.; Kurz, S.; Leucht, F.; Reichel, H.; Lattig, F. Prevalence of sleep deprivation in patients with chronic neck and back pain: A retrospective evaluation of 1016 patients. *J. Pain Res.* **2013**, *6*, 1–6. [CrossRef]
23. Alsaadi, S.M.; McAuley, J.H.; Hush, J.M.; Lo, S.; Bartlett, D.J.; Grunstein, R.R.; Maher, C.G. The Bidirectional Relationship Between Pain Intensity and Sleep Disturbance/Quality in Patients With Low Back Pain. *Clin. J. Pain* **2014**, *30*, 755–765. [CrossRef]
24. Wang, H.-Y.; Fu, T.-S.; Hsu, S.-C.; Hung, C.-I. Association of depression with sleep quality might be greater than that of pain intensity among outpatients with chronic low back pain. *Neuropsychiatr. Dis. Treat.* **2016**, *12*, 1993–1998. [CrossRef]
25. Lee, Y.C.; Chibnik, L.B.; Lu, B.; Wasan, A.D.; Edwards, R.R.; Fossel, A.H.; Helfgott, S.M.; Solomon, D.H.; Clauw, D.J.; Karlson, E.W. The relationship between disease activity, sleep, psychiatric distress and pain sensitivity in rheumatoid arthritis: A cross-sectional study. *Arthritis Res. Ther.* **2009**, *11*, R160. [CrossRef]
26. Kosek, E.; Clauw, D.; Nijs, J.; Baron, R.; Gilron, I.; Harris, R.E.; Mico, J.-A.; Rice, A.S.C.; Sterling, M. Chronic nociplastic pain affecting the musculoskeletal system: Clinical criteria and grading system. *Pain* **2021**, *162*, 2629–2634. [CrossRef] [PubMed]
27. Linton, S.J.; Boersma, K. Early identification of patients at risk of developing a persistent back problem: The predictive validity of the Orebro Musculoskeletal Pain Questionnaire. *Clin. J. Pain* **2003**, *19*, 80–86. [CrossRef] [PubMed]
28. O'Neill, S.; Manniche, C.; Graven-Nielsen, T.; Arendt-Nielsen, L. Association between a composite score of pain sensitivity and clinical parameters in low-back pain. *Clin. J. Pain* **2014**, *30*, 831–838. [CrossRef] [PubMed]
29. Pfingsten, M.; Nagel, B.; Emrich, O.; Seemann, H.; Lindena, G.; Nilges, P.; Kohlmann, T. (Eds.) *Deutscher Schmerzfragebogen*, 3rd ed.; Handbuch: Berlin Germany, 2015.
30. Buysse, D.J.; Reynolds, C.F.; Monk, T.H.; Berman, S.R.; Kupfer, D.J. The Pittsburgh Sleep Quality Index: A new instrument for psychiatric practice and research. *Psychiatry Res.* **1989**, *28*, 193–213. [CrossRef]
31. Lautenbacher, S.; Spernal, J.; Schreiber, W.; Krieg, J.C. Relationship between clinical pain complaints and pain sensitivity in patients with depression and panic disorder. *Psychosom. Med.* **1999**, *61*, 822–827. [CrossRef]
32. Hübscher, M.; Moloney, N.; Leaver, A.; Rebbeck, T.; McAuley, J.H.; Refshauge, K.M. Relationship between quantitative sensory testing and pain or disability in people with spinal pain-a systematic review and meta-analysis. *Pain* **2013**, *154*, 1497–1504. [CrossRef]
33. Clark, J.; Nijs, J.; Yeowell, G.; Goodwin, P.C. What Are the Predictors of Altered Central Pain Modulation in Chronic Musculoskeletal Pain Populations? A Systematic Review. *Pain Physician* **2017**, *20*, 487–500. [CrossRef] [PubMed]
34. Meeus, M.; Nijs, J. Central sensitization: A biopsychosocial explanation for chronic widespread pain in patients with fibromyalgia and chronic fatigue syndrome. *Clin. Rheumatol.* **2007**, *26*, 465–473. [CrossRef] [PubMed]
35. Aoyagi, K.; He, J.; Nicol, A.L.; Clauw, D.J.; Kluding, P.M.; Jernigan, S.; Sharma, N.K. A Subgroup of Chronic Low Back Pain Patients With Central Sensitization. *Clin. J. Pain* **2019**, *35*, 869–879. [CrossRef]
36. Vuilleumier, P.H.; Besson, M.; Desmeules, J.; Arendt-Nielsen, L.; Curatolo, M. Evaluation of anti-hyperalgesic and analgesic effects of two benzodiazepines in human experimental pain: A randomized placebo-controlled study. *PLoS ONE* **2013**, *8*, e43896. [CrossRef]
37. Vaegter, H.B.; Ussing, K.; Johansen, J.V.; Stegemejer, I.; Palsson, T.S.; O'Sullivan, P.; Kent, P. Improvements in clinical pain and experimental pain sensitivity after cognitive functional therapy in patients with severe persistent low back pain. *Pain Rep.* **2020**, *5*, e802. [CrossRef]

38. Wylde, V.; Palmer, S.; Learmonth, I.D.; Dieppe, P. Test-retest reliability of Quantitative Sensory Testing in knee osteoarthritis and healthy participants. *Osteoarthr. Cartil.* **2011**, *19*, 655–658. [CrossRef]
39. Walton, D.M.; Levesque, L.; Payne, M.; Schick, J. Clinical Pressure Pain Threshold Testing in Neck Pain: Comparing Protocols, Responsiveness, and Association With Psychological Variables. *Phys. Ther.* **2014**, *94*, 827–837. [CrossRef]
40. O'Donoghue, G.M.; Fox, N.; Heneghan, C.; Hurley, D.A. Objective and subjective assessment of sleep in chronic low back pain patients compared with healthy age and gender matched controls: A pilot study. *BMC Musculoskelet. Disord.* **2009**, *10*, 122. [CrossRef]
41. Donat, H.; Ozcan, A.; Ozdirenç, M.; Aksakoğlu, G.; Aydinoğlu, S. Age-related changes in pressure pain threshold, grip strength and touch pressure threshold in upper extremities of older adults. *Aging Clin. Exp. Res.* **2005**, *17*, 380–384. [CrossRef] [PubMed]

diagnostics MDPI

Article

Osteomyelitis of the Lower Limb: Diagnostic Accuracy of Dual-Energy CT versus MRI

Giovanni Foti [1,*], Chiara Longo [1], Claudia Sorgato [2], Eugenio Simone Oliboni [1], Cristina Mazzi [3], Leonardo Motta [4], Giulia Bertoli [4] and Stefania Marocco [4]

1 Department of Radiology, IRCCS Sacro Cuore Don Calabria Hospital, Negrar di Valpolicella, 37042 Verona, Italy
2 Department of Diabetology, IRCCS Sacro Cuore Don Calabria Hospital, Negrar di Valpolicella, 37042 Verona, Italy
3 Clinical Research Unit, IRCCS Ospedale Sacro Cuore Don Calabria, Negrar di Valpolicella, 37042 Verona, Italy
4 Department of Infectious, Tropical Diseases and Microbiology, IRCCS Sacro Cuore Don Calabria Hospital, Negrar di Valpolicella, 37042 Verona, Italy
* Correspondence: giovanni.foti@sacrocuore.it

Abstract: Background: MRI is the preferred imaging technique for the identification of osteomyelitis. The key element for diagnosis is the presence of bone marrow edema (BME). Dual-energy CT (DECT) is an alternative tool which is able to identify BME in the lower limb. Purpose: To compare the diagnostic performance of DECT and MRI for osteomyelitis, using clinical, microbiological, and imaging data as reference standards. Materials and Methods: This prospective single-center study enrolled consecutive patients with suspected bone infections undergoing DECT and MRI imaging from December 2020 to June 2022. Four blinded radiologists with various experience levels (range of 3-21 years) evaluated the imaging findings. Osteomyelitis was diagnosed in the presence of BMEs, abscesses, sinus tracts, bone reabsorption, or gaseous elements. The sensitivity, specificity, and AUC values of each method were determined and compared using a multi-reader multi-case analysis. A p value < 0.05 was considered significant. Results: In total, 44 study participants (mean age 62.5 years ± 16.5 [SD], 32 men) were evaluated. Osteomyelitis was diagnosed in 32 participants. For the MRI, the mean sensitivity and specificity were 89.1% and 87.5%, while for the DECT they were 89.0% and 72.9%, respectively. The DECT demonstrated a good diagnostic performance (AUC = 0.88), compared with the MRI (AUC = 0.92) (p = 0.12). When considering each imaging finding alone, the best accuracy was achieved by considering BME (AUC for DECT 0.85 versus AUC of MRI of 0.93, with p = 0.07), followed by the presence of bone erosions (AUC 0.77 for DECT and 0.53 for MRI, with p = 0.02). The inter-reader agreement of the DECT (k = 88) was similar to that of the MRI (k = 90). Conclusion: Dual-energy CT demonstrated a good diagnostic performance in detecting osteomyelitis.

Keywords: chronic pain; osteomyelitis; MRI; dual-energy CT; bone marrow edema

1. Introduction

Osteomyelitis is an infection of the bone which involves the medullary canal [1]. It may present as an acute or chronic inflammatory process secondary to an infection with pyogenic organisms, including bacteria, fungi, and mycobacteria, and may be associated with chronic pain [2]. Foot localization is the most frequent infection site for diabetic patients, and such infection mostly occurs from the contiguous spread of a soft tissue infection from an adjacent skin ulceration or from a post-operative soft tissue defect [3]. In all other localizations, osteomyelitis may be caused by a hematogenous spread, a spread from a contiguous infected source, or a direct implantation or after surgery [4].

Diagnosing osteomyelitis requires a combination of clinical, laboratory, microbiological, and imaging findings [5]. Microbiological diagnosis is based upon the identification of bacteria and the presence of inflammatory cells and osteonecrosis from an uncontaminated sample [6]. Bone biopsies are commonly used for diagnosis, but their diagnostic yield can greatly vary [7]. Even though microbiological identification remains the gold standard for diagnosis, the microbiological accuracy from relevant samples persist to be low, as the culture yields positive results in only 21–28% of the cases [7]. While insufficient material or prior antibiotic therapy may cause false-negative results, false-positive results may arise from contaminants colonizing the skin or wound [1].

Radiographs can be inaccurate in the detection of osteomyelitis, with a pooled sensitivity of 54% and specificity of 68% [8,9]. Furthermore, osseous changes may not be radiographically evident for 7–15 days following the onset of osseous infection [9].

MRI is the preferred technique to identify osteomyelitis and to evaluate the extent of the soft tissue infection [10,11], as well as to plan a surgical resection [12]. MRI is able to identify the BME of the involved bone, representing a key element for diagnosing osteomyelitis. In the evaluation of pedal osteomyelitis, MRI has a high sensitivity (90%) and specificity (ranging from 79% to 83%) and it is the preferred technique to evaluate soft tissue abscesses, with a reported sensitivity of 97% and specificity of 77% [8,9,13–15]. The primary barriers to the use of MRI are limited access and high costs.

Dual-energy CT (DECT) has been extensively used for the identification of BME in traumatic and non-traumatic settings [16–21]. In particular, in non-traumatic patients, DECT showed a sensitivity of 91% and a specificity of 95% in the identification of BME of the ankle [22]. Moreover, recent data suggest that DECT may be proposed for the identification of osteomyelitis, showing a sensitivity of 81% and a specificity ranging from 73% to 81% [23].

The purpose of our study was to investigate the diagnostic performance of DECT compared to MRI for diagnosing osteomyelitis, using microbiological and biopsy data as reference standards for diagnosis.

2. Material and Methods

2.1. Participants

This prospective single-center study was conducted in a large tertiary referral hospital after approval by the institutional review board (IRB). Written informed consent was obtained from all participants. Between December 2020 and June 2022, patients presenting to our institution with a suspected osteomyelitis who also underwent both an MRI and a DECT examination within the space of a week were considered for inclusion in the study. A diagnosis of osteomyelitis was confirmed by a comprehensive multidisciplinary assessment based on clinical, microbiological, and imaging features. The exclusion criteria were: oncologic patients, the lack of imaging examinations, or the absence of clinical and microbiological variables.

2.2. Magnetic Resonance Imaging

MRI was performed with a commercially available 1.5-T unit (Magnetom Avanto Fit; Siemens Healthineers, Erlangen, Germany). Standard 4-mm thick T1-weighted turbo spin-echo (TR/TE/FA = 650.0 ms/18.0 ms/150°) sequences were acquired on the axial and coronal planes, and T2-weighted turbo spin-echo (TR/TE = 4300.0 ms/124.0 ms) sequences on the axial and sagittal planes. Furthermore, proton density fat-saturated sequences (TR/TE/FA = 2320.0 ms/39.0 ms/150°) were acquired on the axial and coronal planes for the detection of bone marrow and soft tissue edema. Finally, a 3D isotropic T1-weighted VIBE sequence (TR/TE/FA = 5.9 ms/2.1 ms/FA 10/NEX 2) was acquired on the axial plane after the intravenous administration of gadolinium (Dotarem) and reconstructed on the coronal and sagittal planes.

2.3. DECT Protocol

All dual-energy CT exams were performed without the intravenous injection of contrast material. A third-generation scanner was employed (Somatom Definition Force,

Siemens Healthineers). A dual-source acquisition technique was used for setting the tube voltages at 80 and 150 kVp with a tin filter. The tube current–time product was set at 1.6:1 (tube A, 220 mAs; tube B, 138 quality reference mAs). Thanks to the implementation of automated attenuation-based tube current modulation (CARE dose 4D; Siemens Healthcare), the radiation burden was similar to that of similar previous studies.

2.4. DECT Post-Processing

Soft-tissue kernel (Qr32) 80 kV and 150 kV set images (thickness 0.75 mm; increment 0.6 mm) were transferred to an offline workstation (SyngoVia® VB40). The virtual non-calcium (VNCa) applications were used to assess bone marrow edema (BME). Color-coded maps superimposed on gray-scale CT images were available in the postprocessing software application. In particular, on 3D imaging, a green-blue-scale was employed, coding the normal bone in blue and the edema in green. In a colored-scale, the 2D images were orientated in the different planes, and edema was coded in green to yellow or in red, according to the cut-off chosen and the type of color-coding adopted (rainbow or violet-green). For each participant, the isotropic image dataset was analyzed using a soft tissue and bone window on the preferred imaging planes.

2.5. Image Analysis

MRI and DECT were analyzed by four independent (R1 to R4) radiologists (GF, EO, CL, and VR, with 15, 11, 4, and 2 years of experience, respectively). The images were analyzed in a random order during three reading sessions separated by 1-month intervals. The readers were blinded to the clinical/microbiological findings. A diagnosis of osteomyelitis was retained based on a comprehensive assessment that included imaging, clinical, and microbiological (bone biopsy or surgery) features.

At MRI, the T1 signal intensity was considered abnormal if the signal of the affected bone marrow had decreased compared with the normal adjacent fatty marrow, while BME was evaluated in fluid-sensitive images (fat-suppressed T2W/proton density-weighted and STIR). Contrast-enhanced T1 imaging was used to confirm the diagnosis, to better delineate the bone abscess or infarction, and to better identify the associated findings in the surroundings tissues, including abscesses or fistulous tracts.

At DECT, the diagnosis of osteomyelitis was defined by the presence of BME of the affected bone segment on color-coded VNCa imaging, with the presence of bone erosion (cortical thinning with blurred margins) or bone resorption around the oedema if far from the cortical bone. In addition, any associated soft tissue findings, including the presence of abscesses or fistulous tracts, with or without gastric elements, were used to corroborate the diagnosis.

For each case and for each imaging tool, the four radiologists rated the patient disease status as follows: 1 = presence of osteomyelitis; 2 = probably osteomyelitis; 3 = non-specific findings; 4 = probably no osteomyelitis; or 5 = no osteomyelitis.

2.6. Clinical Findings and Microbiological Analysis

All patients were evaluated at our Infectious Disease department and a daily clinical examination was ordered for each of them during the time of hospitalization. Clinical characteristics such as local pan, swelling or redness, fever, and functional limitations were evaluated. The demographic characteristics were also registered.

During the hospitalization period, patients underwent either a bone biopsy or surgery for debridement or amputation. The sampled material was analyzed by our Microbiological department.

2.7. Statistical Analysis

The statistical analysis was conducted with STATA software vers. 16 (StataCorp. 2019. Stata Statistical Software: Release 16. College Station, TX, USA: StataCorp LLC) by an experienced statistical analyst (CM, 5 years of experience).

Data available from a previous study performed at our institution, with a similar research design and methodology and similar objectives/hypotheses, were used to define the sample size.

Demographic and clinical data were summarized using descriptive statistics and measures of variability. All parameters were reported with 95% confidence intervals. The statistical models and estimations were adjusted for covariates when necessary. A multi-reader multi-case analysis of the variance was performed using the MRMCoav R package (Version 0.1.3). The sensitivity and specificity were calculated using a binary threshold (score 1 and 2 = osteomyelitis; score 3, 4, or 5 = no presence of osteomyelitis). The multi-observer agreement was calculated by Cohen's K index. Any disagreement was resolved by a consensus review between the specialists.

To further detail the methods, the summary call produces the ANOVA results for a global test of equality of the ROC AUC means across all imaging modalities and tests of pairwise differences, along with the confidence intervals for the differences and intervals for the individual modalities.

The sensitivity, specificity, and ROC areas were calculated for each parameter, and comparisons between the AUCs were performed. Clinical, microbiological, and MRI findings were set as the reference standard for diagnosis.

We also analyzed the diagnostic performance of DECT in the identification of BME alone, given MRI results as the standard of reference.

A multivariable logistic model was used to predict the probability of osteomyelitis, adjusted for the following regressors: age and sex. A p value of <0.05 was considered statistically significant.

3. Results

3.1. Participant Characteristics

In total, 67 patients with suspected osteomyelitis were identified. Twenty-three participants were excluded for the following reasons: lack of CT (n = 15), unsuitable candidates for microbiological confirmation of osteomyelitis (n = 6), and MRI motion artifacts (n = 2). The final study sample was composed of 44 participants reporting osteomyelitis (mean age 62.5 years ± 16.5 [SD]), of which there were 32 men (73%) and 12 women (27%). The participants' clinical data are summarized in Table 1, while a flowchart briefly outlining the participant outcomes shown in Figure 1.

Out of the 44 participants evaluated for the presence of osteomyelitis, 32 (73%) were subsequently confirmed clinically, microbiologically, and at MRI imaging, while 12 (27%) were found to have no signs of osteomyelitis at presentation. For all the cases, there were different segments analyzed, in particular: 30 foots, 9 knee-legs, and 5 hips.

Table 1. Demographic and clinical data of the participants.

Characteristic	No. of Participants (n = 44)
Age (y)	62.5 (18–87) [16.5]
Number of men	32 (72.7%)
Number of women	12 (27.3%)
Osteomyelitis	32 (72.7%)
No osteomyelitis	12 (27.3%)
Side	
Right	21 (47.7%)
Left	23 (52.3%)
Skeletal segment	
Foot	30 (68.1%)
Knee/leg	9 (20.5%)
Hip	5 (11.4%)

Note—Demographic data are presented as mean values with (range) and [standard deviation]. Clinical data are presented as the number of cases with (percentage).

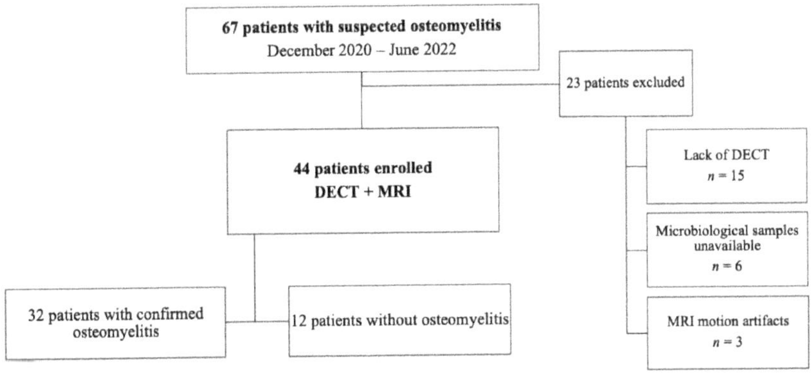

Figure 1. Flowchart of participants. DECT = dual-energy CT; MRI = magnetic resonance imaging.

3.2. Clinical and Microbiological Results

Overall, clinical and microbiological data revealed osteomyelitis in 32 of the 44 participants (73%). Among the remaining 12 participants (27%) for which no osteomyelitis was confirmed, other diagnoses were obtained instead: cellulitis = 7; neuropathic arthropathy = 3; fasciitis = 1; osteonecrosis = 1.

3.3. Imaging Results

The sensitivity and specificity values, AUCs, and delta mean values for the diagnosis of osteomyelitis are reported in Tables 2–4. Figure 2 summarizes the ANOVA results for multi-reader multi-case analysis of ROC AUC across all imaging modalities.

Table 2. Diagnostic performance of four readers at DECT versus MRI for diagnosing presence of osteomyelitis.

	Sensitivity	Specificity	AUC	PPV	NPV
MRI	89.1% * [82.3, 93.9]	87.5% * [71.8, 95.3]	0.88 * [0.78, 0.98]	95.0% [89.4, 98.1]	75.0% [61.6, 85.5]
Reader 1	93.8% [79.2, 99.2]	91.7% [61.5, 99.8]	0.93 [0.84, 1.00]	96.8% [83.3, 99.9]	84.6% [54.6, 98.1]
Reader 2	84.4% [67.2, 94.7]	91.7% [61.5, 99.8]	0.88 [0.78, 0.98]	96.4% [81.7, 99.9]	68.8% [41.3, 89.0]
Reader 3	87.5% [71.0, 96.5]	83.3% [51.6, 97.9]	0.85 [0.73, 0.98]	93.3% [77.9, 99.2]	71.4% [41.9, 91.6]
Reader 4	90.6% [75.0, 98.0]	83.3% [51.6, 97.9]	0.87 [0.75, 0.99]	93.5% [78.6, 99.2]	76.9% [46.2, 95.0]
DECT	89.0% * [82.2, 93.8]	72.9% * [58.2, 84.7]	0.81 * [0.67, 0.95]	89.7% [83.0, 94.4]	71.4% [56.7, 83.4]
Reader 1	93.8% [79.2, 99.2]	75.0% [42.8, 94.5]	0.84 [0.71, 0.98]	90.9% [75.7, 97.7]	81.8% [48.2, 97.7]
Reader 2	84.4% [67.2, 94.7]	75.0% [42.8, 94.5]	0.80 [0.65, 0.94]	90.0% [73.5, 97.9]	64.3% [35.1, 87.2]
Reader 3	93.8% [79.2, 99.2]	66.7% [34.9, 90.1]	0.80 [0.66, 0.95]	88.2% [72.5, 96.7]	80.0% [44.4, 97.5]
Reader 4	81.2% [63.6, 92.8]	75.0% [42.8, 94.5]	0.78 [0.64, 0.93]	89.7% [72.6, 97.8]	60.0% [32.2, 83.7]

Note—Percentages; fraction; 95% CIs in brackets. MRI = magnetic resonance imaging, DECT = dual-energy CT, AUC = area under the receiver operating characteristic (ROC) curve, PPV = positive predictive value, NPV = negative predictive value. * Mean sensitivity, specificity, and AUC of the four readers.

Table 3. Diagnostic performance of four readers at DECT for diagnosing presence of bone marrow edema, giving MRI as gold standard.

	Sensitivity	Specificity	AUC	PPV	NPV
DECT	91.2% * [84.8, 95.5]	82.4% * [69.1, 91.6]	90 * [0.84, 0.96]	92.7% [86.6, 96.6]	79.2% [65.9, 89.2]
Reader 1	90.6% [75.0, 98.0]	83.3% [51.6, 97.9]	0.87 [0.75, 0.99]	93.5% [78.6, 99.2]	76.9% [46.2, 95.0]
Reader 2	87.1% [77, 96]	84% [71, 94]	0.87 [0.80, 0.94]	96.8% [83.3, 99.9]	84.6% [54.6, 98.1]
Reader 3	85% [72, 94]	96% [85, 100]	0.90 [0.84, 0.96]	96.8% [83.3, 99.9]	84.6% [54.6, 98.1]
Reader 4	87% [74, 95]	91% [79, 98]	0.89 [0.83, 0.96]	96.8% [83.3, 99.9]	84.6% [54.6, 98.1]

Note—Percentages; fraction; 95% CIs in brackets. MRI = magnetic resonance imaging, DECT = dual-energy CT, AUC = area under the receiver operating characteristic (ROC) curve, PPV = positive predictive value, NPV = negative predictive value. * Mean sensitivity, specificity, and AUC of the four readers.

Table 4. Diagnostic performance of four readers at DECT versus MRI for diagnosing presence of BMEs, erosions, abscesses, sinus tracts, and gas.

	MRI			DECT		
	Sensitivity	Specificity	AUC	Sensitivity	Specificity	AUC
BME	94.5% * [79.5, 99.6]	91.6% * [61.5, 99.8]	0.93 *	89.1% * [74.5, 97.8]	81.2% * [50.3, 96.8]	0.85 *
Reader 1	93.8% [79.2, 99.2]	100% [73.5, 1.00]	0.97 [0.93, 1.00]	90.6% [75.0, 98.0]	83.3% [51.6, 97.7]	0.87 [0.75, 0.99]
Reader 2	93.8% [79.2, 99.2]	91.7% [61.5, 99.8]	0.93 [0.81, 0.97]	87.5% [71.0, 96.5]	83.3% [51.6, 97.9]	0.85 [0.73, 0.98]
Reader 3	93.8% [79.2, 99.2]	91.7% [61.5, 99.8]	0.93 [0.81, 0.97]	90.6% [75.0, 98.0]	75.0% [42.8, 94.5]	0.82 [0.69, 0.97]
Reader 4	96.9% [83.8, 99.9]	83.3% [51.6, 97.9]	0.90 [0.79, 1.00]	87.5% [71.0, 96.5]	83.3% [51.6, 97.7]	0.85 [0.73, 0.98]
Erosions	49.2% * [40.3, 58.2]	89.4% * [77.3, 96.5]	0.53 *	74.2% * [65.7, 81.5]	79.2% * [65.0, 89.5]	0.77 *
Reader 1	34.4% [18.6, 53.2]	91.7% [61.5, 99.8]	0.37 [0.25, 0.49]	68.8% [50.0, 83.9]	83.3% [51.6, 97.7]	0.76 [0.62, 0.90]
Reader 2	46.9% [29.1, 65.3]	91.7% [61.5, 99.8]	0.31 [0.19, 0.43]	75.0% [56.6, 88.5]	83.3% [51.6, 97.9]	0.79 [0.65, 0.93]
Reader 3	56.3% [37.7, 73.6]	83.3% [51.6, 97.9]	0.70 [0.56, 0.84]	78.1% [60.0, 90.7]	66.7% [34.9, 90.1]	0.72 [0.57, 0.88]
Reader 4	59.4% [40.6, 76.3]	91.7% [61.5, 99.8]	0.75 [0.63, 0.87]	75.0% [56.6, 88.5]	83.3% [51.6, 97.7]	0.79 [0.65, 0.93]
Abscesses	31.2% * [23.4, 40.4]	91.7% * [80.0, 97.7]	0.39 *	26.6% * [19.1, 35.1]	89.6% * [77.3, 96.5]	0.42 *
Reader 1	31.2% [16.1, 50.0]	75.0% [42.8, 94.5]	0.47 [0.31, 0.62]	25.0% [11.5, 43.4]	83.3% [51.6, 97.9]	0.46 [0.32, 0.59]
Reader 2	43.8% [26.4, 62.3]	91.7% [61.5, 99.8]	0.32 [0.20, 0.44]	34.4% [18.6, 53.2]	91.7% [61.5, 99.8]	0.37 [0.25, 0.49]
Reader 3	28.1% [13.7, 46.7]	100% [73.5, 100]	0.36 [0.28, 0.44]	25.0% [11.5, 43.4]	91.7% [61.5, 99.8]	0.42 [0.30, 0.53]
Reader 4	21.9% [9.3, 40.0]	100% [71.5, 100]	0.39 [0.32, 0.46]	21.9% [9.3, 40.0]	91.7% [61.5, 99.8]	0.43 [0.32, 0.54]
Sinus tract	22.7% * [15.7, 30.9]	95.8% * [85.7, 99.5]	0.41 *	21.9% * [15.1, 30.0]	93.8% * [82.8, 98.7]	0.42 *
Reader 1	28.1% [13.7, 46.7]	91.7% [61.5, 99.8]	0.40 [0.29, 0.51]	25.0% [11.5, 43.4]	91.7% [61.5, 99.8]	0.42 [0.31, 0.53]
Reader 2	25.0% [11.5, 43.4]	91.7% [61.5, 99.8]	0.41 [0.31, 0.53]	28.1% [13.7, 46.7]	91.7% [61.5, 99.8]	0.40 [0.29, 0.51]

Table 4. *Cont.*

	MRI			DECT		
	Sensitivity	Specificity	AUC	Sensitivity	Specificity	AUC
Reader 3	25.0% [11.5, 43.4]	100% [73.5, 100]	0.38 [0.30, 0.45]	18.8% [7.2, 36.4]	91.7% [61.5, 99.8]	0.45 [0.34, 0.55]
Reader 4	12.5% [3.5, 29.0]	100% [73.5, 100]	0.44 [0.38, 0.50]	15.6% [5.3, 32.8]	100% [73.5, 100]	0.42 [0.36, 0.49]
Gas	12.5% * [7.3, 19.5]	97.9% * [65.9, 89.2]	0.45 *	15.7% * [9.8, 23.1]	89.6% * [77.3, 96.5]	0.48 *
Reader 1	9.4% [2.0, 25.0]	91.7% [61.5, 99.8]	0.49 [0.40, 0.59]	9.4% [2.0, 25.0]	91.7% [61.5, 99.8]	0.49 [0.40, 0.59]
Reader 2	18.8% [7.2, 36.4]	100% [73.5, 100]	0.40 [0.34, 0.47]	18.8% [7.2, 36.4]	91.7% [61.5, 99.8]	0.45 [0.34, 0.55]
Reader 3	9.4% [2.0, 25.0]	100% [73.5, 100]	0.45 [0.40, 0.50]	15.6% [5.3, 32.8]	83.3% [51.6, 97.9]	0.51 [0.38, 0.63]
Reader 4	12.5% [3.5, 29.0]	100% [73.5, 100]	0.44 [0.38, 0.50]	18.8% [7.2, 36.4]	91.7% [61.5, 99.8]	0.45 [0.34, 0.55]

Note—Percentages; 95% CIs in brackets. MRI = magnetic resonance imaging, DECT = dual-energy CT, AUC = area under the receiver operating characteristic (ROC) curve, BME = bone marrow edema. * Mean sensitivity, specificity, and AUC of the four readers.

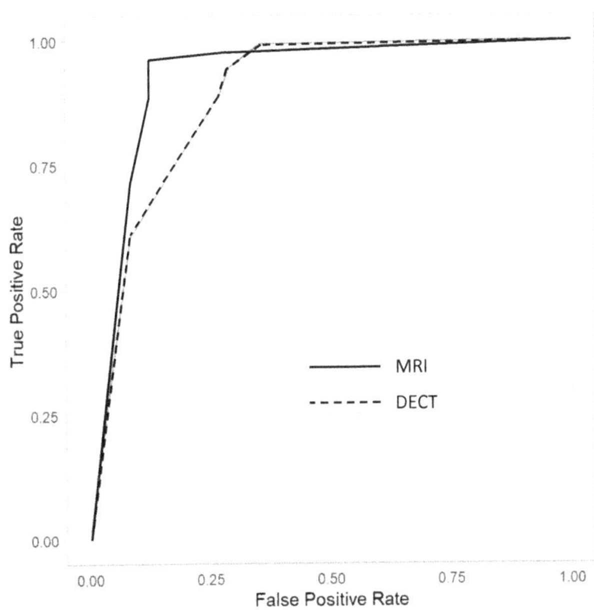

Figure 2. Diagnostic performance of the multi-reader multi-case analysis across all imaging modalities for MRI and DECT. The dashed line-curve represents DECT and the continuous line-curve represents MRI.

DECT showed a good overall performance with respect to MRI. For DECT, the mean sensitivity and specificity were 89.0% (82.2, 93.8) and 72.9% (58.2, 84.7), while for MRI they were 89.1% (82.3, 93.9) and 87.5% (74.8, 95.3), respectively. For DECT, the mean positive and negative predictive values were 89.7% (83.0, 94.4) and 71.4% (56.7, 83.4), while for MRI they were 95.0% (89.4, 98.1) and 75.0% (61.6, 85.6), respectively. For what pertains to the overall performance in diagnosing osteomyelitis, the mean AUC values (as averaged from the four readers) resulted higher for MRI (AUC = 0.88) compared with DECT (AUC = 0.81), with a statistically non-significant difference ($p = 0.12$).

When considering each imaging finding alone, the best accuracy was achieved when considering BMEs (AUC for DECT 0.85 versus AUC of MRI of 0.93, with $p = 0.07$), followed by the presence of bone erosions (AUC 0.77 for DECT and 0.53 for MRI, with $p = 0.02$), abscesses (AUC 0.42 for DECT versus 0.39 for MRI, with $p = 0.43$), sinus tracts (AUC.42 for DECT versus 0.41 for MRI, with $p = 0.45$) and surrounding gaseous elements (AUC 0.48 for DECT versus 0.45 for MRI, with $p = 0.38$).

Concerning the identification of BME alone, using MRI as the reference for diagnosis, DECT had a sensitivity of 91.2% (84.8, 95.5), a specificity of 82.4% (69.1, 91.6), a positive predictive value of 92.7% (86.6, 96.6), and a negative predictive value of 79.2% (65.9, 89.2).

3.4. Inter-Observer Agreement

For osteomyelitis analysis, a very high inter-reader agreement was achieved for DECT (k = 88; 95% CI: 77, 96) and MRI (k = 90; 95% CI: 78, 98).

Figures 3 and 4 show example images of participants for which at least one reader missed diagnosing osteomyelitis.

3.5. Multivariable Logistic Analysis

In multivariable analysis, the diagnosis of osteomyelitis was unrelated to age or sex ($p > 0.05$ for all).

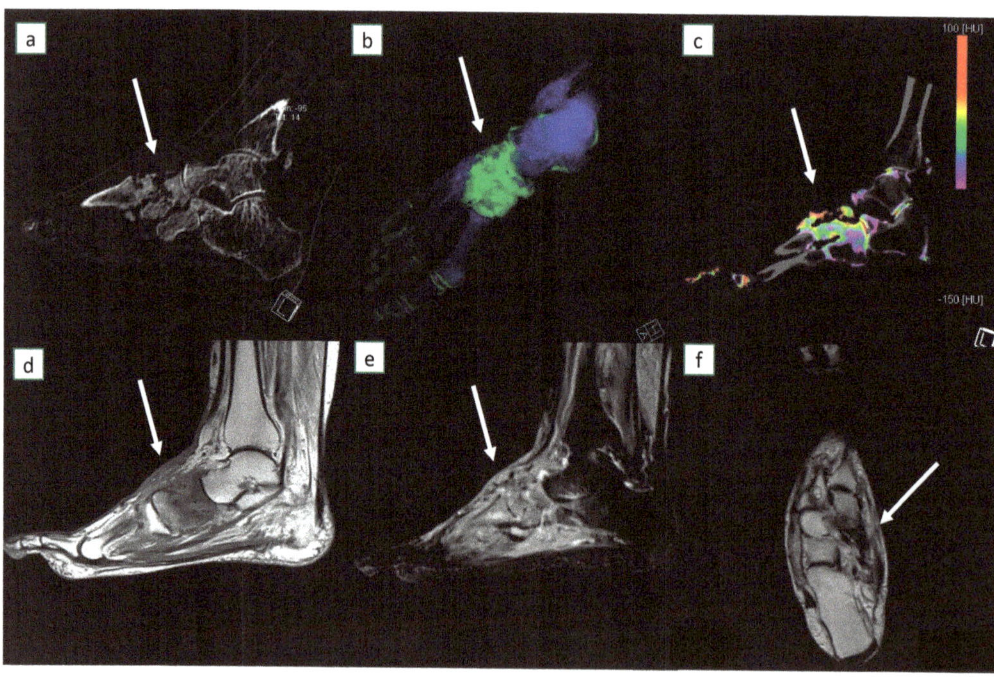

Figure 3. A 45-year-old female presented with acute atraumatic left foot pain and was diagnosed with osteomyelitis at bone biopsy. At dual-energy CT in sagittal plane there is evidence of advanced cortical erosions (**a**). At bone marrow edema analysis on 3D map (**b**) and sagittal 2D reconstruction image (**c**), diffuse bone marrow edema (arrows) can be identified around the midfoot. MRI sagittal T1 sequence (**d**), STIR sagittal (**e**), and T1 axial (**f**) images confirm the corresponding diffuse marrow edema (arrows) and extensive soft tissue edema.

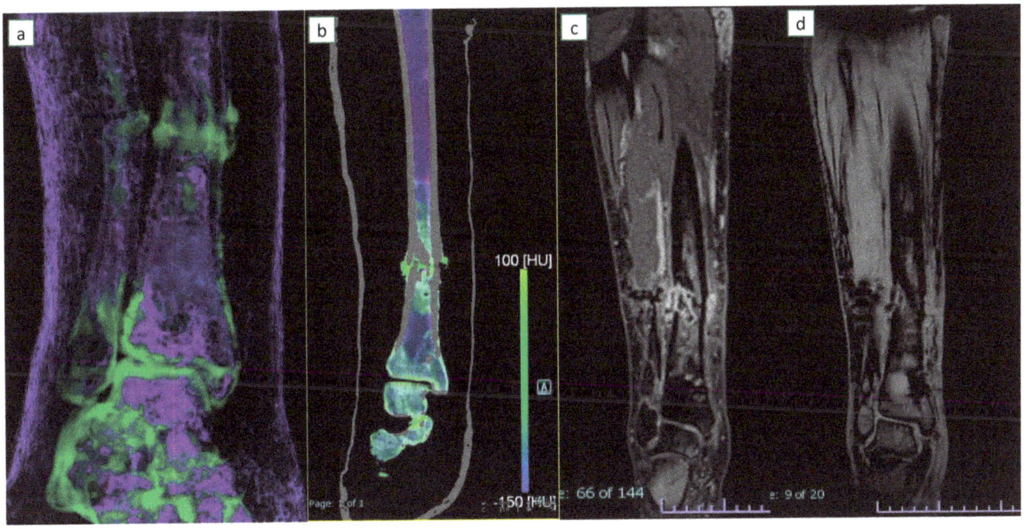

Figure 4. A 52-year-old female with osteomyelitis on tibial exposed fracture. On coronal 3D (**a**) and 2D (**b**) dual-energy CT images, severe bone marrow edema is identified around the fracture line. Additional edema is also present on the adjacent soft tissues. On the corresponding coronal MRI T1-weighted image after contrast material administration (**c**), additional edema with a sequestrum is depicted around the fracture foci. The corresponding T1-weighted image without contrast material (**d**) was considered non-diagnostic because of some metal-induced artifacts from a previous surgical fixation.

4. Discussion

4.1. Discussion of Background

The DECT reports for the diagnosis of osteomyelitis, made using multiple imaging parameters, were compared with the MRI reports, with evidence of a similar diagnostic accuracy of osteomyelitis in the lower limb as with MRI ($p = 0.12$).

Osteomyelitis is associated with high morbidity and high healthcare costs and may require aggressive surgery or amputation. Thus, the prompt diagnosis is of great importance in guiding appropriate medical and surgical treatments. MRI is the most reliable imaging tool for the evaluation of osteomyelitis due to its high sensitivity and specificity performance. At MRI, STIR hyperintensity with corresponding T1-weighted hypointensity characterizes the typical bone marrow signaling abnormalities. However, false positive cases were described because of the confluent intramedullary patterns in T1W images. In addition, normal T1 signals have been reported in skeletal segments with confirmed osteomyelitis at the pathology examination, possibly reflecting a necrotic bone with fatty marrow. In this clinical setting, the associated anatomical findings, including ulcers, abscesses, and bone erosions, can play a crucial role to help the diagnosis.

4.2. Role of DECT and Comparison with Previous Studies

DECT has been successfully used to identify BMEs in traumatic and non-traumatic settings. Furthermore, DECT has been applied for the evaluation of several districts, including the hip, the knee, and the foot. One of the major strength points of DECT is its ability to yield high-resolution isotropic images that can also be reconstructed with the bone of soft tissue kernel. These images may help in highlighting fine anatomic details both in the bone and adjacent tissues.

In a recent study evaluating DECT for diagnosing osteomyelitis, among 26 positive cases, the sensitivity ranged from 53.8% (by reading VNCa images alone) to 80.8% with the combined use of VNCa and standard CT images [23]. In the above-mentioned study, the specificity values ranged from 84.9% to 71.2% and decreased when evaluating both VNCa and standard images together. However, most patients were negative according to the reference standard; the reason for the decreased accuracy in the reading of both BME maps and standard images may be attributable in the inclusion of several different bone segments in both the upper and lower limbs. In clinical practice, the shape of the bone, the presence of cortical bone thickening, or the presence of reduced mineral density may interfere with the diagnosis of BME [24].

Our results confirm that DECT is accurate in diagnosing osteomyelitis of the lower limb, yielding similar accuracy values with respect to MRI, with an overall AUC of 0.81, and with 89.0% and 72.9% sensitivity and specificity, respectively. To achieve a higher statistical validity, we performed a multi-reader multi-case analysis. Overall, the results were similar among the four radiologists, despite the different experiences of the readers. Such agreement confirms that DECT may be considered a reliable imaging tool in this setting.

In our opinion, and in accordance with other recently published reports, the evaluation of both BME maps and standard high-resolution images is essential for a correct osteomyelitis diagnosis [23].

Thanks to DECT color-coded images, it is possible to identify the presence of BME, a nonspecific marker of chronic pain, and one of the key imaging findings for the diagnosis of osteomyelitis in the lower limb [19,20,25]. In clinical practice, BME, as detected with an MRI, is used for the identification and demarcation of osteomyelitis foci [10,26–28].

In this study, DECT correctly identified the presence of BMEs in most patients, with an average sensitivity and specificity of 91.2% and 82.4%, (AUC = 0.90), with respect to MRI. These values are in line with those previously reported for other skeletal segments (ankle and knee) [22,29,30].

4.3. Discussion of Specific Imaging Parameters

On the other hand, BME is a nonspecific marker of bone damage and can be detected in other pathological conditions. For this reason, other imaging parameters evaluated on standard high-resolution CT images, both with bone and soft tissue windows, can play a crucial role to achieve diagnosis, and, above all, to rule out other differentials (such as stress fractures or osteo-chondral lesions). In our study, the parameter "bone erosions at the site of infection" allowed the diagnosis of the presence of osteomyelitis only in 8/44 cases but helped to increase the diagnostic likelihood and reduce the inter-observer agreement. Of fundamental importance, when bone erosions are not present, the diagnosis of osteomyelitis is improbable (specificity of 79.2% with NPV of 53.5%).

On the other hand, all other imaging parameters, when considered alone, achieved diagnostic accuracy values that are inferior to those of BME. Among these parameters, gaseous elements can represent a key finding; when present, these are typically associated with infection and can be clearly depicted on CT. However, gaseous elements were present only in six patients in our series. Fistulous tracts and soft tissue abscesses represent other important imaging findings that may help radiologists in this setting. As a matter of fact, when using a non-contrast scan, thanks to the improved soft tissues contrast resolution, DECT can be applied to identify soft tissue's involvement [31]. Nevertheless, for the evaluation of these parameters, DECT is still of limited value when compared with the contrast-enhanced MRI. Even if an additional contrast-enhanced CT scan could raise the detection rate of abscesses and fistulous tracts, and possibly ameliorate the overall accuracy of CT, it is our belief that acquiring an unenhanced CT represents one of the major strengths of DECT itself.

4.4. Strenghts and Drawbacks of DECT

While MRIs still represents the reference standard for diagnosis, DECTs may play a role in patients unable to undergo an MRI, or when am MRI is not readily available. Numerous patients with suspect osteomyelitis may suffer from chronic invalidating diseases (diabetes, vascular stenosis, neuropathy), and renal impairment might represent a limitation for both

CT and MR contrast-enhanced studies. Conversely, DECT is readily available and the scanning time is very short, reducing the potential concerns regarding motion artifacts. Moreover, additional features of DECT may be useful for differential diagnoses, such as in the identification of gout or thanks to the reduction in peri-prosthetic artifacts in patients with metal hardware [32–34]. Our study population did not include any patients with metal hardware so that a comparison of MRI versus DECT in reducing metal artifacts was not carried out. However, in our experience, the detection of BME may be limited by the presence of metal hardware, both at MRI and DECT imaging. On the other hand, in the subgroup of patients enrolled in this study who also had their hardware previously removed, metal-induced artifacts were better controlled on DECT than on MRI.

Furthermore, it should be underlined that morphological changes in the bone and soft tissues can be easily identified on the standard CT. As a matter of fact, the possible use of CT for diagnosing osteomyelitis has been proposed in previous studies that compared MRI and CT; Chandnani et al. showed a lower performance of single-energy CT when compared to MRI [15]. In another study by Gold et al., CT was useful in the detection of sequestrum, while MR imaging was helpful in defining the extent of the inflammatory process and in distinguishing osteomyelitis from cellulitis [35]. However, technological advancements allowed significant improvements for CT imaging [15,35]. Actually, in a more recent systematic review exploring the capacity of imaging tests to diagnose osteomyelitis, 81 studies were considered, showing that single-energy CT has a sensitivity of 69.7% and a specificity of 90.2% in detecting osteomyelitis [36].

The possibility of identifying BME represents an important additional feature of DECT [28,37]. However, bone marrow edema itself can be misleading as non-specific and can be observed in association with other non-infectious phenomena [38]. For this reason, we coupled morphological parameters and our results showed that the coexistence of multiple findings in the same patient can increase the diagnostic accuracy.

Nonetheless, DECT may be associated with a higher radiation exposure. In our series, patients were relatively old (62.5 yo). In spite of that, thanks to the use of a software for dose modulation, and the acquisition of a single scan of the lower limb, the radiation burden should not represent a major concern in our population. Conversely, MRI should be preferred for young patients, especially if repeated checks could be expected in the management and follow-up.

4.5. Limitations and Conclusions

Our study has some limitations. Firstly, we enrolled a relatively limited number of patients, although previous studies comparing DECT and MRI were carried out, on average, on comparable numbers. Secondly, we performed only a qualitative assessment of BME and associated imaging parameters. Furthermore, we did not perform a quantitative assessment of DECT numbers in the areas of BME to avoid the use of different cut-offs for the diagnosis of BME in the different segments analyzed. Finally, different segments were assessed in this study, namely the hip, knee, leg, and foot, potentially representing a source of confounding variables. However, the imaging appearance of osteomyelitis was similar across these districts, and we registered a higher prevalence of feet localization in comparison to other segments. Other limitations include the lack of specific imaging-clinical correlation and the inability to rule out the presence of overlapping diseases associated with BME, such as stress fractures or BME syndromes.

In conclusion, DECT showed a high diagnostic performance in the diagnosis of osteomyelitis. In our view, DECT might represent a useful alternative for the diagnosis of osteomyelitis when MRI is not available, or patients have contraindications to its execution.

Author Contributions: Conceptualization, G.F., C.S., L.M. and S.M.; Methodology, G.F., C.L., E.S.O., C.M., G.B. and S.M.; Software, E.S.O. and C.M.; Validation, G.F. and E.S.O.; Investigation, C.L. and E.S.O.; Resources, C.S. and S.M.; Data curation, C.S., C.M., L.M. and G.B.; Writing—original draft, G.F. and C.L. All authors have read and agreed to the published version of the manuscript.

Funding: This work partly received funds from the Italian Ministry of Health: "Ricerca Corrente".

Institutional Review Board Statement: The study was conducted in accordance with the Declaration of Helsinki, and approved by the Institutional Review Board (or Ethics Committee of Verona and Rovigo Area (protocol code 3761 CESC and date of approval 20 April 2022).

Informed Consent Statement: Informed consent was obtained from all subjects involved in the study. Written informed consent has been obtained from the patient(s) enrolled in this study and for publication of the paper.

Data Availability Statement: Additional data are unavailable due to privacy or ethical restrictions.

Conflicts of Interest: The authors declare no conflict of interest.

References

1. Alaia, E.F.; Chhabra, A.; Simpfendorfer, C.S.; Cohen, M.; Mintz, D.N.; Vossen, J.A.; Zoga, A.C.; Fritz, J.; Spritzer, C.E.; Armstrong, D.G.; et al. MRI nomenclature for musculoskeletal infection. *Skelet. Radiol.* **2021**, *50*, 2319–2347. [CrossRef] [PubMed]
2. Schmitt, S.K. Osteomyelitis. *Infect. Dis. Clin. N. Am.* **2017**, *31*, 325–338. [CrossRef] [PubMed]
3. Ledermann, H.P.; Morrison, W.B.; Schweitzer, M.E. MR image analysis of pedal osteomyelitis: Distribution, patterns of spread, and frequency of associated ulceration and septic arthritis. *Radiology* **2002**, *223*, 747–755. [CrossRef]
4. Resnick, D. *Diagnosis of Bone and Joint Disorders*, 4th ed.; W.B. Saunders Company: Philadephia, PA, USA, 2002.
5. Glaudemans, A.W.; Jutte, P.C.; Cataldo, M.A.; Cassar-Pullicino, V.; Gheysens, O.; Borens, O.; Trampuz, A.; Wörtler, K.; Petrosillo, N.; Winkler, H.; et al. Consensus document for the diagnosis of peripheral bone infection in adults: A joint paper by the EANM, EBJIS, and ESR (with ESCMID endorsement). *Eur. J. Nucl. Med. Mol. Imaging* **2019**, *46*, 957–970. [CrossRef] [PubMed]
6. Lipsky, B.A.; Berendt, A.R.; Cornia, P.B.; Pile, J.C.; Peters, E.J.; Armstrong, D.G.; Deery, H.G.; Embil, J.M.; Joseph, W.S.; Karchmer, A.W.; et al. 2012 Infectious Diseases Society of America clinical practice guideline for the diagnosis and treatment of diabetic foot infections. *Clin. Infect. Dis. Off. Publ. Infect. Dis. Soc. Am.* **2012**, *54*, e132–e173. [CrossRef]
7. Hirschfeld, C.B.; Kapadia, S.N.; Bryan, J.; Jannat-Khah, D.P.; May, B.; Vielemeyer, O.; Esquivel, E.L. Impact of diagnostic bone biopsies on the management of non-vertebral osteomyelitis: A retrospective cohort study. *Medicine* **2019**, *98*, e16954. [CrossRef]
8. Schweitzer, M.E.; Daffner, R.H.; Weissman, B.N.; Bennett, D.L.; Blebea, J.S.; Jacobson, J.A.; Morrison, W.B.; Resnik, C.S.; Roberts, C.C.; Rubin, D.A.; et al. ACR Appropriateness Criteria on suspected osteomyelitis in patients with diabetes mellitus. *J. Am. Coll. Radiol.* **2008**, *5*, 881–886. [CrossRef]
9. Dinh, M.T.; Abad, C.L.; Safdar, N. Diagnostic accuracy of the physical examination and imaging tests for osteomyelitis underlying diabetic foot ulcers: Meta-analysis. *Clin. Infect. Dis. Off. Publ. Infect. Dis. Soc. Am.* **2008**, *47*, 519–527. [CrossRef]
10. Donovan, A.; Schweitzer, M.E. Use of MR imaging in diagnosing diabetes-related pedal osteomyelitis. *Radiographics* **2010**, *30*, 723–736. [CrossRef] [PubMed]
11. Kotecha, H.M.; Lo, H.S.; Vedantham, S.; Shin, H.; Cerniglia, C.A. Abbreviated MRI of the foot in patients with suspected osteomyelitis. *Emerg. Radiol.* **2020**, *27*, 9–16. [CrossRef]
12. McCarthy, E.; Morrison, W.B.; Zoga, A.C. MR Imaging of the Diabetic Foot. *Magn. Reson. Imaging Clin. N. Am.* **2017**, *25*, 183–194. [CrossRef] [PubMed]
13. Kapoor, A.; Page, S.; Lavalley, M.; Gale, D.R.; Felson, D.T. Magnetic resonance imaging for diagnosing foot osteomyelitis: A meta-analysis. *Arch. Intern. Med.* **2007**, *167*, 125–132. [CrossRef] [PubMed]
14. Beltran, J.; Noto, A.M.; McGhee, R.B.; Freedy, R.M.; McCalla, M.S. Infections of the musculoskeletal system: High-field-strength MR imaging. *Radiology* **1987**, *164*, 449–454. [CrossRef] [PubMed]
15. Chandnani, V.P.; Beltran, J.; Morris, C.S.; Khalil, S.N.; Mueller, C.F.; Burk, J.M.; Bennett, W.F.; Shaffer, P.B.; Vasila, M.S.; Reese, J. Acute experimental osteomyelitis and abscesses: Detection with MR imaging versus CT. *Radiology* **1990**, *174*, 233–236. [CrossRef]
16. Baffour, F.I.; Glazebrook, K.N.; Morris, J.M.; Michalak, G.J.; Fletcher, J.G.; Leng, S.; McCollough, C.H. Clinical utility of virtual noncalcium dual-energy CT in imaging of the pelvis and hip. *Skelet. Radiol.* **2019**, *48*, 1833–1842. [CrossRef]
17. Jang, S.W.; Chung, B.M.; Kim, W.T.; Gil, J.R. Nondisplaced fractures on hip CT: Added value of dual-energy CT virtual non-calcium imaging for detection of bone marrow edema using visual and quantitative analyses. *Acta Radiol.* **2019**, *60*, 1465–1473. [CrossRef] [PubMed]
18. Kellock, T.T.; Nicolaou, S.; Kim, S.S.; Al-Busaidi, S.; Louis, L.J.; O'Connell, T.W.; Ouellette, H.A.; McLaughlin, P.D. Detection of Bone Marrow Edema in Nondisplaced Hip Fractures: Utility of a Virtual Noncalcium Dual-Energy CT Application. *Radiology* **2017**, *284*, 798–805. [CrossRef]
19. Foti, G.; Faccioli, N.; Silva, R.; Oliboni, E.; Zorzi, C.; Carbognin, G. Bone marrow edema around the hip in non-traumatic pain: Dual-energy CT vs MRI. *Eur. Radiol.* **2020**, *30*, 4098–4106. [CrossRef]
20. Chen, Z.; Chen, Y.; Zhang, H.; Jia, X.; Zheng, X.; Zuo, T. Diagnostic accuracy of dual-energy computed tomography (DECT) to detect non-traumatic bone marrow edema: A systematic review and meta-analysis. *Eur. J. Radiol.* **2022**, *153*, 110359. [CrossRef]

21. Ghazi Sherbaf, F.; Sair, H.I.; Shakoor, D.; Fritz, J.; Schwaiger, B.J.; Johnson, M.H.; Demehri, S. DECT in Detection of Vertebral Fracture–associated Bone Marrow Edema: A Systematic Review and Meta-Analysis with Emphasis on Technical and Imaging Interpretation Parameters. *Radiology* **2021**, *300*, 110–119. [CrossRef]
22. Foti, G.; Guerriero, M.; Faccioli, N.; Fighera, A.; Romano, L.; Zorzi, C.; Carbognin, G. Identification of bone marrow edema around the ankle joint in non-traumatic patients: Diagnostic accuracy of dual-energy computed tomography. *Clin. Imaging* **2021**, *69*, 341–348. [CrossRef]
23. Yan, Y.Y.; Ouellette, H.A.; Saththianathan, M.; Munk, P.L.; Mallinson, P.I.; Sheikh, A. The Role of a Virtual Noncalcium Dual-Energy CT Application in the Detection of Bone Marrow Edema in Peripheral Osteomyelitis. *Can. Assoc. Radiol. J. J. Assoc. Can. Radiol.* **2022**, *73*, 549–556. [CrossRef] [PubMed]
24. Foti, G.; Beltramello, A.; Catania, M.; Rigotti, S.; Serra, G.; Carbognin, G. Diagnostic accuracy of dual-energy CT and virtual non-calcium techniques to evaluate bone marrow edema in vertebral compression fractures. *Radiol. Med.* **2019**, *124*, 487–494. [CrossRef] [PubMed]
25. Foti, G.; Serra, G.; Iacono, V.; Zorzi, C. Identification of Traumatic Bone Marrow Oedema: The Pearls and Pitfalls of Dual-Energy CT (DECT). *Tomography* **2021**, *7*, 424–433. [CrossRef] [PubMed]
26. Erdman, W.A.; Tamburro, F.; Jayson, H.T.; Weatherall, P.T.; Ferry, K.B.; Peshock, R.M. Osteomyelitis: Characteristics and pitfalls of diagnosis with MR imaging. *Radiology* **1991**, *180*, 533–539. [CrossRef]
27. Morrison, W.B.; Schweitzer, M.E.; Batte, W.G.; Radack, D.P.; Russel, K.M. Osteomyelitis of the foot: Relative importance of primary and secondary MR imaging signs. *Radiology* **1998**, *207*, 625–632. [CrossRef]
28. Lee, Y.J.; Sadigh, S.; Mankad, K.; Kapse, N.; Rajeswaran, G. The imaging of osteomyelitis. *Quant. Imaging Med. Surg.* **2016**, *6*, 184–198. [CrossRef]
29. Foti, G.; Catania, M.; Caia, S.; Romano, L.; Beltramello, A.; Zorzi, C.; Carbognin, G. Identification of bone marrow edema of the ankle: Diagnostic accuracy of dual-energy CT in comparison with MRI. *Radiol. Med.* **2019**, *124*, 1028–1036. [CrossRef]
30. Booz, C.; Nöske, J.; Albrecht, M.H.; Lenga, L.; Martin, S.S.; Wichmann, J.L.; Huizinga, N.A.; Eichler, K.; Nour-Eldin, N.E.; Vogl, T.J.; et al. Traumatic bone marrow edema of the calcaneus: Evaluation of color-coded virtual non-calcium dual-energy CT in a multi-reader diagnostic accuracy study. *Eur. J. Radiol.* **2019**, *118*, 207–214. [CrossRef]
31. Deng, K.; Sun, C.; Liu, C.; Ma, R. Initial experience with visualizing hand and foot tendons by dual-energy computed tomography. *Clin. Imaging* **2009**, *33*, 384–389. [CrossRef] [PubMed]
32. Foti, G.; Fighera, A.; Campacci, A.; Natali, S.; Guerriero, M.; Zorzi, C.; Carbognin, G. Diagnostic Performance of Dual-Energy CT for Detecting Painful Hip Prosthesis Loosening. *Radiology* **2021**, *300*, 641–649. [CrossRef] [PubMed]
33. Foti, G.; Longo, C.; D'Onofrio, M.; Natali, S.; Piovan, G.; Oliboni, E.; Iacono, V.; Guerriero, M.; Zorzi, C. Dual-Energy CT for Detecting Painful Knee Prosthesis Loosening. *Radiology* **2022**, 211818. [CrossRef]
34. Zou, Z.; Yang, M.; Wang, Y.; Zhang, B. Gout of ankle and foot: DECT versus US for crystal detection. *Clin. Rheumatol.* **2021**, *40*, 1533–1537. [CrossRef] [PubMed]
35. Gold, R.H.; Hawkins, R.A.; Katz, R.D. Bacterial osteomyelitis: Findings on plain radiography, CT, MR, and scintigraphy. *AJR Am. J. Roentgenol.* **1991**, *157*, 365–370. [CrossRef]
36. Llewellyn, A.; Jones-Diette, J.; Kraft, J.; Holton, C.; Harden, M.; Simmonds, M. Imaging tests for the detection of osteomyelitis: A systematic review. *Health Technol. Assess.* **2019**, *23*, 1. [CrossRef]
37. Johnson, P.W.; Collins, M.S.; Wenger, D.E. Diagnostic utility of T1-weighted MRI characteristics in evaluation of osteomyelitis of the foot. *Am. J. Roentgenol.* **2009**, *192*, 96–100. [CrossRef] [PubMed]
38. Jang, Y.H.; Park, S.; Park, Y.U.; Kwack, K.S.; Jeon, S.W.; Lee, H.Y. Multivariate analyses of MRI findings for predicting osteomyelitis of the foot in diabetic patients. *Acta Radiol.* **2020**, *61*, 1205–1212. [CrossRef] [PubMed]

diagnostics

MDPI

Article

Feasibility of the 30 s Sit-to-Stand Test in the Telehealth Setting and Its Relationship to Persistent Symptoms in Non-Hospitalized Patients with Long COVID

Rodrigo Núñez-Cortés [1,2], Cristina Flor-Rufino [3,*], Francisco Miguel Martínez-Arnau [1], Anna Arnal-Gómez [1,3], Claudia Espinoza-Bravo [4], David Hernández-Guillén [3,5] and Sara Cortés-Amador [1,3]

1 Physiotherapy in Motion Multispeciality Research Group (PTinMOTION), Department of Physiotherapy, University of Valencia, 46010 Valencia, Spain
2 Department of Physical Therapy, Faculty of Medicine, University of Chile, Santiago 8240000, Chile
3 Department of Physiotherapy, Faculty of Physiotherapy, University of Valencia, 46010 Valencia, Spain
4 Day Hospital Unit, Hospital Clínico la Florida, Santiago 8240000, Chile
5 Group of Physiotherapy in the Aging Process: Social and Health Care Strategies (PT_AGE), Department of Physiotherapy, Faculty of Physiotherapy, University of Valencia, 46010 Valencia, Spain
* Correspondence: cristina.flor@uv.es; Tel.: +34-662-257-112

Abstract: Fatigue, dyspnea and pain are the main limitations of patients with long COVID. The aim of this study was to determine the feasibility of the 30 s sit-to-stand (30s-STS) test in the telehealth setting and its relationship to persistent symptoms in a sample of non-hospitalized patients with long COVID. A cross-sectional study was conducted in community patients with long COVID. Data collection and assessments were performed by videoconference and consisted of the fatigue assessment scale (FAS), London activity of daily living scale (LCADL), post-COVID-19 functional status (PCFS) and European quality of life questionnaire (EQ-5D-5L), including the pain/discomfort dimension. The 30s-STS test was performed using a standardized protocol adapted for remote use, and the modified Borg scale (0–10) was used to assess dyspnea and lower limb fatigue immediately after the test. The feasibility of the 30s-STS test was assessed by the proportion of eligible participants who were able to complete the test. Safety was assessed by the number of adverse events that occurred during the test. Seventy-nine participants were included (median age: 44 years, 86.1% women). Performance in the 30s-STS test was 11.5 ± 3.2 repetitions with 60.8% of the sample below reference values. All eligible participants were able to complete the test. No adverse events were reported during the evaluation. Participants with lower 30s-STS performance had more fatigue and dyspnea, worse quality of life, more severe pain/discomfort, and worse functional status ($p < 0.05$). A significant correlation was obtained between LCADL and dyspnea, reported on the Borg scale (0–10) post 30s-STS ($r = 0.71$; $p < 0.001$). In conclusion, the 30s-STS test proved to be a feasible test to implement in the telehealth setting and is related to fatigue, dyspnea, quality of life and pain in non-hospitalized patients with long COVID. Clinicians may use this test when assessment of the physical sequelae of COVID-19 in the face-to-face setting is not possible.

Keywords: telemedicine; functional capacity; rehabilitation; SARS-CoV-2; pain

1. Introduction

Since the onset of the COVID-19 pandemic in December 2019, more than 640 million cases have been confirmed worldwide according to the World Health Organization (WHO) [1]. In addition, the restrictions adopted to control the quick spread of COVID-19 have had negative consequences on the overall health of the population (e.g., the practice of physical activity levels have been affected) [2]. Previous research has reported that 81% of COVID-19 cases show a mild presentation of the disease, 14% moderate and the remaining

5% trigger a critical situation [3,4]. Post-COVID-19 sequelae may be present in more than 60% of infected people [5], with female sex being a risk factor for the development of some persistent symptoms [6].

In recent months, research has focused on the post-infection stages, as it has been reported that, in some patients, symptomatology may reappear and persist for months or even years after infection [7,8]. This persistent condition is named "Long COVID" [6] and it can affect different organs and body systems, with a wide range of signs and symptoms. The most commonly reported symptoms are fatigue, dyspnea and pain [9], with no differences between hospitalized and non-hospitalized patients [5]. These sequelae can affect physical performance, activities of daily living, and lead to a loss of health-related quality of life [10]. Thus, an evaluation and follow-up of individuals who have suffered COVID-19 is considered desirable in order to detect sequelae and implement treatment if necessary [11,12].

In this context, the assessment of patients' functional performance after COVID-19 has become a challenge for clinicians' decision-making. The 6 min walk test (6MWT) is considered the gold standard for functional performance assessment. However, the 6MWT requires technical performance conditions that are not easy to meet in the telerehabilitation setting, such as a 20–30 m corridor [13]. In contrast, the 30 s sit-to-stand (30s-STS) is a quick and easy-to-use, low-cost clinical test of functional capacity, which has been validated in vulnerable populations such as older adults [14] or oncological patients [15]. The 30s-STS is a time-based assessment in which participants are asked to stand and sit from a chair as many times as possible for 30 s with their arms crossed over their chest [14]. In general, the 30s-STS is better tolerated than the 1-min STS [16], and performance requires greater cardiorespiratory endurance than the five times STS [17].

Due to the outbreak of COVID-19, many rehabilitation programs were adapted from face-to-face to remote models [18,19]. Thus, compared to face-to-face programs, telehealth programs can eliminate geographic and socioeconomic barriers by improving access for participants in rural and transportation-challenged areas, and are a suitable alternative for clinical assessment and intervention during pandemics [18,20,21]. For example, a recent meta-analysis identified that home-based cardiac rehabilitation significantly improves functional capacity and health-related quality of life, compared to usual care, being a potential alternative for patients who are not suitable for in-center cardiac rehabilitation [22]. In addition, a recent systematic review concluded that the risk of adverse events during home rehabilitation appears to be very low in cardiac patients [23]. In this context, the STS test may also be performed safely at home, provided that patients are not at risk of desaturation [24]. Traditionally, the 30s-STS has been used to assess lower limb strength, muscle power or physical function [25–27]. However, since the performance of the test requires some cardiorespiratory demand [17], it could also be an alternative to assess lower limb fatigue and dyspnea on physical exertion, which are both very prevalent symptoms in patients with long COVID. Therefore, the use of the 30s-STS in a telehealth context could be interesting, especially for assessing patients who did not have early access to rehabilitation programs, such as people who have suffered a mild COVID-19 infection and yet experienced persistence of COVID-19 symptoms months after the initial episode. Consequently, the objective of this study was to determine the feasibility of the 30s-STS test in the telehealth setting and its relationship to persistent symptoms such as fatigue, dyspnea and pain in a sample of non-hospitalized patients with long COVID.

2. Materials and Methods

2.1. Design and Participants

We conducted a cross-sectional study that collected data from consecutive community patients with long COVID admitted to a telerehabilitation program implemented at the University of Valencia (Valencia, Spain) between October 2021 and May 2022. Participants were recruited through social networks and by contact with long COVID associations in the autonomous communities of Comunidad Valenciana, Madrid, Castilla la Mancha,

Cataluña, Galicia, Cantabria and Aragon. Inclusion criteria were as follows: (i) age between 20 and 60 years old; (ii) positive PCR test results from nasal and pharyngeal swab sample; (iii) presence of at least one of the following persistent COVID-19-related symptoms: fatigue, dyspnea, or functional limitation for at least 6 weeks after infection; (iv) having a device with Internet access (e.g., smartphone, computer or tablet). Exclusion criteria were: (i) severe case of COVID-19 (i.e., history of hospitalization, severe pneumonia or pulmonary thromboembolism); (ii) other concomitant acute or chronic pulmonary or cardiac pathologies; (iii) presence of more severe symptoms requiring monitorization by clinical staff (i.e., desaturation on exertion, unsteadiness, hemodynamic instability).

This study was approved by the Ethics Committee of the University of Valencia (Registration number: 15737788), and all patients provided written informed consent. The research was conducted in accordance with the ethical principles of the Declaration of Helsinki. This study was conducted in accordance with the Guidelines for Strengthening the Reporting of Observational Studies in Epidemiology (STROBE) [28].

2.2. Data Collection

The evaluation was conducted by 1:1 videoconference in real time using Zoom Communication software (Zoom Video Communications, Inc., San Jose, CA, USA). Data were collected by four PhD physiotherapists (C.F-R., F.M.M-A., A.A.-G. and D.H-G.) with more than five years of clinical experience. All evaluators received prior training to standardize the evaluation. The assessment was performed in the patient's environment, using the device of their choice (computer, smartphone or tablet), and data protection was ensured by storing the information anonymously, with access restricted to research staff only. Data regarding age, sex, time post-infection, symptoms related to long COVID, and smoking history were collected by structured interview.

The level of fatigue was assessed using the fatigue assessment scale (FAS) [29], which consists of 10 items evaluating both physical and mental fatigue, with 5 questions, respectively. Each item is scored on a scale of 1 "never" to 5 "always," with a higher score (which ranged between 10 and 50) indicating a higher level of fatigue. This instrument has proven to be valid and reliable for fatigue assessment [29].

Dyspnea was assessed using the Spanish version of the London chest activity of daily living scale (LCADL) [30], which is a valid questionnaire that evaluates the degree of limitation in activities of daily living due to dyspnea in patients with chronic respiratory diseases. The LCADL comprises 15 items that consider self-care, household, physical and leisure activities, and each question is scored from 0 to 5. A higher score indicates a greater degree of limitation in activities of daily living due to dyspnea [30].

Health-related quality of life was assessed using the 5-dimensional European quality of life questionnaire (EQ-5D-5L) [31], which provides an index score ranging from 0 (death) to 1 (full health), and a self-reported rating of current general health status based on a visual analogue scale ranging from 0 "the worst health you can imagine" to 100 "the best health you can imagine". Pain or discomfort were rated using a 5-choice categorical scale: (1) "No pain or discomfort"; (2) "Slight pain or discomfort"; (3) "Moderate pain or discomfort"; (4) "Severe pain or discomfort"; (5) "Extreme pain or discomfort".

Finally, functional status was assessed with the Spanish version of the Post-COVID-19 functional status scale (PCFS) [32], which is a 6-grade ordinal scale: grade 0 (no functional limitations); grade 1 (negligible functional limitations); grade 2 (slight functional limitations); grade 3 (moderate functional limitations); grade 4 (severe functional limitations); and grade 5 (death). The feasibility of the 30s-STS test was assessed by the proportion of eligible participants who were able to complete the test. Reasons for not completing the test were also recorded. Safety was assessed by the number of adverse events of any type (serious or minor) that occurred during the performance of the 30s-STS test.

The 30s-STS test was performed in the participant's home environment using a standardized protocol adapted for remote use [15]. First, the clinician explained the 30s-STS test and ensured that the patient understood how to perform it. Adequate Internet connection was also checked. Then, participants were instructed to place a sturdy chair against the wall. Participants were asked to position themselves in the center of the device's camera view to obtain the best visibility for the clinician. If available, participants were asked to use a chair without armrests. The 30s-STS test was performed only once, since it is considered to have good test–retest reliability [33]. Patients were instructed to cross their arms over their chest and complete as many standing cycles as possible in 30 s. The instructions were to stand until fully upright and then sit until the buttocks touched the chair, without aid of their hands [27]. During the test they were verbally encouraged [27]. To compare functional performance in the 30s-STS test with reference values in healthy populations, the sex- and age-specific centile curves reported by Warden et al. [34] were used. To categorize low and normal functional performance in the 30s-STS test, the lower limit of the standard deviation of the mean number of repetitions according to age and sex was used as the cutoff point. The modified Borg scale (0–10) was used to assess dyspnea and lower limb fatigue immediately after the 30s-STS test [35]. The Borg scale score ranges from 0 to 10, where 0 corresponds to the absence of dyspnea or physical exertion and 10 corresponds to the maximum degree of dyspnea or physical exertion.

2.3. Statistical Analysis

Sample size calculation was performed with G*Power, version 3.1.9.2 (Universität Düsseldorf, Germany). A moderate effect size (d = 0.7) was estimated from a clinically relevant 4-point difference in fatigue (FAS score) [36] (difference between two independent means, n1 $\neq$ n2). Considering a statistical power of 80%, two tails, and α err prob = 0.05, the minimum required sample size was 68 patients. Statistical analysis was performed with Statistical Package for the Social Sciences (SPSS) version 22.0 (IBM Corporation, Armonk, NY, USA). Normality of the data was determined with the Shapiro–Wilk test. Considering the distribution of the data, parametric or nonparametric, the results were presented as mean and standard deviation or as median and interquartile range (IQR), respectively. Comparison between the low and normal performance groups in the 30s-STS according to baseline values was performed using the chi-square test for categorical variables (sex, PCFS and pain/discomfort), the Mann–Whitney U-test for nonparametric variables (post-infection time and dyspnea), and the independent samples *t*-test for variables with normal distribution. A correlation analysis using Spearman's correlation coefficient was applied to assess the association between lower limb fatigue and dyspnea, measured with the Borg scale (0–10) post 30s-STS, and the FAS and LCADL, respectively. The significance level was set at 0.05 for all statistical analyses.

3. Results

A total of 79 participants met the eligibility criteria (Figure 1).

The median age was 44 (range: 24–52) years, and 68 (86.1%) participants were women. Time passed after COVID-19 infection ranged from 2 to 28 months, with a median of 17 months. In the total sample, 72.2% of cases had moderate to extreme pain, with high levels of dyspnea and fatigue (Table 1).

Performance in the 30s-STS test was 11.5 $\pm$ 3.2 repetitions and 48 (60.8%) cases performed below the reference values according to age and sex (Figure 2).

Table 1. Baseline characterization of patients (*n* = 79).

Characteristics	Values
Age (years)	44 (24–52)
Sex *n* (%)	
Men	11 (13.9)
Women	68 (86.1)
Post infection time (months)	17 (2–28)
Symptoms *n* (%)	
Fatigue	74 (93.7)
Dyspnea	23 (29.1)
Cognition problems	23 (29.1)
Myalgia	23 (29.1)
Headache	5 (6.3)
Cough	4 (5.1)
Smoking history *n* (%)	77 (97.5)
PCFS *n* (%)	
Grade 1	1 (1.3)
Grade 2	6 (7.6)
Grade 3	40 (50.6)
Grade 4	32 (40.5)
Grade 5	0 (0)
EQ-5D-5L	
Index score (0–1)	0.60 ± 0.23
Visual analogue scale	47.3 ± 17.1
Pain/discomfort *n* (%)	
I have no pain or discomfort	7 (8.9)
I have slight pain or discomfort	15 (19.0)
I have moderate pain or discomfort	37 (46.8)
I have severe pain or discomfort	19 (24.1)
I have extreme pain or discomfort	1 (1.3)
LCADL (10–75)	25.5 (15–68)
LCADL (%)	33.3 (20–90)
FAS (10–50)	34.7 ± 8.4
30s-STS (repetitions)	11.5 ± 3.2

Abbreviation: 30s-STS, 30 s sit-to-stand; EQ-5D-5L, European quality of life–5 dimensions–5 levels; FAS, fatigue assessment scale; LCADL, London chest activity of daily living; PCDS, Post-COVID-19 functional status. Values are mean (standard deviation), median (min-max) or *n* (%).

No adverse events were reported during the evaluation. All patients were able to complete the test; only two participants reported mild dizziness at the end of the test. Significant differences in LCADL (p = 0.001) and FAS (p = 0.004) were obtained when comparing the low and normal functional performance groups in the 30s-STS according to reference values. Moreover, participants with lower 30s-STS performance had worse quality of life on the EQ5D index score (mean difference = −0.22, 95% confidence interval: −0.32 to −0.14, $p < 0.001$), on the visual analogue scale (mean difference = −13.9, 95% confidence interval: −21.1 to −6.7, $p < 0.001$), more severe pain/discomfort (χ^2 = 13.1, p = 0.011), and more severe PCFS (χ^2 = 11.1, p = 0.011). There were no differences with respect to age and time post infection ($p > 0.05$) (Table 2).

The median (IQR) fatigue and dyspnea reported on the Borg scale (0–10) after the 30s-STS test were 6.0 (5.0) and 3.0 (5.0), respectively. A low and significant correlation was obtained between FAS and lower limb fatigue reported on the Borg scale (0–10) post-30s-STS (r = 0.24, p = 0.034). A high and significant correlation was obtained between LCADL and dyspnea reported on the Borg scale (0–10) post-30s-STS (r = 0.71, $p < 0.001$). The distribution of dyspnea and fatigue data for each scale are shown in Supplementary Material (Figure S1).

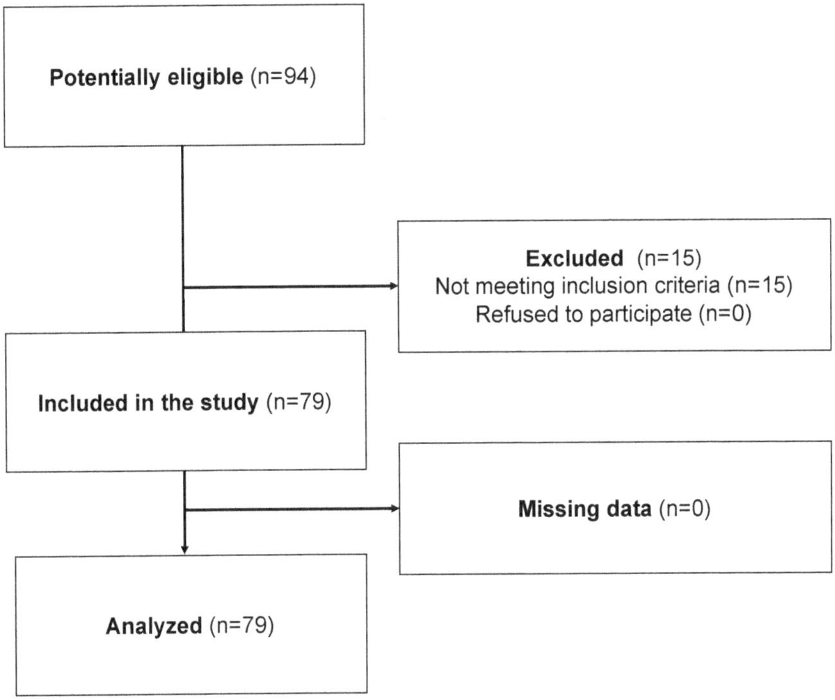

Figure 1. Flow-chart.

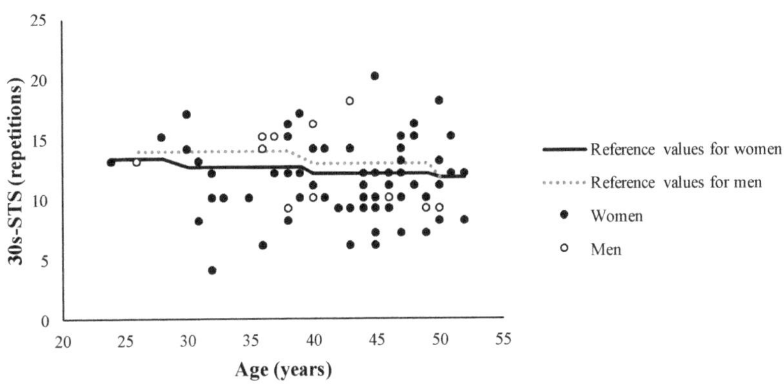

Figure 2. Functional performance of women and men long COVID patients vs. sex- and age-specific reference values. The reference values correspond to the sex- and age-specific zenith curves reported by Warden et al. [34] (i.e., the lower limit of the standard deviation of the mean number of repetitions in 30 s-sit-to-stand).

Table 2. Comparison between low and normal physical performance.

Characteristics	Low 30s-STS (n = 48)	Normal 30s-STS (n = 31)	p-Value
Age (years)	44 (9)	43 (10)	0.879
Post infection time (months)	17 (12)	18 (19)	0.948
PCFS n (%)			
Grade 1	0 (0)	1 (3.2)	
Grade 2	1 (2.1)	5 (16.1)	
Grade 3	22 (45.8)	18 (58.1)	0.011 *
Grade 4	25 (52.1)	7 (22.6)	
Grade 5	0 (0)	0 (0)	
EQ-5D-5L			
Index score (0–1)	0.51 ± 0.2	0.74 ± 0.2	<0.001 ***
Visual analogue scale	41.9 ± 14.8	55.8 ± 17.1	<0.001 ***
Pain/discomfort n (%)			
No pain or discomfort	1 (2.1)	6 (19.4)	
Slight pain or discomfort	6 (12.5)	9 (29.0)	
Moderate pain or discomfort	25 (52.1)	12 (38.7)	0.011 *
Severe pain or discomfort	15 (31.3)	4 (12.9)	
Extreme pain or discomfort	1 (2.1)	0 (0)	
LCADL (0–75)	33 (16.8)	20 (10)	<0.001 ***
LCADL (%)	44 (22.3)	26.7 (13.3)	<0.001 ***
FAS (10–50)	38 (13)	31 (12)	0.001 **
Dyspnea post 30s-STS (0–10)	4 (4)	2 (4)	0.029 *
Fatigue post 30s-STS (0–10)	7 (3)	3 (5)	<0.001 ***

Values are median (IQR) or mean ± SD. Abbreviation: 30s-STS, 30 s sit-to-stand; EQ-5D-5l, European quality of life–5 dimensions–5 levels; FAS, fatigue assessment scale; LCADL, London chest activity of daily living; PCDS, Post-COVID-19 functional status. * Statistically significant difference ($p < 0.05$); ** Statistically significant difference ($p < 0.01$); *** Statistically significant difference ($p < 0.001$).

4. Discussion

The 30s-STS test proved to be a feasible test to implement in the telehealth setting when assessing physical function and its relationship to persistent symptoms such as fatigue, dyspnea, quality of life and pain/discomfort in a sample of community patients with long COVID. Functional tests (e.g., 30s-STS) performed via teleassessment are reliable, valid and feasible for measuring the performance of healthy young adults in clinical practice [37]. Considering that all the cases included in our study were able to perform the test and no adverse events were recorded, our results indicate that the 30s-STS may also be an excellent option for telehealth assessment of the main symptoms of prolonged COVID (e.g., fatigue, dyspnea, functional impairment and pain), especially in pandemics, when equipment, time and space requirements may be limited. Therefore, rehabilitation clinicians may perform the 30s-STS test with confidence when they aim to identify cases with greater physical sequelae [15,24].

Our results are similar to those published by Bowman et al. [15], who evaluated the feasibility and safety of 30s-STS via telehealth in the oncology population, with a 94% test completion rate and no reported safety incidents. Furthermore, in this investigation they found a moderate correlation between the 30s-STS and self-reported physical activity level, providing evidence of convergent validity [15]. Interestingly, performance in the number of repetitions of the 30s-STS in our population (median = 11.5 repetitions) was lower than the one reported by Bowman et al. [15] (median 13.5 repetitions) even when our sample was, according to median age, 18 years younger. These findings show that the physical sequelae following COVID-19 were also significant in non-hospitalized cases, regardless of severity.

More than half of the cases had poor functional performance (i.e., 30s-STS below the reference values), which was associated with increased levels of fatigue, dyspnea and pain/discomfort. In fact, the difference between groups was greater than the minimal important difference established for FAS (4-point) [36], LCADLtotal (range: −2.1 and −5.9 points), and for LCADL%total (−2 and −6 points) in patients with chronic respiratory diseases (Table 2) [38]. On the other hand, the modified Borg scale used to assess lower limb fatigue and dyspnea after the 30s-STS test showed a significant association with the validated scales for these symptoms, FAS and LCADL, respectively. This test has been commonly used as an indicator of lower limb muscle strength/power in patients with chronic conditions [25–27]. However, taking into account that the number of repetitions in the 30s-STS has a moderate correlation with the distance walked in the six-minute walk test and therefore requires some physical and cardiorespiratory demand [17], our results indicate that this test may also be applied to assess symptoms of fatigue and dyspnea after physical exertion, which are very frequent in patients with long COVID [9].

Patients with low 30s-STS performance according to reference values also had worse quality of life and more severe functional status on PCFS. In addition, participants with low 30s-STS performance had a higher severity of pain/discomfort. In fact, more than 85% of them had moderate to extreme pain/discomfort, in contrast to participants with normal 30s-STS performance, of which only 51.6% had this condition. Persistent pain is one of the most common symptoms in long COVID and addressing it could be key to improving functional performance as well [39].

The COVID-19 pandemic has forced healthcare teams to innovate and implement new strategies for monitoring patients in need of rehabilitation [19]. Thus, the 30s-STS test can also be used to prescribe exercise in telehealth programs or when geographic or economic barriers prevent assessment of COVID-19 physical sequelae. For example, functional performance assessment through telehealth could improve access to follow-up of physical sequelae for people living in rural areas, having financial or transport problems, insufficient social assistance or being unable to take time off work, which are common barriers to rehabilitation programs [18]. Telehealth also presents an opportunity to safely benefit vulnerable populations (e.g., home-based rehabilitation). However, new approaches are needed to achieve a sense of connection similar to that of face-to-face care in terms of practical teaching, training and human connection [19]. Particularly, improving functional performance using the 30s-STS test has also been a goal of telerehabilitation programs for people with COVID-19 and post-COVID-19 conditions. For example, exercises performed through telerehabilitation can specifically improve performance in the 30s-STS test [40]. Thus, this test can be used for both screening and assessment of post-treatment changes. Additionally, a functional assessment test prior to the start of the rehabilitation program could allow an accurate exercise prescription at home [41]. The 30s-STS has the potential to be delivered safely through telehealth [15], reducing the delivery cost and improving patient access and autonomy [40–42].

The main limitation of this study was that the chair used for the assessment was not standardized for all participants, as it varied from household to household. This could limit comparison with baseline data and therefore the results should be interpreted with caution. In addition, the device for evaluation varied among each participant. On the other hand, we were unable to control cardiorespiratory variables such as oxygen saturation or heart rate. Finally, we recognize that there may be a selection bias because recruitment of participants was by disclosure and voluntary participation. However, our study has a pragmatic focus and may provide guidance to clinicians when assessing and prescribing exercise to their patients via telehealth. Future studies should evaluate the possibility of a more comprehensive assessment of functional performance via telehealth, including, for example, step test or timed up and go, as well as cardiorespiratory function [24]. In addition, inter-rater reliability testing remains necessary for this type of assessment in patients with long COVID.

5. Conclusions

The 30s-STS test proved to be a feasible test to implement in the telehealth setting and has shown a relation to fatigue, dyspnea, quality of life and pain/discomfort in a sample of community patients with long COVID. Clinicians may use this test to prescribe exercise in telehealth programs or when geographic or economic barriers prevent assessment of the physical sequelae of COVID-19.

Supplementary Materials: The following supporting information can be downloaded at: https://www.mdpi.com/article/10.3390/diagnostics13010024/s1, Figure S1. Association between exertional fatigue and dyspnea after 30s-STS and validated dyspnea and fatigue questionnaires (FAS and LCADL).

Author Contributions: R.N.-C., S.C.-A., F.M.M.-A. and C.E.-B. conceived and designed the study; R.N.-C. and C.F.-R. drafted the article; S.C.-A., F.M.M.-A., A.A.-G., C.F.-R. and D.H.-G. acquired the data; R.N.-C. analyzed the data; S.C.-A., F.M.M.-A., A.A.-G., C.E.-B. and D.H.-G. revised the manuscript for key intellectual content; all the authors approved the last version to be submitted. All authors have read and agreed to the published version of the manuscript.

Funding: This research received no external funding.

Institutional Review Board Statement: This study was approved by the Ethics Committee of the University of Valencia (Registration number: 15737788), and all patients gave written informed consent. The research was conducted in accordance with the ethical principles of the Declaration of Helsinki.

Informed Consent Statement: Informed consent was obtained from all subjects involved in the study. Written informed consent has been obtained from the patient(s) to publish this paper.

Data Availability Statement: Not applicable.

Acknowledgments: The authors thank all participants in the study.

Conflicts of Interest: The authors declare no conflict of interest.

References

1. World Health Organization. Coronavirus (COVID-19) Dashboard. Available online: https://covid19.who.int/ (accessed on 16 September 2022).
2. Di Stefano, V.; Ornello, R.; Gagliardo, A.; Torrente, A.; Illuminato, E.; Caponnetto, V.; Frattale, I.; Golini, R.; Di Felice, C.; Graziano, F.; et al. Social Distancing in Chronic Migraine during the Covid-19 Outbreak: Results from a Multicenter Observational Study. *Nutrients* **2021**, *13*, 1361. [CrossRef] [PubMed]
3. Ozma, M.A.; Maroufi, P.; Khodadadi, E.; Köse, Ş.; Esposito, I.; Ganbarov, K.; Dao, S.; Esposito, S.; Dal, T.; Zeinalzadeh, E.; et al. Clinical Manifestation, Diagnosis, Prevention and Control of SARS-CoV-2 (COVID-19) during the Outbreak Period. *Infez. Med.* **2020**, *28*, 153–165.
4. Wu, Z.; McGoogan, J.M. Characteristics of and Important Lessons from the Coronavirus Disease 2019 (COVID-19) Outbreak in China: Summary of a Report of 72314 Cases from the Chinese Center for Disease Control and Prevention. *J. Am. Med. Assoc.* **2020**, *323*, 1239–1242. [CrossRef] [PubMed]
5. Fernández-de-las-Peñas, C.; Palacios-Ceña, D.; Gómez-Mayordomo, V.; Florencio, L.L.; Cuadrado, M.L.; Plaza-Manzano, G.; Navarro-Santana, M. Prevalence of Post-COVID-19 Symptoms in Hospitalized and Non-Hospitalized COVID-19 Survivors: A Systematic Review and Meta-Analysis. *Eur. J. Intern. Med.* **2021**, *92*, 55–70. [CrossRef] [PubMed]
6. Fernández-De-las-peñas, C.; Martín-Guerrero, J.D.; Pellicer-Valero, Ó.J.; Navarro-Pardo, E.; Gómez-Mayordomo, V.; Cuadrado, M.L.; Arias-Navalón, J.A.; Cigarán-Méndez, M.; Hernández-Barrera, V.; Arendt-Nielsen, L. Female Sex Is a Risk Factor Associated with Long-Term Post-COVID Related-Symptoms but Not with COVID-19 Symptoms: The LONG-COVID-EXP-CM Multicenter Study. *J. Clin. Med.* **2022**, *11*, 413. [CrossRef] [PubMed]
7. Spruit, M.A.; Holland, A.E.; Singh, S.J.; Tonia, T.; Wilson, K.C.; Troosters, T. COVID-19: Interim Guidance on Rehabilitation in the Hospital and Post-Hospital Phase from a European Respiratory Society- And American Thoracic Society-Coordinated International Task Force. *Eur. Respir. J.* **2020**, *56*, 2002197. [CrossRef]
8. Callard, F.; Perego, E. How and Why Patients Made Long Covid. *Soc. Sci. Med.* **2021**, *268*, 113426. [CrossRef]
9. Michelen, M.; Manoharan, L.; Elkheir, N.; Cheng, V.; Dagens, A.; Hastie, C.; O'Hara, M.; Suett, J.; Dahmash, D.; Bugaeva, P.; et al. Characterising Long COVID: A Living Systematic Review. *BMJ Glob. Health* **2021**, *6*, e005427. [CrossRef]
10. Malik, P.; Patel, K.; Pinto, C.; Jaiswal, R.; Tirupathi, R.; Pillai, S.; Patel, U. Post-Acute COVID-19 Syndrome (PCS) and Health-Related Quality of Life (HRQoL)—A Systematic Review and Meta-Analysis. *J. Med. Virol.* **2022**, *94*, 253–262. [CrossRef]

11. Zhao, Y.; Shang, Y.; Song, W.; Li, Q.; Xie, H.; Xu, Q.; Jia, J.; Li, L.; Mao, H.; Zhou, X.; et al. Follow-up Study of the Pulmonary Function and Related Physiological Characteristics of COVID-19 Survivors Three Months after Recovery. *EClinicalMedicine* **2020**, *25*, 100463. [CrossRef]
12. Núñez-Cortés, R.; Malhue-Vidal, C.; Gath, F.; Valdivia-Lobos, G.; Torres-Castro, R.; Cruz-Montecinos, C.; Martinez-Arnau, F.M.; Pérez-Alenda, S.; López-Bueno, R.; Calatayud, J. The Impact of Charlson Comorbidity Index on the Functional Capacity of COVID-19 Survivors: A Prospective Cohort Study with One-Year Follow-Up. *Int. J. Environ. Res. Public Health* **2022**, *19*, 7473. [CrossRef] [PubMed]
13. Holland, A.E.; Spruit, M.A.; Troosters, T.; Puhan, M.A.; Pepin, V.; Saey, D.; McCormack, M.C.; Carlin, B.W.; Sciurba, F.C.; Pitta, F.; et al. An Official European Respiratory Society/American Thoracic Society Technical Standard: Field Walking Tests in Chronic Respiratory Disease. *Eur. Respir. J.* **2014**, *44*, 1428–1446. [CrossRef] [PubMed]
14. Jones, C.J.; Rikli, R.E.; Beam, W.C. A 30-s Chair-Stand Test as a Measure of Lower Body. *Res. Q. Exerc. Sport* **2013**, *70*, 37–41.
15. Bowman, A.; Denehy, L.; Benjemaa, A.; Crowe, J.; Bruns, E.; Hall, T.; Traill, A.; Edbrooke, L. Feasibility and Safety of the 30-Second Sit-to-Stand Test Delivered via Telehealth: An Observational Study. *PM&R* **2022**, 1–10. [CrossRef]
16. Zanini, A.; Aiello, M.; Cherubino, F.; Zampogna, E.; Azzola, A.; Chetta, A.; Spanevello, A. The One Repetition Maximum Test and the Sit-to-Stand Test in the Assessment of a Specific Pulmonary Rehabilitation Program on Peripheral Muscle Strength in COPD Patients. *Int. J. Chronic Obstr. Pulm. Dis.* **2015**, *10*, 2423–2430. [CrossRef]
17. Yee, X.S.; Ng, Y.S.; Allen, J.C.; Latib, A.; Tay, E.L.; Abu Bakar, H.M.; Ho, C.Y.J.; Koh, W.C.C.; Kwek, H.H.T.; Tay, L. Performance on Sit-to-Stand Tests in Relation to Measures of Functional Fitness and Sarcopenia Diagnosis in Community-Dwelling Older Adults. *Eur. Rev. Aging Phys. Act.* **2021**, *18*, 1. [CrossRef]
18. Stefanakis, M.; Batalik, L.; Papathanasiou, J.; Dipla, L.; Antoniou, V.; Pepera, G. Exercise-Based Cardiac Rehabilitation Programs in the Era of COVID-19: A Critical Review. *Rev. Cardiovasc. Med.* **2021**, *22*, 1143–1155. [CrossRef]
19. Epstein, E.; Patel, N.; Maysent, K.; Taub, P.R. Cardiac Rehab in the COVID Era and beyond: MHealth and Other Novel Opportunities. *Curr. Cardiol. Rep.* **2021**, *23*, 42. [CrossRef]
20. Winnige, P.; Filakova, K.; Hnatiak, J.; Dosbaba, F.; Bocek, O.; Pepera, G.; Papathanasiou, J.; Batalik, L.; Grace, S.L. Validity and Reliability of the Cardiac Rehabilitation Barriers Scale in the Czech Republic (Crbs-Cze): Determination of Key Barriers in East-Central Europe. *Int. J. Environ. Res. Public Health* **2021**, *18*, 13113. [CrossRef]
21. Nso, N.; Nassar, M.; Mbome, Y.; Emmanuel, K.E.; Lyonga Ngonge, A.; Badejoko, S.; Akbar, S.; Landry, I.; Alfishawy, M.; Munira, M.; et al. Comparative Assessment of the Long-Term Efficacy of Home-Based versus Center-Based Cardiac Rehabilitation. *Cureus* **2022**, *14*, e23495. [CrossRef]
22. Imran, H.M.; Baig, M.; Erqou, S.; Taveira, T.H.; Shah, N.R.; Morrison, A.; Choudhary, G.; Wu, W.C. Home-Based Cardiac Rehabilitation Alone and Hybrid with Center-Based Cardiac Rehabilitation in Heart Failure: A Systematic Review and Meta-Analysis. *J. Am. Heart Assoc.* **2019**, *8*, e012779. [CrossRef] [PubMed]
23. Stefanakis, M.; Batalik, L.; Antoniou, V.; Pepera, G. Safety of Home-Based Cardiac Rehabilitation: A Systematic Review. *Heart Lung* **2022**, *55*, 117–126. [CrossRef] [PubMed]
24. Holland, A.E.; Malaguti, C.; Hoffman, M.; Lahham, A.; Burge, A.T.; Dowman, L.; May, A.K.; Bondarenko, J.; Graco, M.; Tikellis, G.; et al. Home-Based or Remote Exercise Testing in Chronic Respiratory Disease, during the COVID-19 Pandemic and beyond: A Rapid Review. *Chron. Respir. Dis.* **2020**, *17*, 1479973120952418. [CrossRef]
25. Jerez-Mayorga, D.; Delgado-Floody, P.; Intelangelo, L.; Campos-Jara, C.; Arias-Poblete, L.; García-Verazaluce, J.; Garcia-Ramos, A.; Chirosa, L.J. Behavior of the Muscle Quality Index and Isometric Strength in Elderly Women. *Physiol. Behav.* **2020**, *227*, 113145. [CrossRef]
26. Roldán-Jiménez, C.; Bennett, P.; Cuesta-Vargas, A.I. Muscular Activity and Fatigue in Lower-Limb and Trunk Muscles during Different Sit-to-Stand Tests. *PLoS ONE* **2015**, *10*, e0141675. [CrossRef] [PubMed]
27. Núñez-Cortés, R.; Cruz-Montecinos, C.; Martinez-Arnau, F.; Torres-Castro, R.; Zamora-Risco, E.; Pérez-Alenda, S.; Andersen, L.L.; Calatayud, J.; Arana, E. 30 s Sit-to-Stand Power Is Positively Associated with Chest Muscle Thickness in COVID-19 Survivors. *Chron. Respir. Dis.* **2022**, *19*, 14799731221114263. [CrossRef]
28. von Elm, E.; Altman, D.G.; Egger, M.; Pocock, S.J.; Gøtzsche, P.C.; Vandenbroucke, J.P. The Strengthening the Reporting of Observational Studies in Epidemiology (STROBE) Statement: Guidelines for Reporting Observational Studies. *Int. J. Surg.* **2014**, *12*, 1495–1499. [CrossRef]
29. Michielsen, H.J.; De Vries, J.; Van Heck, G.L. Psychometric Qualities of a Brief Self-Rated Fatigue Measure: The Fatigue Assessment Scale. *J. Psychosom. Res.* **2003**, *54*, 345–352. [CrossRef]
30. Vilaró, J.; Gimeno, E.; Férez, N.S.; Hernando, C.; Díaz, I.; Ferrer, M.; Roca, J.; Alonso, J. Daily Living Activity in Chronic Obstructive Pulmonary Disease: Validation of the Spanish Version and Comparative Analysis of 2 Questionnaires. *Med. Clin.* **2007**, *129*, 326–332. [CrossRef]
31. Herdman, M.; Badia, X.; Berra, S. El EuroQol-5D: Una Alternativa Sencilla Para La Medición de La Calidad de Vida Relacionada Con La Salud En Atención Primaria. *Atención Primaria* **2001**, *28*, 425–429. [CrossRef]
32. Sacristán-Galisteo, C.; del Corral, T.; Ríos-León, M.; Martín-Casas, P.; Plaza-Manzano, G.; de-Uralde-Villanueva, I.L. Construct Validity of the Spanish Version of the Post-COVID-19 Functional Status Scale and Validation of the Web-Based Form in COVID-19 Survivors. *PLoS ONE* **2022**, *17*, e0269274. [CrossRef] [PubMed]

33. Tiedemann, A.; Lord, S.R.; Sherrington, C. The Development and Validation of a Brief Performance-Based Fall Risk Assessment Tool for Use in Primary Care. *J. Gerontol. Ser. A Biol. Sci. Med. Sci.* **2010**, *65*, 896–903. [CrossRef] [PubMed]
34. Warden, S.J.; Liu, Z.; Moe, S.M. Sex- and Age-Specific Centile Curves and Downloadable Calculator for Clinical Muscle Strength Tests to Identify Probable Sarcopenia. *Phys. Ther. Rehabil. J.* **2022**, *102*, pzab299. [CrossRef] [PubMed]
35. Wilson, R.C.; Jones, P.W. A Comparison of the Visual Analogue Scale and Modified Borg Scale for the Measurement of Dyspnoea during Exercise. *Clin. Sci.* **1989**, *76*, 277–282. [CrossRef]
36. De Kleijn, W.P.E.; De Vries, J.; Wijnen, P.A.H.M.; Drent, M. Minimal (Clinically) Important Differences for the Fatigue Assessment Scale in Sarcoidosis. *Respir. Med.* **2011**, *105*, 1388–1395. [CrossRef]
37. Güngör, F.; Ovacık, U.; Ertan Harputlu, Ö.; Yekdaneh, A.A.; Kurt, Í. Tele-Assessment of Core Performance and Functional Capacity: Reliability, Validity, and Feasibility in Healthy Individuals. *J. Telemed. Telecare* **2022**, *2*, 1357633X221117335. [CrossRef]
38. Almeida Gulart, A.; de Araujo, C.L.P.; Bauer Munari, A.; Schneider, B.F.; Dal Lago, P.; Mayer, A.F. Minimal Important Difference for London Chest Activity of Daily Living Scale in Patients with Chronic Obstructive Pulmonary Disease. *Physiotherapy* **2020**, *107*, 28–35. [CrossRef]
39. Khoja, O.; Passadouro, B.S.; Mulvey, M.; Delis, I.; Astill, S.; Tan, A.L.; Sivan, M. Clinical Characteristics and Mechanisms of Musculoskeletal Pain in Long COVID. *J. Pain Res.* **2022**, *15*, 1729–1748. [CrossRef]
40. Vieira, A.G.S.; Pinto, A.C.P.N.; Garcia, B.M.S.P.; Eid, R.A.C.; Mól, C.G.; Nawa, R.K. Telerehabilitation Improves Physical Function and Reduces Dyspnoea in People with COVID-19 and Post-COVID-19 Conditions: A Systematic Review. *J. Physiother.* **2022**, *68*, 90–98. [CrossRef]
41. Lundell, S.; Holmner, Å.; Rehn, B.; Nyberg, A.; Wadell, K. Telehealthcare in COPD: A Systematic Review and Meta-Analysis on Physical Outcomes and Dyspnea. *Respir. Med.* **2015**, *109*, 11–26. [CrossRef]
42. Salawu, A.; Green, A.; Crooks, M.G.; Briexy, N.; Ross, D.H.; Sivan, M. A Proposal for Multidisciplinary Tele-Rehabilitation in the Assessment and Rehabilitation of COVID-19 Survivors. *Int. J. Environ. Res. Public Health* **2020**, *17*, 4890. [CrossRef] [PubMed]

diagnostics

MDPI

Article

Myofascial Pain Syndrome in Women with Primary Dysmenorrhea: A Case-Control Study

Ana Serrano-Imedio [1,2], Cesar Calvo-Lobo [3,*], Coraima Casañas-Martin [1,2], Alejandro Garrido-Marin [2,4,5] and Daniel Pecos-Martin [1]

1 Grupo de Investigación en Fisioterapia y Dolor, Departamento de Fisioterapia, Facultad de Enfermería y Fisioterapia, Universidad de Alcalá, 28801 Alcalá de Henares, Spain
2 CARMASALUD Clinical and Research Center, 28037 Madrid, Spain
3 Facultad de Enfermería, Fisioterapia y Podología, Universidad Complutense de Madrid, 28040 Madrid, Spain
4 Department of Physiotherapy, Faculty of Biomedical and Health Sciences, Universidad Europea de Madrid, 28670 Madrid, Spain
5 Medical Services, Getafe C.F., 28905 Getafe, Spain
* Correspondence: cescalvo@ucm.es

Abstract: There is limited information on myofascial trigger points (MTrPs) and specific symptoms of chronic pelvic pain and, more specifically, dysmenorrhea. The objective of this study was to determine whether patients suffering from primary dysmenorrhea present alterations in mechanosensitivity and pain patterns, and greater presence of MTrPs in the abdominal and pelvic floor muscles. A case-control study was carried out with a total sample of 84 participants distributed based on primary dysmenorrhea and contraceptive treatment. The sample was divided into four groups each comprising 21 women. Data on pain, quality of life, and productivity and work absenteeism were collected; three assessments were made in different phases of the menstrual cycle, to report data on pressure pain threshold, MTrP presence, and referred pain areas. One-way ANOVA tests showed statistically significant differences ($p < 0.01$) between the groups, for the Physical Health domain and the total score of the SF-12 questionnaire, and for all the domains of the McGill questionnaire; but no significant differences were found in the data from the WPAI-GH questionnaire. Statistically significant data ($p < 0.01$) were found for mechanosensitivity in the abdominal area and limbs, but not for the lumbar assessment, within the group, with very few significant intergroup differences. The frequency of active MTrPs is higher in the groups of women with primary dysmenorrhea and during the menstrual phase, with the prevalence of myofascial trigger points of the iliococcygeus muscle being especially high in all examination groups (>50%) and higher than 70% in women with primary dysmenorrhea, in the menstrual phase, and the internal obturator muscle (100%) in the menstrual phase. Referred pain areas of the pelvic floor muscles increase in women with primary dysmenorrhea.

Keywords: primary dysmenorrhea; myofascial pain syndrome; myofascial trigger points; mechanosensitivity; pain pressure threshold

1. Introduction

Dysmenorrhea is considered one of the most prevalent gynecological disorders in women of reproductive age [1,2], reaching prevalence rates of up to 97% of the population in some locations [3], and ranging in Spain from 61.9% to 84.7% of the population [4,5]. Dysmenorrhea can be classified as secondary dysmenorrhea when pathological causes of the uterus or pelvis are responsible for the pain, the most frequent being endometriosis and pelvic inflammatory disorders, in addition to other causes, such as adenomyosis, uterine fibroids (myomas) or polyps, ovarian cysts, uterine malformations, pelvic adhesions, cervical stenosis of the uterus, pelvic congestion syndrome, and irritable bowel syndrome [1,6–8].

Primary dysmenorrhea (PD) is determined by a set of symptoms that appears to be associated with menstruation in the absence of relevant organic pathology that explains it, and that presents pain described as moderate or severe and that is fundamentally associated with an increase in the production of prostaglandins (PGs) at the endometrial level [2]. The etiology of PD is characterized by an increase in the synthesis and release of PGs, which cause hypercontractability of the myometrium with respect to the normal dynamics of the menstrual uterus. Hypercontractibility causes uterine ischemia and hypoxia and, consequently, an accumulation of metabolites and acids, which are also responsible for pain [5,9–12]. This increased contractility is mediated by the local release of nociceptive substances in response to hormonal stimuli. There is also a sensitization of nerve endings to nociceptive stimuli [5]. The increased volume of menstrual flow due to ovulatory cycles increases the release of uterine PGs, which stimulates uterine contraction, increasing the tone, frequency, and intensity of contractions and causing colic-like pain [5]. However, Akman et al., found that in young women with PD, there are no differences in pain regardless of whether the cycles are ovulatory or anovulatory [13]. In addition, historically, menstrual pain was related to psychological factors [14]. However, these theories have lost credibility as biochemical knowledge has increased, assuming that psychological problems are more a consequence than a cause [15,16].

This condition of cyclical and chronic pain also means a decrease in both the quality of life of patients [17] and in their academic and/or professional development, presenting itself as the main cause of absenteeism [1,18]. Despite these data and the high prevalence of menstrual pain, underdiagnosis and the absence or inadequacy of treatment are prominent problems in the majority of cases [8]. Data indicate that only one in three women consults a health professional for menstrual pain, and the vast majority also consult pharmacists instead of doctors or nurses [19]. This could be one of the reasons why the most common forms of treatment are pharmacological; for example, with analgesics aimed at alleviating symptoms at the time of menstruation [10,19], or through contraceptives aimed at reducing endometrial activity throughout the menstrual cycle [20]. Despite presenting greater side-effects relative to more conservative forms of treatment, they continue to be used more frequently because they provide greater relief of symptoms [21].

Studies on conservative forms of treatment other than pharmaceuticals remain highly limited and heterogeneous, complicating the search for therapeutic alternatives. There have been studies examining physiotherapy as a treatment for the management of PD, and in recent years studies have aimed at treating MTrPs in this type of patient [22–24].

The myofascial component is considered one of the most common diagnoses in clinical practice for chronic pelvic pain (CPP) [25], including PD in the classification of the *International Association for the Study of Pain* (IASP) as a condition of CPP [26]. Focusing on myofascial pain syndrome (MPS) shows that it shares clinical characteristics with PD that extend beyond pain, such as the fact that it causes autonomic symptoms [27], emotional disorders [28], or changes in mood [29], in addition to considering the central sensitization associated with both [29,30].

The diagnosis of MTrPs has been widely debated and studied in recent years [31–33]. Diagnosis has been based on clinical history and physical examination by palpation, and following the widely extended criteria described in 1999 by Travell and Simons; these are the presence of a tender point within a palpable taut band in skeletal muscle, exhibiting a local spasm response to sudden palpation of this taut band, and causing referred pain in response to stimulation or compression of the MTrPs [34,35].

Both active MTrPs and latent MTrPs induce peripheral and even central sensitization mechanisms [35,36] and, therefore, are related to a decrease in pain pressure thresholds (PPTs) [37]. Another of the characteristics of MTrPs is referred pain [38], with the areas of representation of referred pain being the rectus abdominis, external oblique, internal oblique, adductor magnus, gluteal, and quadratus lumborum muscles, very similar to menstrual pain [7–9,27,39–41].

MTrPs can be present in any skeletal muscle, including the pelvic floor (PF), where they can refer pain to the urethra, vagina, rectum, coccyx, sacrum, lower back, lower abdomen, and posterior thighs, as well as muscles in other body locations such as the back or hip; all of these cause pain to the pelvic area [39,42]. MTrPs may also be responsible for other symptoms compatible with some gynecological, gastrointestinal, and urological disorders or conditions [42,43]. We found studies in which the presence of MTrPs in the abdominal and pelvic musculature may be highly prevalent in patients with CPP [42,44–46].

In the urological field, the main clinical entities that refer to the relationship, in some aspect of their symptomatology, with MPS are interstitial cystitis [47–52] and chronic prostatitis [45,51–56]. In both pathologies, the assessment and treatment of MTrPs is both abdominal musculature and SP musculature [45,47–55]. The main improvement in both cases were in pain and quality of life [45,50]. In the case of prostatitis, improvements were seen not only in those aspects, but also in urinary problems and sexual dysfunction [53,54,56].

Although fewer studies have been published in this regard, in the coloproctological sphere the relationship between PF myofascial pathology and anorectal pain is highlighted [57], and Ashrafi et al., reported the presence of MTrPs in abdominal and lumbopelvic musculature with functional constipation problems [58].

Within gynecology, dyspareunia, endometriosis, and dysmenorrhea are the disorders most frequently associated with the presence of MTrPs. Although there are no studies on the prevalence of MTrPs in each specific pathology, we do have data that estimate their prevalence rate in CPP to be between 22% and 94%, most being gynecological disorders [42].

Regarding PD in particular, Yacubovich et al., considered that the data on the prevalence of MTrPs in adolescent women with PD in the abdominal and lumbar musculature are high, triple the number of MTrPs found in women with PD compared with women without PD. For this reason, it should be taken into account in exploration and treatment [59].

In the study by Gaubeca et al., dry needling treatment was performed on women with PD on the abdominal muscles [22] and, in the study by Huang et al., invasive treatment was also performed on this muscle, although in this case it was a lidocaine infiltration [23]. In both studies, improvements in pain reduction of up to 3 points on the visual analog scale (VAS) were found, which were also maintained in the medium and long term [22,23]. A study by Langford et al., found improvements in patients with CPP after infiltration of lidocaine over MTrPs of the levator ani muscles [60]; and extant studies that compared the effects of lidocaine, botulinum toxin, and dry needling on MTrPs show similar results [61,62]. A 2013 systematic review on the use of botulinum toxin demonstrated relief in patients with CPP secondary to muscle spasm of PF muscles [63].

Although the main clinical practice guidelines indicate the need to explore the location of the pain in CPP—referring to the exploration of the PF muscles—only a recent study by Espinosa et al., provided treatment for MTrPs of this musculature through manual techniques in women with PD, also achieving clinical improvements [24]. Myofascial pain syndrome was studied by Travell and Simons [27], and other urological disorders such as prostatitis and interstitial cystitis have a high prevalence of MTrPs; their examination offers broader descriptions of referred pain [43,45,49–51].

There is a lack of scientifically based resources in clinical practice that can guide the development of physiotherapy treatment for MPS in women with CPP who, in many cases, in a pelviperineal evaluation, manifest referred pain from the PF muscles that they identify as their menstrual pain. Therefore, assessing the responsibility of the MTrPs in this musculature, as well as expanding the maps of referred pain that they reproduce, may offer conservative therapeutic alternatives with fewer side-effects than the main forms of treatment currently benefiting women with PD, improving their quality of life and reducing the socioeconomic and psychological impacts of this gynecological disorder. Therefore, the objective of our study was to determine whether patients suffering from PD show an alteration in local mechanosensitivity—which could be related to the presence of MTrPs in the abdominal and PF muscles—compared to women without PD. We also aimed to obtain new maps of referred pain that can elaborate on the current maps.

2. Material and Methods

We performed a cross-sectional descriptive study of cases and controls that assessed four groups. The evaluator was blind with respect to the condition of participants. This study meets the criteria of The Strengthening the Reporting of Observational Studies in Epidemiology (STROBE) [64], and was approved by the Research Ethics and Animal Experimentation Committee of the University of Alcalá (IEC Code: CEID/HU/2017/01).

The sample was obtained using a consecutive sampling method between October 2018 and May 2021. The study participants were recruited and assessed at the CARMASALUD Clinical and Research Center, located in Madrid, Spain.

The target population was women of childbearing age over 18 years of age. The participants had to have a regular menstrual cycle that was no longer than 35 days [65,66], and they were considered to have dysmenorrhea if they had a VAS greater than 3/10 at the time of the first assessment [22,23]. The women participated in the study voluntarily and provided written informed consent.

Women whose menstrual cycle was irregular or longer than 35 days were excluded from the study, as were women suffering from secondary dysmenorrhea (i.e., the menstrual pain was related to some gynecological pathology that caused pain, such as endometriosis or adenomyosis); those suffering from chronic pelvic pain unrelated to their menstrual cycle [22,23]; those diagnosed with fibromyalgia, since they are considered to be patients suffering from a central sensitization process where pressure pain thresholds are altered [67]; and those who had taken analgesics in the 12 h prior to the assessment, considering that, based on the pharmacokinetics of the analgesics administered, after this 12 h period, the effects of the drug no longer persist, and the drugs do not interfere with the perception of pain or compliance with questionnaires [68].

2.1. Procedures, Variables and Assessments

Sociodemographic and clinical data were collected through a personalized questionnaire filled out by the women themselves. They self-completed the 12-item Short Form Survey (SF-12) [69], the Mc Gill pain questionnaire [70–73], and the VAS [73].

The first evaluation was performed within the first 3 days of menstruation, in which, in addition to self-completing the questionnaires, algometry was used to record PPT values, and a manual exploration was carried out by palpation on the study musculature (i.e., the PF musculature) performed vaginally, using gloves. The muscles evaluated were: rectus abdominis, external oblique, internal oblique, quadratus lumborum, gluteus maximus, gluteus medius, gluteus medius, gluteus minimus, adductor magnus, piriformis, bulbospongiosus, ischiocavernosus, transverse perineal, puborectus, pubococcygeus, iliococcygeus, coccygeus, obturator internus, and external anal sphincter. This palpatory examination was performed to confirm the presence or absence of MTrPs. The women in the study shaded the areas of referred pain they felt during the examination on a body representation map. The second evaluation was based on the duration of the menstrual cycle of each of the women; we sought to perform the second evaluation at the time of ovulation, 14 days before the end of the menstrual cycle, given the periovulatory phase in women without contraceptive, or intermenstrual treatment in those who were under contraceptive treatment. In said intervention, the VAS was completed again, and we recorded once more the PPT, the presence of MTrPs, and the pain as referred to in the body representation map. The third and last interventions were carried out 1 week later, during which only VAS and PPT data were collected. The professional who performed the examinations was a physiotherapist with expertise in urogynecological physiotherapy and myofascial pain and with more than 10 years of experience.

The diagnosis of MTrPs was made by manual palpation following the diagnostic criteria described by Travell and Simons in 1999 [27], revised and recommended in a recent

Delphi study [33]: presence of a taut band within the explored muscle; presence of a nodule or hypersensitive area to palpation located within the tense band of the explored muscle; and presence of referred pain appearing after sustained compression on the trigger point.

The indications to the participants were: "It may be that some of the points where we apply pressure cause pain; in that case, if the pain is recognized as your usual pain, you should check the box for active MTrPs, and if the pain is not recognized as usual during your menstruation, you should check the box for latent MTrPs. In some cases, in addition to the pain in the pressure area, you may notice that your pain refers to other areas; in that case, shade in the areas in the body representation map to which it spreads".

2.2. Sample Size Calculation

A priori sample size calculation was carried out based on a pilot study using the same methodology, since there were no previous similar studies, by F-test for repeated measures analysis of variance (ANOVA; intra-between interaction) using G*Power 3.1.9.2 software for Windows, based on the main outcome measure of the pressure pain threshold (kg/cm^2) in the lumbar region just below L5 from a pilot study with 4 groups (n = 20; 5 women comprised the group without dysmenorrhea and without contraceptives; 5 women comprised the group without dysmenorrhea and contraceptives; 5 women comprised the dysmenorrhea and no contraceptives group; and 5 women comprised the dysmenorrhea and contraceptives group) and 3 measurement times (proliferative phase, ovulation phase, and luteal phase), showing a partial eta^2 of $\eta^2 = 0.048$ corrected for Greenhouse–Geisser. Assuming an effect size of f = 0.22, an error probability α of 0.01, power (1-β error probability) of 0.90, correlation between repeated measurements of 0.5, and a correction for non-sphericity of 1, a total sample size of 84 participants (n = 21 women per group) was needed to achieve a true power of 0.91.

2.3. Statistical Analysis

Statistical analysis was performed using SPSS Statistics software v. 27.0 (IBM, Chicago, IL, USA; 2021).

According to the a priori sample size calculation parameters, statistical significance was set at $p < 0.01$ for a 99% confidence interval (CI). For quantitative data, the Shapiro–Wilk test was used to assess normal distribution. Although some data were not normally distributed, F-tests are robust in terms of type I error and regardless of manipulated conditions, and are considered a valid option for nonparametric distributions [74]. In addition, the mean $\pm$ standard deviation (SD), with 99% CIs, was applied to describe these quantitative data. First, ANOVA was applied to compare the differences between groups of descriptive data and questionnaire results at a single measurement time. Second, a two-way ANOVA was performed for repeated measures over time (at the menstrual, ovulation, and luteal phases of the menstrual cycle) as a within-subject factor and group (group without dysmenorrhea and no contraceptives; group without dysmenorrhea and with contraceptives; dysmenorrhea and no contraception group; and dysmenorrhea and contraception group) as a between-group factor to compare VAS and PPT outcomes [74]. The significance of the Greenhouse–Geisser correction was considered when the Mauchly test rejected sphericity [75]. In addition, post hoc comparisons were made by the Bonferroni correction. The effect size of the F-tests was analyzed using the coefficients of eta squared (η^2) and interpreted as a small effect size for the $\eta^2 = 0.01$ coefficient, a medium effect size for $\eta^2 = 0.06$, and a large effect size for $\eta^2 = 0.14$ [76]. Effect size for post hoc comparisons was determined using Cohen's d ($d = 2t/\sqrt{gdl}$) and interpreted as very small effect size ($d < 0.20$), small effect size (d = 0.20–0.49), medium effect size (d = 0.50–0.79), and large effect size ($d > 0.8$) [75–77]. These data were represented by linear graphs using means with 99% CIs. A p-value < 0.01 was considered statistically significant for a 99% CI, and was completed with the F statistic for all ANOVA analyses and adjusted for Greenhouse–Geisser corrections [75]. Finally, the categorical data were described by frequencies and percentages (n[%]) and compared by the chi square test (χ^2) [78]. The statistical differences were visualized as bar graphs indicating the distribution of frequencies.

3. Results

A total of 90 women decided to participate in the study. Six women dropped out of the study, resulting in a final sample of 84 participants, who were divided into the following groups: women with dysmenorrhea and with contraceptive treatment (WDWC) (n = 21), women with dysmenorrhea without contraceptive treatment (WDNC) (n = 21), women without dysmenorrhea with contraceptive treatment (NDWC) (n = 21), and women without dysmenorrhea and without contraceptive treatment (NDNC) (n = 21). This process is outlined in the flowchart in Figure 1.

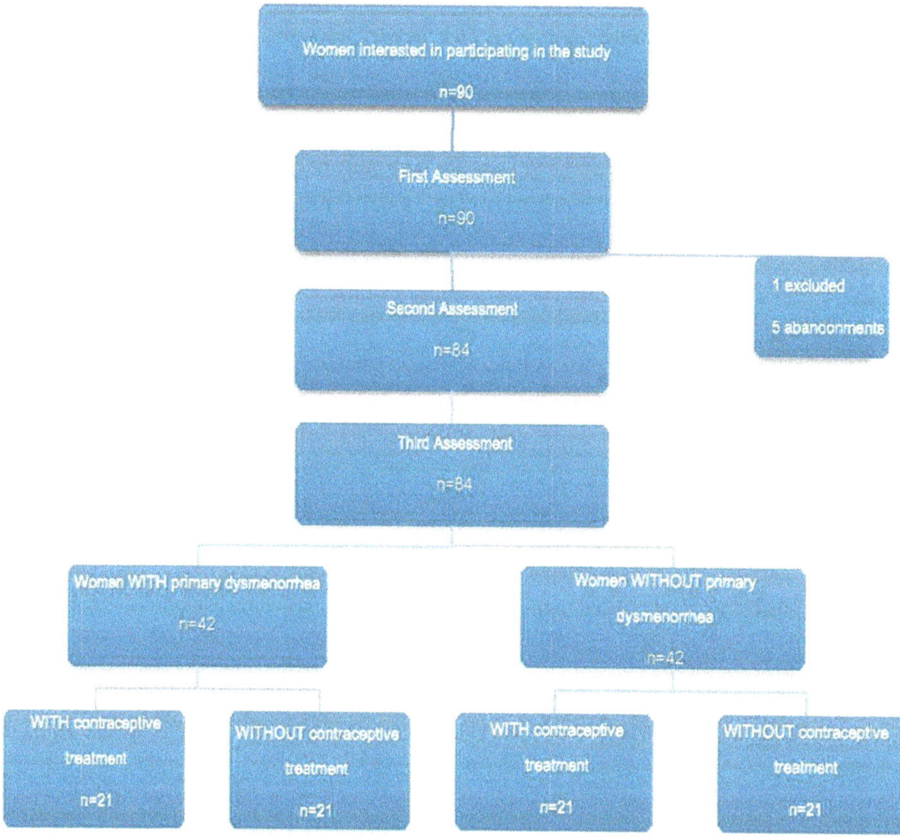

Figure 1. Flowchart.

3.1. Demographics

The total sample consisted of 84 participants with a mean ± SD age of 31.20 ± 7.65 years, weight of 58.22 ± 6.50 kg, height of 1.64 ± 0.04 m, and a BMI of 21.50 ± 2.25 kg/m^2. The one-way ANOVA did not show statistically significant differences ($p > 0.01$) between the groups, with an effect size that varied from small to medium ($\eta^2 = 0.041$–0.124) for any of the sociodemographic variables (Table 1).

Table 1. Demographics.

	Total Mean ± SD (99% CI, n = 84)	NDNC Mean ± SD (99% CI, n = 21)	NDWC Mean ± SD (99% CI, n = 21)	WDNC Mean ± SD (99% CI, n = 21)	WDWC Mean ± SD (99% CI, n = 21)	*p*-Value * F (η^2)
Age (years)	31.20 ± 7.65 (28.99–33.40)	35.47 ± 9.36 (29.65–41.29)	30.57 ± 5.57 (27.11–34.03)	30.71 ± 7.65 (25.96–35.46)	28.04 ± 5.97 (28.99–33.40)	$p = 0.013$ F = 3.792 $\eta^2 = 0.124$
Weight (kg)	58.22 ± 6.50 (56.35–60.09)	61.08 ± 8.42 (55.84–66.31)	57.23 ± 4.04 (54.72–59.75)	56.80 ± 5.68 (53.27–60.34)	57.76 ± 6.60 (53.65–61.86)	$p = 0.129$ F = 1.944 $\eta^2 = 0.068$
Height (m)	1.64 ± 0.04 (1.63–1.65)	1.64 ± 0.04 (1.61–1.67)	1.65 ± 0.03 (1.63–1.67)	1.63 ± 0.03 (1.60–1.65)	1.65 ± 0.05 (1.61–1.68)	$p = 0.334$ F = 1.151 $\eta^2 = 0.041$
BMI (Kg/m^2)	21.51 ± 2.25 (20.87–22.16)	22.61 ± 3.26 (20.59–24.64)	20.93 ± 1.79 (19.82–22.05)	21.31 ± 1.28 (20.52–22.11)	21.20 ± 1.96 (19.98–22.42)	$p = 0.070$ F = 2.441 $\eta^2 = 0.084$

Abbreviations: BMI: body mass index. NDNC: non-dysmenorrhea non-contraceptives group; NDWC: non-dysmenorrhea, with contraceptives group; WDNC: with dysmenorrhea non-contraceptives group; WDWC: with dysmenorrhea with contraceptives group. SD: standard deviation; A $p < 0.01$ with a 99% confidence interval was considered statistically significant. * One-way ANOVA was used.

A share of 50% of the study participants were not under contraceptive treatment and, of this 50%, more than half, 29.76%, were taking oral contraceptives; 13.10% were using the vaginal ring and 7.14% had an IUD implanted. Half of the sample reported back pain on some occasion, and 28.57% reported pelvic pain at times unrelated with menstruation. Statistically significant data ($p < 0.01$) were found for gastrointestinal disturbances such as diarrhea, constipation, nausea, vomiting, or discomfort, which appeared in 63.10% of participants during menstruation, with only 15.48% suffering from them outside the menstrual bleeding period. Dyspareunia was found in 29.76% of women and 69.05% considered they had menstrual pain. Statistically significant data ($p < 0.001$) were found for menstrual treatment, with 35.71% of participants not needing treatment to relieve menstrual symptoms. The most widely used treatment to alleviate these symptoms was medication, which was used in 30.95% of cases, followed by the combination of heat and medication, used by 28.57% of participants. The remaining variables from the qualitative clinical descriptive analysis did not show statistically significant differences ($p > 0.001$). These data are shown in Table 2.

Table 2. Qualitative clinical descriptive data.

		Total (n = 84)	NDNC (n = 21)	NDWC (n = 21)	WDNC (n = 21)	WDWC (n = 21)	*p*-Value * χ^2
		n (%)	n (%)	n (%)	n (%)	n (%)	
Contraceptive treatment	YES	42 (50)	0 (0)	21 (100)	0 (0)	21 (100)	$\mathbf{p < 0.001}$
	NO	42 (50)	21 (100)	0 (0)	21 (100)	0 (0)	$\chi^2 = 80.188$
Type of contraceptive treatment	NO TRT	42 (50)	21 (100)	0 (0)	21 (100)	0 (0)	
	RING	11 (13.10)	0 (0)	7 (33.33)	0 (0)	4 (19.05)	$\mathbf{p < 0.001}$
	IUD	6 (7.14)	0 (0)	2 (9.52)	0 (0)	4 (19.05)	$\chi^2 = 83.765$
	COCs	25 (29.76)	0 (0)	12 (57.14)	0 (0)	13 (61.90)	
Low back pain	YES	42 (50)	9 (42.86)	9 (42.86)	16 (76.19)	8 (9.52)	$p = 0.05$
	NO	42 (50)	12 (57.14)	12 (57.14)	5 (23.81)	13 (61.90)	$\chi^2 = 7.81$
Pelvic pain	YES	24 (28.57)	5 (23.81)	6 (7.14)	8 (9.52)	5 (23.81)	$p = 0.706$
	NO	60 (71.43)	16 (76.19)	15 (71.43)	13 (61.90)	16 (76.19)	$\chi^2 = 1.400$
GI symptoms during menstruation	YES	53 (63.10)	15 (71.43)	7 (33.33)	17 (20.24)	14 (66.67)	$\mathbf{p < 0.01}$ *
	NO	31 (36.90)	6 (7.14)	14 (66.67)	4 (19.05)	7 (33.33)	$\chi^2 = 11.606$

Table 2. *Cont.*

		Total (n = 84)	NDNC (n = 21)	NDWC (n = 21)	WDNC (n = 21)	WDWC (n = 21)	*p*-Value * χ^2
		n (%)	n (%)	n (%)	n (%)	n (%)	
Common GI symptoms	YES	13 (15.48)	4 (19.05)	5 (23.81)	1 (4.76)	3 (14.28)	$p = 0.364$
	NO	71 (84.52)	17 (20.24)	16 (76.19)	20 (95.24)	18 (85.71)	$\chi^2 = 3.185$
Dyspareunia	YES	25 (29.76)	6 (7.14)	7 (33.33)	6 (7.14)	6 (7.14)	$p = 0.982$
	NO	59 (70.24)	15 (71.43)	14 (66.67)	15 (71.43)	15 (71.43)	$\chi^2 = 0.171$
Menstrual pain	YES	58 (69.05)	9 (42.86)	7 (33.33)	21 (100)	21 (100)	$\boldsymbol{p < 0.001}$ *
	NO	26 (30.95)	12 (57.14)	14 (66.67)	0 (0)	0 (0)	$\chi^2 = 34.659$
Menstrual Pain Treatment	Heat	2 (2.38)	0 (0)	1 (4.76)	1 (4.76)	0 (0)	
	Medication	26 (30.95)	7 (33.33)	3 (14.28)	8 (9.52)	8 (9.52)	$p < 0.144$
	Heat and medication	24 (28.57)	2 (9.52)	1 (4.76)	10 (47.62)	11 (52.38)	$\chi^2 = 17.147$
	Kinesiotape	2 (2.38)	0 (0)	1 (4.76)	0 (0)	1 (4.76)	

Abbreviations: GI: gastrointestinal; NDNC: non-dysmenorrhea non-contraceptive group; NDWC: non-dysmenorrhea with contraceptives group; WDNC: with dysmenorrhea non-contraceptives group; WDWC: with dysmenorrhea with contraceptives group. A $p < 0.01$ (**Bold**) was considered statistically significant. * One-way ANOVA was used.

3.2. *Quality of Life*

One-way ANOVA revealed statistically significant differences ($p < 0.01$) between the groups, with a large effect size ($\eta^2 = 0.168$–0.180) for the Physical Health domain and a high total SF-12 score (Table 3). However, no significant differences were found ($p > 0.01$) between the groups, with a medium effect size ($\eta^2 = 0.104$–0.106) for the Mental Health domain of the SF-12 questionnaire.

Post hoc comparisons between groups for the Physical Health domain of the SF-12 questionnaire showed statistically significant differences ($p = 0.001$), with a large effect size ($d = 1.191$–1.206) for the NDWC vs. WDNC comparison, showing a higher percentage for the Physical Health domain in the NDWC group compared with the WDNC group. Similarly, these post hoc comparisons for the total score of the SF-12 questionnaire showed statistically significant differences ($p < 0.01$), with a large effect size ($d = 1.260$–1.274) for the NDWC vs. WDNC comparison, showing a higher score the total SF-12 score in the NDWC group relative to the WDNC group. The rest of the post hoc comparisons showed no significant differences.

3.3. *Pain*

3.3.1. The McGill Pain Questionnaire

Statistically significant differences ($p < 0.01$) were found between the groups, with a large effect size ($\eta^2 = 0.262$–0.459) for all domains of the McGill Pain Questionnaire (PRI-S, PRI-A, PRI-E, PRI-Total, Number of words, and PPI), as shown in Table 4.

The post hoc comparisons showed a significantly higher score in the NDNC group for the PRI-E ($p < 0.01$), with a large effect size ($d = 1.090$). The WDNC group had a significantly higher score than other groups in all domains (PRI-S, PRI-A, PRI-E, PRI-Total, Number of words, and PPI; $p < 0.01$), with a large effect size ($d = 0.953$–1.652). Similarly, post hoc comparisons between the NDWC and WDNC groups and between the NDWC and WDWC groups showed significant differences ($p < 0.01$) in all domains, with a higher score for the WDNC and WDWC groups, with a large effect size. ($d = 1.442$–2.410 and $d = 1.269$–2.163, respectively). The WDWC group had a significantly higher score than the NDCA group for the domains PRI-S, PRI-Total, and Number of words, with a large effect size ($d = 1.033$–1.055). The WDNC had a significantly higher score than the WDWC group in the PPI domain only ($p < 0.01$), with a large effect size ($d = 0.974$).

Table 3. Questionnaire SF-12.

	Total	NDNC	NDWC	WDNC	WDWC		Post-Hoc *P* (d Cohen) a-NDNC vs. NDWC b-NDNC vs. WDNC c-NDNC vs. WDWC d-NDWC vs. WDNC e-NDWC vs. WDWC f-WDNC vs. WDWC
	Mean ± SD (99% CI, n = 84)	**Mean ± SD (99% CI, n = 21)**	**Mean ± SD (99% CI, n = 21)**	**Mean ± SD (99% CI, n = 21)**	**Mean ± SD (99% CI, n = 21)**	***p*-Value * *F* (η^2)**	
Physical Health	18.07 ± 1.81 (17.54–18.59)	18.09 ± 2.02 (16.83–19.35)	18.95 ± 1.20 (18.20–19.69)	16.85 ± 2.15 (15.52–18.19)	18.38 ± 1.02 (17.74–19.01)	***p* = 0.001** * F = 5.860 $\eta^2 = 0.180$	a-p = 0.606 d = 0.517 b-p = 0.113 d = 0.594 c-p = 1.000 d = 0.181 d-***p* = 0.001** d = 1.206 e-p = 1.000 d = 0.511 f-p = 0.025 d = 0.909
Physical Health (%)	86.36 ± 12.98 (82.63–90.10)	86.52 ± 14.43 (77.55–95.48)	92.61 ± 8.58 (87.28–97.95)	77.71 ± 15.46 (68.11–87.31)	88.61 ± 7.28 (84.09–93.14)	***p* = 0.001** * F = 5.805 $\eta^2 = 0.179$	a-p = 0.619 d = 0.513 b-p = 0.117 d = 0.589 c-p = 1.000 d = 0.182 d-***p* = 0.001** d = *1.191* e-p = 1.000 d = 0.502 f-p = 0.025 d = 0.902
Mental Health	20.90 ± 3.13 (20.00–21.80)	20.04 ± 3.98 (17.57–22.51)	22.61 ± 2.13 (21.29–23.94)	20.38 ± 2.97 (18.53–22.22)	20.57 ± 2.71 (18.88–22.25)	p = 0.31 F = 3.105 $\eta^2 = 0.104$	a-p = 0.044 d = 0.805 b-p = 1.000 d = 0.096 c-p = 1.000 d = 0.155 d-p = 0.113 d = 0.862 e-p = 0.187 d = 0.836 f-p = 1.000 d = 0.066
Mental Health (%)	71.00 ± 14.90 (66.71–75.28)	66.90 ± 18.88 (55.18–78.62)	79.19 ± 10.12 (72.90–85.47)	68.42 ± 14.04 (59.70–77.15)	69.47 ± 12.94 (61.43–77.51)	p = 0.029 F = 3.153 $\eta^2 = 0.106$	a-p = 0.041 d = 0.811 b-p = 1.000 d = 0.091 c-p = 1.000 d = 0.158 d-p = 0.104 d = 0.880 e-p = 0.187 d = 0.836 f-p = 1.000 d = 0.077
Total	38.97 ± 3.92 (37.84–40.10)	38.14 ± 4.74 (35.19–41.08)	41.57 ± 2.80 (39.83–43.31)	37.23 ± 3.92 (34.80–39.67)	38.95 ± 2.65 (37.30–40.60)	***p* = 0.002** * F = 5.54 $\eta^2 = 0.172$	a-p = 0.018 d = 0.881 b-p = 1.000 d = 0.209 c-p = 1.000 d = 0.210 d-***p* = 0.001** d = 1.274 e-p = 0.132 d = 0.961 f-p = 0.782 d = 0.514

Table 3. *Cont.*

	Total **Mean ± SD (99% CI, n = 84)**	NDNC **Mean ± SD (99% CI, n = 21)**	NDWC **Mean ± SD (99% CI, n = 21)**	WDNC **Mean ± SD (99% CI, n = 21)**	WDWC **Mean ± SD (99% CI, n = 21)**	***p*-Value * *F* (η^2)**	**Post-Hoc *P* (d Cohen) a-NDNC vs. NDWC b-NDNC vs. WDNC c-NDNC vs. WDWC d-NDWC vs. WDNC e-NDWC vs. WDWC f-WDNC vs. WDWC**
Total (%)	77.05 ± 11.15 (73.84–80.26)	74.71 ± 13.57 (66.28–83.14)	84.38 ± 7.93 (79.45–89.30)	72.19 ± 11.14 (65.27–79.10)	76.95 ± 7.63 (72.21–81.69)	***p* = 0.002** * F = 5.396 $\eta^2 = 0.168$	a-p = 0.020 d = 0.870 b-p = 1.000 d = 0.202 c-p = 1.000 d = 0.203 d-***p* = 0.002** d = 1.260 e-p = 0.137 d = 0.954 f-p = 0.843 d = 0.498

Abbreviations: NDNC: non-dysmenorrhea non-contraceptive group; NDWC: non-dysmenorrhea with contraceptives group; WDNC: with dysmenorrhea non-contraceptives group; WDWC: with dysmenorrhea with contraceptives group. SF-12: Short Form 12 Health Survey. SD: standard deviation; A $p < 0.01$ with a 99% confidence interval (**Bold**) was considered statistically significant. * One-way ANOVA was used.

Table 4. The McGill Pain Questionnaire.

	Total Mean ± SD (99% CI, n = 84)	NDNC Mean ± SD (99% CI, n = 21)	NDWC Mean ± SD (99% CI, n = 21)	WDNC Mean ± SD (99% CI, n = 21)	WDWC Mean ± SD (99% CI, n = 21)	*p*-Value * F (η^2)	Post-Hoc *P* (d Cohen) a-NDNC vs. NDWC b-NDNC vs. WDNC c-NDNC vs. WDWC d-NDWC vs. WDNC e-NDWC vs. WDWC f-WDNC vs. WDWC
PRI-S	14.92 ± 10.34 (11.95–17.90)	11.61 ± 8.89 (6.08–17.13)	5.61 ± 6.93 (1.31–9.92)	22.52 ± 9.02 (16.92–28.12)	19.95 ± 6.77 (15.74–24.15)	**p = 0.000** * F = 19.879 $\eta^2 = 0.427$	a-p = 0.102 d = 0.752 b-p = **0.000** d = 1.218 c-p = **0.007** d = 1.055 d-p = **0.000** d = 2.102 e-p = **0.000** d = 2.093 f-p = 1.000 d = 0.326
PRI-A	1.17 ± 1.48 (0.75–1.60)	0.76 ± 0.83 (0.24–1.27)	0.19 ± 0.40 (−0.05–0.44)	2.14 ± 1.87 (0.97–3.30)	1.61 ± 1.53 (0.66–2.57)	**p = 0.000** * F = 9.462 $\eta^2 = 0.262$	a-p = 0.944 d = 0.874 b-p = **0.005** d = 0.953 c-p = 0.212 d = 0.690 d-p = **0.000** d = 1.442 e-p = **0.004** d = 1.269 f-p = 1.000 d = 0.310
PRI-E	1.85 ± 1.28 (1.48–2.22)	1.61 ± 0.97 (1.01–2.22)	0.61 ± 0.86 (0.08–1.15)	2.95 ± 1.07 (2.28–3.61)	2.23 ± 0.94 (1.65–2.82)	**p = 0.000** * F = 22.007 $\eta^2 = 0.452$	a-p = **0.007** d = 1.090 b-p = **0.000** d = 1.312 c-p = 0.246 d = 0.649 d-p = **0.000** d = 2.410 e-p = **0.000** d = 1.798 f-p = 0.114 d = 0.714
PRI-Total	17.96 ± 12.34 (14.41–21.51)	14.09 ± 10.46 (7.59–20.59)	6.33 ± 7.85 (1.45–11.21)	27.47 ± 9.97 (21.28–33.66)	23.95 ± 8.43 (18.71–29.18)	**p = 0.000** * F = 22.649 $\eta^2 = 0.459$	a-p = 0.048 d = 0.839 b-p = **0.000** d = 1.309 c- p = **0.005** d = 1.037 d-p = **0.000** d = 2.356 e-p = **0.000** d = 2.163 f-p = 1.000 d = 0.381
N° of words	8.38 ± 4.61 (7.05–9.70)	7.19 ± 4.26 (4.54–9.83)	4.38 ± 4.34 (1.68–7.07)	11.09 ± 3.46 (8.94–13.24)	10.85 ± 2.63 (9.22–12.49)	**p = 0.000** * F = 15.478 $\eta^2 = 0.367$	a-p = 0.103 d = 0.653 b-p = **0.007** d = 1.004 c-p = **0.013** d = 1.033 d-p = **0.000** d = 1.709 e-p = **0.000** d = 1.803 f-p = 1.000 d = 0.078

Table 4. *Cont.*

	Total	NDNC	NDWC	WDNC	WDWC		**Post-Hoc *P* (d Cohen)** **a-NDNC vs. NDWC** **b-NDNC vs. WDNC** **c-NDNC vs. WDWC** **d-NDWC vs. WDNC** **e-NDWC vs. WDWC** **f-WDNC vs. WDWC**
	Mean ± SD (99% CI, n = 84)	**Mean ± SD (99% CI, n = 21)**	**Mean ± SD (99% CI, n = 21)**	**Mean ± SD (99% CI, n = 21)**	**Mean ± SD (99% CI, n = 21)**	***p*-Value * F (η^2)**	
PPI	1.63 ± 1.01 (1.33–1.92)	1.19 ± 0.51 (0.87–1.50)	0.90 ± 0.62 (0.51–1.29)	2.66 ± 1.15 (1.94–3.38)	1.76 ± 0.62 (1.37–2.14)	$\mathbf{p = 0.000}$ * F = 21.343 $\eta^2 = 0.445$	a-p = 1.000 d = 0.510 b-$\mathbf{p = 0.000}$ d = 1.652 c-p = 0.112 d = 1.004 d-$\mathbf{p = 0.000}$ d = 1.905 e-$\mathbf{p = 0.003}$ d = 1.387 f-$\mathbf{p = 0.002}$ d = 0.974

Abbreviations: NDNC: non-dysmenorrhea non-contraceptive group; NDWC: non-dysmenorrhea with contraceptives group; PPI: Pain Intensity Index; PRI: Pain Assessment Index; PRI-A: Pain Rating Index–Affective; PRI-E: Pain Assessment Index–Evaluative; PRI-S: Pain Rating Index–Sensory; WDNC: with dysmenorrhea non-contraceptives group; WDWC: with dysmenorrhea with contraceptives group. SD: standard deviation; A $p < 0.01$ with a 99% confidence interval (**Bold**) was considered statistically significant. * One-way ANOVA was used.

3.3.2. Visual Analog Scale

Regarding between-group comparisons, the two-way ANOVA test (3 measurement moments × 4 groups) of repeated measures showed statistically significant differences ($p < 0.001$; $F = 58.519$; $\eta^2 = 0.687$) between the groups, with a large effect size for pain intensity measurements using the VAS (Figure 2). Post hoc comparisons of VAS score between groups in the menstrual phase showed statistically significant differences ($p \leq 0.001$) with a large effect size ($d = 2.052$–3.776), indicating a lower intensity of pain in the NDNC group with respect to the WDNC group, in the NDNC group with respect to the WDWC group, and in the NDWC group with respect to the WDNC group; however, a greater pain intensity in the NDWC group vs. the WDWC group was found. The remaining post hoc comparisons, in the ovulatory phase and the luteal phase, indicated no further significant differences.

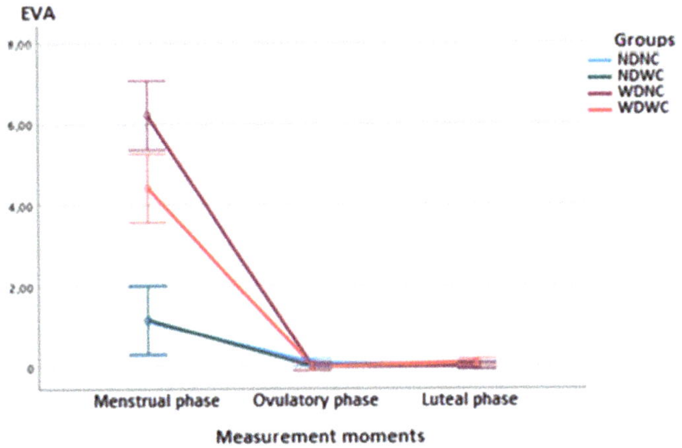

Figure 2. Linear graphs of the means completed with the error bars at 99% of the Cl, for the pain intensity variable (VAS scale) that show the differences between the groups (NDNC, NDWC, WDNC, WDWC) and the measurement moments (menstrual phase, ovulatory phase, and luteal phase).

Regarding intra-group comparisons, the ANOVA test showed statistically significant differences ($p < 0.001$; $F = 377.092$; $\eta^2 = 0.827$) between the different measurement moments, with a large effect size for pain intensity measurements using the VAS. Post hoc comparisons for pain intensity of the NDNC and NDWC groups showed statistically significant differences ($p < 0.01$), with a large effect size ($d = 1.367$–1.763), indicating greater pain intensity in the menstrual phase relative to the ovulatory and luteal phases. Post hoc comparisons in the WDNC and WDWC groups showed statistically significant differences ($p < 0.001$), with a large effect size ($d = 3.299$–5.196), also reflecting a greater intensity of pain in the menstrual vs ovulatory and luteal phases.

3.4. *Mechanosensitivity*

3.4.1. Between-Group Comparisons

Regarding between-group comparisons, the two-way ANOVA test (3 measurement moments × 4 groups) of repeated measures did not show statistically significant differences ($p > 0.01$; $F = 1.160$; $\eta^2 = 0.019$) between the groups, with a small effect size for PPT measurements in the abdominal region and L5 (Figure 3). Post hoc comparisons of right abdominal PPT between groups at different measurement phases (menstruation, ovulation, and luteal) revealed no statistically significant differences.

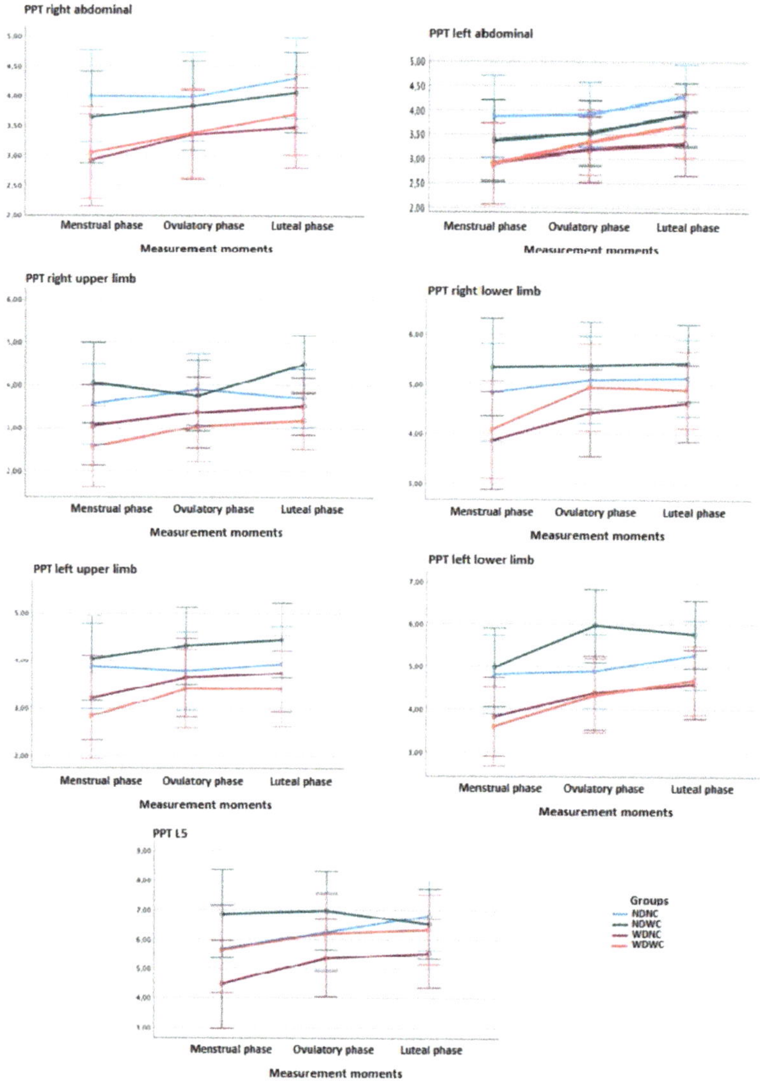

Figure 3. Linear graphs of the means completed with the error bars at 99% of the Cl, for the variable pressure pain threshold (PPT) that show the differences in the different measurement zones between the groups and the measurement moments (menstrual phase, ovulatory phase and luteal phase).

For measurements in areas furthest from the upper and lower extremity pain, repeated measures two-way ANOVA (3 time-points × 4 groups) showed no statistically significant difference ($p > 0.01$, $F = 1.389$; $\eta^2 = 0.032$) between groups, with a small effect size, as shown in Figure 3. Post hoc comparisons of the PPT in the right upper limb between the NDWC and WDWC groups in the luteal phase showed significant differences ($p < 0.01$) with a large effect size ($d = 1.133$), and post hoc comparisons of PPT in the left lower limb between groups in the ovulatory phase showed significant differences ($p < 0.01$), with a large effect size ($d = 0.944$–1.049), indicating a lower intensity of pain in the NDWC vs. WDNC group and in the NDWC vs. WDWC group.

3.4.2. Within-Group Comparisons

Regarding the intra-group comparisons, the ANOVA test revealed significant differences ($p < 0.001$; $F = 14.381$; $\eta^2 = 0.152$) between the different measurement moments, with a small effect size for the PPT measurements in the right abdominal region and L5. Significant differences ($p < 0.001$; $F = 11.627$; $\eta^2 = 0.127$) were also found between the different measurement moments, with a small effect size for the PPT measurements in the left abdominal region (Figure 3).

Post hoc comparisons for the PPT in the right abdominal area of the NDNC, NDWC, and WDNC groups indicated no significant differences between the measurement time-points. Significant differences ($p < 0.01$) were found for the PPT in the right abdominal region in the WDWC group, with a medium effect size ($d = 0.556$), indicating a greater intensity of the PPT in the menstrual vs. the luteal phase, but not the ovulatory phase. The rest of the post hoc comparisons for all groups in the left abdominal region and L5 did not reveal any further significant differences (Figure 3).

For the measurements in regions farthest from the pain in the upper and lower extremities, no significant differences were found ($p > 0.01$; $F = 5.996$; $\eta^2 = 0.054$) between the different measurement time-points, with a small effect size for upper limb PDU measurements. However, significant differences were found ($p = 0.001$, $F = 8.313$, $\eta^2 = 0.094$) between the measurement time-points, with a medium effect size for right lower-limb PDU measurements, and those in the left lower limb ($p < 0.001$; $F = 18.175$; $\eta^2 = 0.185$), with a large effect size.

Post hoc comparisons indicated significant differences for PPT in the extremities. In the right upper limb, the significant data were in the NDWC group ($p < 0.01$), with a medium effect size ($d = 0.574$), indicating a higher PPT in the ovulatory vs. luteal phase. Post hoc comparisons for these PPT of the NDNC, WDNC, and WDWC groups showed no significant differences between the measurement time-points for the right upper limb. For the PPT of the right lower limb of the WDNC group, a significantly lower PPT was found ($p = 0.01$) in the menstrual vs. luteal phase, with a small effect size ($d = 0.474$). Similarly, a significantly lower PPT in the WDWC group was found ($p < 0.01$) in the menstrual vs. luteal phase, with a medium effect size ($d = 0.593$). In the lower left limb of the NDWC group, a significantly lower PPT in the NDWC group was found ($p < 0.01$) in the menstrual vs. ovulatory phase, with a medium effect size ($d = 0.559$). Similarly, a significantly lower PPT in the WDWC group was found ($p < 0.01$) in the menstrual vs. luteal phase, with a large effect size ($d = 0.953$) (Figure 3).

3.5. *Presence of MTrPs*

The prevalence of MTrPs in the muscles during the menstrual phase is shown in Tables 5 and 6. A significantly higher prevalence of MTrPs in the rectus abdominis muscle was found ($p < 0.01$) in the WDNC and WDWC groups (52.38% and 61.90%, respectively). A significantly higher prevalence of active MTrPs in the gluteus maximus was found in the WDWC group (23.80%). A significantly higher prevalence of active MTrPs in the ischiocavernosus muscle was found in the WDNC and WDWC groups, whereas MTrPs were absent in the NDNC and NDWC groups. Furthermore, a significantly higher prevalence of active MTrPs in the pubococcygeus muscle was found in the WDNC and WDWC groups (66.66%). The remaining muscles studied showed no significant differences, although the iliococcygeus muscle presented active MTrPs in more than half of the total sample (69.04%).

The prevalence of MTrPs in the muscles during the periovulatory or intermenstrual phases is shown in Tables 7 and 8. A significantly higher prevalence of MTrPs was found in the WDNC and WDWC groups for the ischiocavernosus muscle (66.66% and 71.4%, respectively). A high prevalence of active MTrPs in the iliococcygeus muscle was also found in the WDNC and WDWC groups (85.71%); MTrPs were present in 60.71% of the total sample. Furthermore, there is a greater presence of latent MTrPs in the external anal sphincter in the WDWC group.

Table 5. Presence of MTrPs in the external musculature evaluated in the menstrual phase.

Muscles	Presence of MTrPs	Total (n = 84)	NDNC (n = 21)	NDWC (n = 21)	WDNC (n = 21)	WDWC (n = 21)	*p*-Value * χ^2
		n (%)	n (%)	n (%)	n (%)	n (%)	
Rectus abdominis	Does not have Active Latent	7 (8.33) 28 (33.33) 49 (58.33)	4 (19.04) 2 (9.52) 15 (71.42)	3 (14.28) 2 (9.52) 16 (76.19)	0 11 (52.38) 10 (47.61)	0 13 (61.90) 8 (38.09)	$\boldsymbol{p < 0.001}$ * $\chi^2 = 25.510$
External oblique	Does not have Active Latent	13 (15.47) 10 (11.90) 61 (72.61)	6 (28.57) 3 (14.28) 12 (57.14)	4 (19.04) 0 17 (80.95)	2 (9.52) 5 (23.80) 14 (66.66)	1 (4.76) 2 (9.52) 18 (85.71)	$p = 0.082$ $\chi^2 = 11.230$
Internal oblique	Does not have Active Latent	34 (40.47) 23 (27.38) 27 (32.14)	13 (61.90) 1 (4.76) 7 (33.33)	11 (52.38) 4 (19.04) 6 (28.57)	3 (14.28) 10 (47.61) 8 (38.09)	7 (33.33) 8 (38.09) 6 (28.57)	$p = 0.015$ $\chi^2 = 15.827$
Adductor magnus	Does not have Active Latent	6 (7.14) 4 (4.76) 74 (88.09)	3 (14.28) 0 18 (85.71)	0 0 21 (100)	1 (4.76) 3 (14.28) 17 (80.95)	2 (9.52) 1 (4.76) 18 (85.71)	$p = 0.132$ $\chi^2 = 9.820$
Gluteus maximus	Does not have Active Latent	17 (20.23) 7 (8.33) 60 (71.42)	5 (23.80) 0 16 (76.19)	9 (42.85) 1 (4.76) 11 (52.38)	2 (9.52) 1 (4.76) 18 (85.71)	1 (4.76) 5 (23.80) 15 (71.42)	$\boldsymbol{p < 0.01}$ * $\chi^2 = 19.280$
Gluteus medius	Does not have Active Latent	9 (10.71) 8 (9.52) 67 (79.76)	4 (19.04) 0 17 (80.95)	3 (14.28) 0 18 (85.71)	0 5 (23.80) 16 (76.19)	2 (9.52) 3 (14.28) 16 (76.19)	$p = 0.042$ $\chi^2 = 13.053$
Gluteus minimus	Does not have Active Latent	13 (15.47) 5 (5.95) 66 (78.57)	5 (23.80) 1 (4.76) 15 (71.42)	5 (23.80) 0 16 (76.19)	2 (9.52) 3 (14.28) 16 (76.19)	1 (4.76) 1 (4.76) 19 (90.47)	$p = 0.219$ $\chi^2 = 8.269$
Quadratus lumborum	Does not have Active Latent	4 (4.76) 24 (28.57) 56 (66.66)	3 (14.28) 3 (14.28) 15 (71.42)	0 4 (19.04) 17 (80.95)	1 (4.76) 9 (42.85) 11 (52.38)	0 8 (38.09) 13 (61.90)	$p = 0.067$ $\chi^2 = 11.762$
Piriformis	Does not have Active Latent	4 (4.76) 28 (33.33) 52 (61.90)	1 (4.76) 4 (19.04) 16 (76.19)	1 (4.76) 4 (19.04) 16 (76.19)	0 12 (57.14) 9 (42.85)	2 (9.52) 8 (38.09) 11 (52.38)	$p = 0.082$ $\chi^2 = 11.209$

Abbreviations: NDNC: non-dysmenorrhea non-contraceptive group; NDWC: non-dysmenorrhea with contraceptives group; WDNC: with dysmenorrhea non-contraceptives group; WDWC: with dysmenorrhea with contraceptives group. A $p < 0.01$ with a 99% confidence interval (**Bold**) was considered statistically significant. * One-way ANOVA was used.

Table 6. Presence of MTrPs in the pelvic floor muscles evaluated in the menstrual phase.

Muscles	Presence of MTrPs	Total (n = 84)	NDNC (n = 21)	NDWC (n = 21)	WDNC (n = 21)	WDWC (n = 21)	*p*-Value * χ^2
		n (%)	n (%)	n (%)	n (%)	n (%)	
Ischiocavernosus	Does not have Active Latent	27 (32.14) 7 (8.33) 50 (59.52)	10 (47.61) 0 11 (52.38)	12 (57.14) 0 9 (42.85)	2 (9.52) 3 (14.28) 16 (76.19)	3 (14.28) 4 (19.04) 14 (66.66)	$\boldsymbol{p < 0.01}$ * $\chi^2 = 20.680$
Bulbospongiosus	Does not have Active Latent	39 (46.42) 4 (4.76) 41 (48.80)	13 (61.90) 0 8 (38.09)	13 (61.90) 1 (4.76) 7 (33.33)	8 (38.09) 1 (4.76) 12 (57.14)	5 (23.80) 2 (9.52) 14 (66.66)	$p = 0.125$ $\chi^2 = 9.990$
Transverse perineal	Does not have Active Latent	37 (44.04) 5 (5.95) 42 (50)	12 (57.14) 0 9 (42.85)	12 (57.14) 0 9 (42.85)	7 (33.33) 1 (4.76) 13 (61.90)	6 (28.57) 4 (19.04) 11 (52.38)	$p = 0.043$ $\chi^2 = 12.972$

Table 6. *Cont.*

Muscles	Presence of MTrPs	Total (n = 84)	NDNC (n = 21)	NDWC (n = 21)	WDNC (n = 21)	WDWC (n = 21)	*p*-Value * χ^2
		n (%)	n (%)	n (%)	n (%)	n (%)	
Puborectalis	Does not have	12 (14.28)	6 (28.57)	4 (19.04)	1 (4.76)	1 (4.76)	$p = 0.268$ $\chi^2 = 7.610$
	Active	28 (33.33)	5 (23.80)	6 (28.57)	9 (42.85)	8 (38.09)	
	Latent	44 (52.38)	10 (47.61)	11 (52.38)	11 (52.38)	12 (57.14)	
Pubococcygeus	Does not have	6 (7.14)	5 (23.80)	0	0	1 (4.76)	$\mathbf{p = 0.001}$ * $\chi^2 = 22.140$
	Active	41 (48.80)	7 (33.33)	6 (28.57)	14 (66.66)	14 (66.66)	
	Latent	37 (44.04)	9 (42.85)	15 (71.42)	7 (33.33)	6 (28.57)	
Iliococcygeus	Does not have	1 (1.19)	1 (4.76)	0	0	0	$p = 0.035$ $\chi^2 = 13.539$
	Active	58 (69.04)	12 (57.14)	11 (52.38)	20 (95.23)	15 (71.42)	
	Latent	25 (29.76)	8 (38.09)	10 (47.61)	1 (4.76)	6 (28.57)	
Obturator internus	Does not have	0	0	0	0	0	$p = 0.110$ $\chi^2 = 6.024$
	Active	35 (41.66)	6 (28.57)	6 (28.57)	11 (52.38)	12 (57.14)	
	Latent	49 (58.33)	15 (71.42)	15 (71.42)	10 (47.61)	9 (42.85)	
Coccygeus	Does not have	32 (38.09)	9 (42.85)	8 (38.09)	8 (38.09)	7 (33.33)	$p = 0.274$ $\chi^2 = 7.532$
	Active	13 (15.47)	3 (14.28)	0	4 (19.04)	6 (28.57)	
	Latent	39 (46.42)	9 (42.85)	13 (61.90)	9 (42.85)	8 (38.09)	
Anal sphincter	Does not have	58 (69.04)	12 (57.14)	16 (76.19)	15 (71.42)	15 (71.42)	$p = 0.774$ $\chi^2 = 3.268$
	Active	5 (5.95)	1 (4.76)	1 (4.76)	2 (9.52)	1 (4.76)	
	Latent	21 (25)	8 (38.09)	4 (19.04)	4 (19.04)	5 (23.80)	

Abbreviations: NDNC: non-dysmenorrhea non-contraceptive group; NDWC: non-dysmenorrhea with contraceptives group; MTrP: myofascial trigger points; WDNC: with dysmenorrhea non-contraceptives group; WDWC: with dysmenorrhea with contraceptives group. A $p < 0.01$ (**Bold**) was considered statistically significant. * One-way ANOVA was used.

Table 7. Presence of MTrPs in the external muscles evaluated in the ovulatory phase.

Muscles	Presence of MTrPs	Total (n = 84)	NDNC (n = 21)	NDWC (n = 21)	WDNC (n = 21)	WDWC (n = 21)	*p*-Value * χ^2
		n (%)	n (%)	n (%)	n (%)	n (%)	
Rectus abdominis	Does not have	13 (15.47)	6 (28.57)	3 (14.28)	1 (4.76)	3 (14.28)	$p = 0.073$ $\chi^2 = 11.554$
	Active	3 (3.57)	3 (14.28)	0	4 (19.04)	6 (28.57)	
	Latent	58 (69.04)	12 (57.14)	18 (85.71)	16 (76.19)	12 (57.14)	
External oblique	Does not have	20 (23.80)	7 (33.33)	5 (23.80)	3 (14.28)	5 (23.80)	$p = 0.216$ $\chi^2 = 8.310$
	Active	2 (2.38)	0	0	0	2 (9.52)	
	Latent	62 (73.80)	14 (66.66)	16 (76.19)	18 (85.71)	14 (66.66)	
Internal oblique	Does not have	55 (65.47)	17(80.95)	18 (85.71)	10 (47.61)	10 (47.61)	$p = 0.021$ $\chi^2 = 14.959$
	Active	10 (11.90)	0	2 (9.52)	3 (14.28)	5 (23.80)	
	Latent	19 (22.61)	4 (19.04)	1 (4.76)	8 (38.09)	6 (28.57)	
Adductor magnus	Does not have	14 (16.66)	5 (23.80)	5 (23.80)	0	4 (19.04)	$p = 0.177$ $\chi^2 = 8.944$
	Active	1 (1.19)	0	0	0	1 (4.76)	
	Latent	69 (82.14)	16 (76.19)	16 (76.19)	21 (100)	16 (76.19)	
Gluteus maximus	Does not have	19 (22.61)	6 (28.57)	7 (33.33)	3 (14.28)	3 (14.28)	$p = 0.683$ $\chi^2 = 3.951$
	Active	5 (5.95)	1 (4.76)	1 (4.76)	2 (9.52)	1 (4.76)	
	Latent	60 (71.42)	14 (66.66)	13 (61.90)	16 (76.19)	17 (80.95)	
Gluteus medius	Does not have	20 (23.80)	4 (19.04)	9 (42.85)	3 (14.28)	4 (19.04)	$p = 0.379$ $\chi^2 = 6.407$
	Active	5 (5.95)	1 (4.76)	1 (4.76)	1 (4.76)	2 (9.52)	
	Latent	59 (70.23)	16 (76.19)	11 (52.38)	17 (80.95)	15 (71.42)	

Table 7. *Cont.*

Muscles	Presence of MTrPs	Total (n = 84)	NDNC (n = 21)	NDWC (n = 21)	WDNC (n = 21)	WDWC (n = 21)	*p*-Value * χ^2
		n (%)	n (%)	n (%)	n (%)	n (%)	
Gluteus minimus	Does not have	16 (19.04)	5 (23.80)	6 (28.57)	2 (9.52)	3 (14.28)	$p = 0.500$ $\chi^2 = 4.875$
	Active	4 (4.76)	1 (4.76)	0	1 (4.76)	2 (9.52)	
	Latent	64 (76.19)	15 (71.42)	15 (71.42)	18 (85.71)	16 (76.19)	
Quadratus lumborum	Does not have	10 (11.90)	4 (19.04)	2 (9.52)	3 (14.28)	1 (4.76)	$p = 0.082$ $\chi^2 = 11.209$
	Active	15 (17.85)	4 (19.04)	1 (4.76)	2 (9.52)	8 (38.09)	
	Latent	59 (70.23)	13 (61.90)	18 (85.71)	16 (76.19)	12 (57.14)	
Piriformis	Does not have	17 (20.23)	5 (23.80)	3 (14.28)	7 (33.33)	2 (9.52)	$p = 0.358$ $\chi^2 = 6.616$
	Active	21 (25)	3 (14.28)	5 (23.80)	6 (28.57)	7 (33.33)	
	Latent	46 (54.76)	13 (61.90)	13 (61.90)	8 (38.09)	12 (57.14)	

Abbreviations: NDNC: non-dysmenorrhea non-contraceptive group; NDWC: non-dysmenorrhea with contraceptives group; WDNC: with dysmenorrhea non-contraceptives group; WDWC: with dysmenorrhea with contraceptives group. A $p < 0.01$ was considered statistically significant. * One-way ANOVA was used.

Table 8. Presence of MTrPs in the pelvic floor muscles evaluated in the ovulatory phase.

Muscles	Presence of MTrPs	Total (n = 84)	NDNC (n = 21)	NDWC (n = 21)	WDNC (n = 21)	WDWC (n = 21)	*p*-Value * χ^2
		n (%)	n (%)	n (%)	n (%)	n (%)	
Ischiocavernosus	Does not have	39 (46.42)	14 (66.66)	14 (66.66)	7 (3333)	4 (19.04)	$\mathbf{p < 0.01}$ * $\chi^2 = 16.969$
	Active	4 (4.76)	1 (4.76)	1 (4.76)	0	2 (9.52)	
	Latent	41 (48.80)	6 (28.57)	6 (28.57)	14 (66.66)	15 (71.42)	
Bulbospongiosus	Does not have	56 (66.66)	17 (80.95)	17 (80.95)	13 (61.90)	9 (42.85)	$p = 0.052$ $\chi^2 = 12.476$
	Active	1 (1.19)	0	0	1 (4.76)	0	
	Latent	27 (32.14)	4 (19.04)	4 (19.04)	7 (33.33)	12 (57.14)	
Transverse perineal	Does not have	52 (61.90)	13 (61.90)	16 (76.19)	11 (52.38)	12 (57.14)	$p = 0.600$ $\chi^2 = 4.573$
	Active	5 (5.95)	2 (9.52)	0	1 (4.76)	2 (9.52)	
	Latent	27 (32.14)	6 (28.57)	5 (23.80)	9 (42.85)	7 (33.33)	
Puborectalis	Does not have	18 (21.42)	4 (19.04)	10 (47.61)	1 (4.76)	3 (14.28)	$p = 0.030$ $\chi^2 = 14.000$
	Active	22 (26.19)	6 (28.57)	2 (9.52)	8 (38.09)	6 (28.57)	
	Latent	44 (52.38)	11 (52.38)	9 (42.85)	12 (57.14)	12 (57.14)	
Pubococcygeus	Does not have	21 (25)	6 (28.57)	8 (38.09)	6 (28.57)	1 (4.76)	$p = 0.116$ $\chi^2 = 10.210$
	Active	35 (41.66)	6 (28.57)	6 (28.57)	10 (47.61)	13 (61.90)	
	Latent	28 (33.33)	9 (42.85)	7 (33.33)	5 (23.80)	7 (33.33)	
Iliococcygeus	Does not have	15 (17.85)	6 (28.57)	8 (38.09)	1 (4.76)	0	$\mathbf{p < 0.001}$ * $\chi^2 = 25.286$
	Active	51 (60.71)	7 (33.33)	8 (38.09)	18 (85.71)	18 (85.71)	
	Latent	18 (21.42)	8 (38.09)	5 (23.80)	2 (9.52)	3 (14.28)	
Obturator internus	Does not have	6 (7.14)	2 (9.52)	4 (19.04)	0	0	$p = 0.049$ $\chi^2 = 12.659$
	Active	28 (33.33)	4 (19.04)	5 (23.80)	8 (38.09)	11 (52.38)	
	Latent	50 (59.52)	15 (71.42)	12 (57.14)	13 (61.90)	10 (11.90)	
Coccygeus	Does not have	39 (46.42)	12 (57.14)	10 (47.61)	12 (57.14)	5 (23.80)	$p = 0.55$ $\chi^2 = 12.314$
	Active	7 (8.33)	0	1 (4.76)	1 (4.76)	5 (23.80)	
	Latent	38 (45.23)	9 (42.85)	10 (47.61)	8 (38.09)	11 (52.38)	
Anal sphincter	Does not have	69 (82.14)	17 (80.95)	21 (100)	17 (80.95)	14 (66.66)	$\mathbf{p < 0.01}$ * $\chi^2 = 18.435$
	Active	5 (5.95)	3 (14.28)	0	2 (9.52)	0	
	Latent	10 (11.90)	1 (4.76)	0	2 (9.52)	7 (33.33)	

Abbreviations: NDNC: non-dysmenorrhea non-contraceptive group; NDWC: non-dysmenorrhea with contraceptives group; MTrPs: myofascial trigger points; WDNC: with dysmenorrhea non-contraceptives group; WDWC: with dysmenorrhea with contraceptives group. A $p < 0.01$ (**Bold**) was considered statistically significant. * One-way ANOVA was used.

3.6. Referred Pain Areas

Rectus Abdominis Muscle

Statistically significant results were found during the menstrual phase for the areas of referred pain in the flank (64.29%), iliac fossa (40.48%), pubis (11.90%), and groin (8.33%), with a higher frequency of these areas of referred pain in the WDNC group. In the rest of the referred pain areas, and in all referred pain areas during the ovulatory phase, no significant results were found for the rectus abdominis muscle. Figure 4 shows a graphical simulation of the representation of the referred pain, showing with greater intensity of color the zones where it was referred with greater frequency and, with less intensity, those with less frequency.

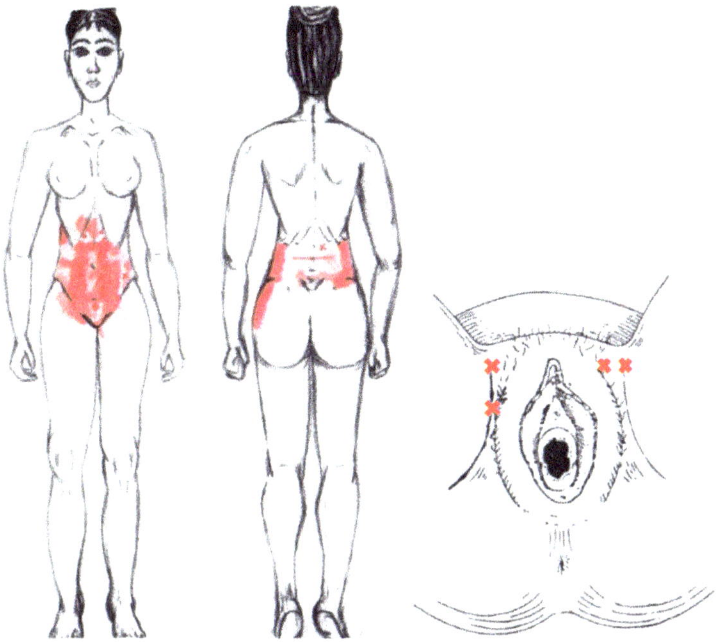

Figure 4. Graphical simulation of referred pain areas of the rectus abdominis muscle.

The frequency at the areas of referred rectus abdominis muscle pain in the menstrual phase and in the ovulatory phase is shown in Tables 9 and 10, respectively.

3.7. External Oblique Muscle

No significant results were found during either the menstrual or ovulatory phase in any of the areas of referred pain for the external oblique muscle. Figure 5 shows a graphical simulation of the representation of the referred pain zones, showing with greater intensity of color the zones where it was referred with greater frequency and, with less intensity, those with less frequency.

The frequency at the areas of referred external oblique muscle pain in the menstrual phase and in the ovulatory phase is shown in Tables 9 and 10, respectively.

Table 9. Pain reproduced at specific sites after palpation in 84 participants during menstrual phase.

Muscles	Self-Reported Pain Site																		
	Flank n (%)	Iliac Fossa n (%)	Hypogastrium n (%)	Mesogastrium n (%)	Epigastrium n (%)	Anterior Part Lower Limb n (%)	Posterior Part Lower Limb n (%)	Pubis n (%)	Groin n (%)	Gluteus n (%)	Lumbar n (%)	Coccyx n (%)	Sacrum n (%)	Internal Part Lower Limb n (%)	Vulva n (%)	Vagina n (%)	Urethra n (%)	Anus n (%)	Rectum n (%)
Rectus Abdominis	54 (64.29)	34 (40.48)	68 (80.95)	61 (72.62)	24 (28.57)	1 (1.19)	0 (0)	10 (11.90)	7 (8.33)	1 (1.19)	4 (4.76)	0 (0)	0 (0)	0 (0)	0 (0)	0 (0)	0 (0)	0 (0)	0 (0)
External Oblique	56 (66.67)	60 (71.43)	7 (8.33)	4 (4.76)	0 (0)	4 (4.76)	1 (1.19)	3 (3.57)	4 (4.76)	0 (0)	4 (4.76)	0 (0)	0 (0)	0 (0)	0 (0)	0 (0)	0 (0)	0 (0)	0 (0)
Internal Oblique	1 (1.19)	12 (14.29)	24 (28.57)	0 (0)	0 (0)	10 (11.90)	0 (0)	10 (11.90)	14 (16.67)	0 (0)	0 (0)	1 (1.19)	1 (1.19)	0 (0)	0 (0)	0 (0)	0 (0)	0 (0)	0 (0)
Adductor Magnus	0 (0)	0 (0)	1 (1.19)	0 (0)	0 (0)	7 (8.33)	3 (3.57)	2 (2.38)	2 (2.38)	0 (0)	0 (0)	1 (1.19)	0 (0)	75 (89.29)	0 (0)	0 (0)	0 (0)	0 (0)	0 (0)
Gluteus Maximus	0 (0)	1 (1.19)	0 (0)	0 (0)	0 (0)	5 (5.95)	1 (1.19)	0 (0)	0 (0)	64 (76.19)	12 (14.29)	3 (3.57)	4 (4.76)	9 (10.71)	0 (0)	0 (0)	0 (0)	0 (0)	0 (0)
Gluteus Medius	1 (1.19)	1 (1.19)	1 (1.19)	0 (0)	0 (0)	4 (4.76)	9 (10.71)	1 (1.19)	3 (3.57)	74 (88.10)	5 (5.95)	3 (3.57)	4 (4.76)	0 (0)	1 (1.19)	0 (0)	0 (0)	0 (0)	0 (0)
Gluteus Minimus	0 (0)	1 (1.19)	1 (1.19)	0 (0)	0 (0)	9 (10.71)	15 (17.86)	1 (1.19)	2 (2.38)	70 (83.33)	5 (5.95)	0 (0)	0 (0)	1 (1.19)	0 (0)	0 (0)	0 (0)	0 (0)	0 (0)
Quadratus Lumborum	3 (3.57)	3 (3.57)	5 (5.95)	1 (1.19)	1 (1.19)	1 (1.19)	2 (2.38)	2 (2.38)	2 (2.38)	20 (23.81)	75 (89.29)	1 (1.19)	8 (9.52)	0 (0)	0 (0)	0 (0)	0 (0)	0 (0)	0 (0)
Piriformis	1 (1.19)	7 (8.33)	11 (13.10)	1 (1.19)	0 (0)	6 (7.14)	10 (11.90)	10 (11.90)	17 (20.24)	48 (57.14)	6 (7.14)	11 (13.10)	9 (10.71)	2 (2.38)	16 (19.05)	3 (3.57)	2 (2.38)	8 (9.52)	0 (0)

Table 10. Pain reproduced at specific sites after palpation in 84 participants during ovulatory phase.

	Self-Reported Pain Site																	
Muscles n (%)	**Flank n (%)**	**Iliac Fossa n (%)**	**Hypogastrium n (%)**	**Mesogastrium n (%)**	**Epigastrium n (%)**	**Anterior Part Lower Limb n (%)**	**Pubis n (%)**	**Groin n (%)**	**Vulva n (%)**	**Sacrum n (%)**	**Lumbar n (%)**	**Internal Part Lower Limb n (%)**	**Coccyx n (%)**	**Posterior Part Lower Limb n (%)**	**Gluteus n (%)**	**Vagina n (%)**	**Urethra n (%)**	**Anus n (%)**	**Rectum n (%)**
Rectus Abdominis	15 (17.86)	25 (29.76)	56 (66.67)	50 (59.52)	14 (16.67)	1 (1.19)	1 (1.19)	4 (4.76)	1 (1.19)	1 (1.19)	5 (5.95)	0 (0)	0 (0)	0 (0)	0 (0)	0 (0)	0 (0)	0 (0)	0 (0)
External Oblique	43 (51.19)	56 (66.67)	5 (5.95)	2 (2.38)	2 (2.38)	5 (5.95)	0 (0)	1 (1.19)	0 (0)	1 (1.19)	2 (2.38)	0 (0)	0 (0)	0 (0)	0 (0)	0 (0)	0 (0)	0 (0)	0 (0)
Internal Oblique	0 (0)	10 (11.90)	11 (13.10)	0 (0)	0 (0)	4 (4.76)	6 (7.14)	4 (4.76)	0 (0)	0 (0)	0 (0)	1 (1.19)	0 (0)	0 (0)	0 (0)	0 (0)	0 (0)	0 (0)	0 (0)
Adductor Magnus	0 (0)	0 (0)	1 (1.19)	0 (0)	0 (0)	8 (9.52)	0 (0)	2 (2.38)	0 (0)	0 (0)	0 (0)	65 (77.38)	0 (0)	0 (0)	0 (0)	0 (0)	0 (0)	0 (0)	0 (0)
Gluteus Maximus	2 (2.38)	2 (2.38)	1 (1.19)	0 (0)	0 (0)	9 (10.71)	1 (1.19)	1 (1.19)	0 (0)	3 (3.57)	17 (20.24)	1 (1.19)	1 (1.19)	3 (3.57)	64 (76.19)	0 (0)	0 (0)	0 (0)	0 (0)
Gluteus Medius	1 (1.19)	1 (1.19)	0 (0)	0 (0)	0 (0)	6 (7.14)	1 (1.19)	1 (1.19)	0 (0)	1 (1.19)	6 (7.14)	0 (0)	0 (0)	7 (8.33)	61 (71.62)	0 (0)	0 (0)	0 (0)	0 (0)
Gluteus Minimus	0 (0)	1 (1.19)	2 (2.38)	0 (0)	0 (0)	8 (9.52)	0 (0)	0 (0)	0 (0)	2 (2.38)	9 (10.71)	1 (1.19)	1 (1.19)	7 (8.33)	62 (73.81)	0 (0)	0 (0)	0 (0)	0 (0)
Quadratus Lumborum	1 (1.19)	4 (4.76)	0 (0)	0 (0)	0 (0)	0 (0)	1 (1.19)	2 (2.38)	0 (0)	4 (4.76)	72 (85.71)	0 (0)	0 (0)	3 (3.57)	18 (21.43)	0 (0)	0 (0)	0 (0)	0 (0)
Piriformis	1 (1.19)	8 (9.52)	7 (8.33)	1 (1.19)	0 (0)	3 (3.57)	9 (10.71)	11 (13.10)	17 (20.24)	2 (2.38)	4 (4.76)	2 (2.38)	4 (4.76)	6 (7.14)	47 (55.95)	4 (4.76)	0 (0)	10 (11.90)	3 (3.57)

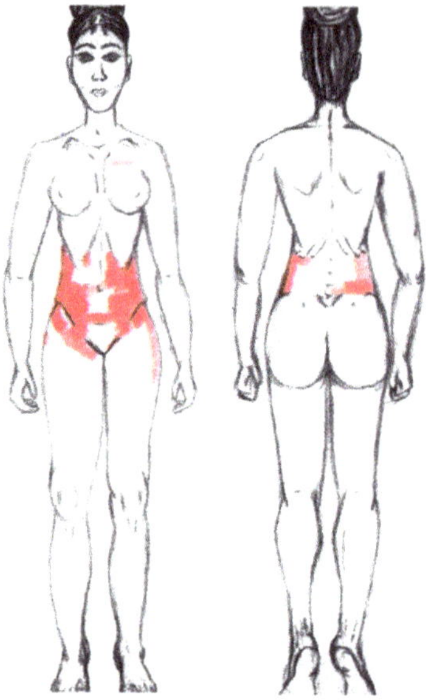

Figure 5. Graphical simulation of referred pain areas of the external oblique muscle.

3.8. Internal Oblique Muscle

A significantly higher frequency of the referred pain areas of the pubis (11.90%) and groin (16.67%) were found in the WDNC group. In the rest of the referred pain areas and in all referred pain areas during the ovulatory phase, no significant results were found for the internal oblique muscle. Figure 6 shows a graphical simulation of the representation of the referred pain zones, showing with greater intensity of color the zones where it was referred with greater frequency and, with less intensity, those with less frequency.

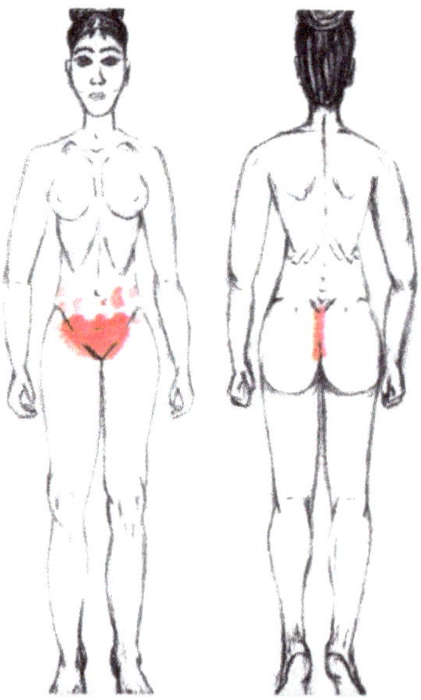

Figure 6. Graphical simulation of referred pain areas of the internal oblique muscle.

The frequency at the areas of referred internal oblique muscle pain in the menstrual phase and in the ovulatory phase is shown in Tables 9 and 10, respectively.

3.9. Adductor Magnus Muscle

No significant results were found in either the menstrual or ovulatory phase in any of the areas of referred pain for the adductor magnus muscle. Figure 7 shows a graphical simulation of the representation of the referred pain zones, showing with greater intensity of color the zones where it was referred more frequently and, with less intensity, those with less frequency.

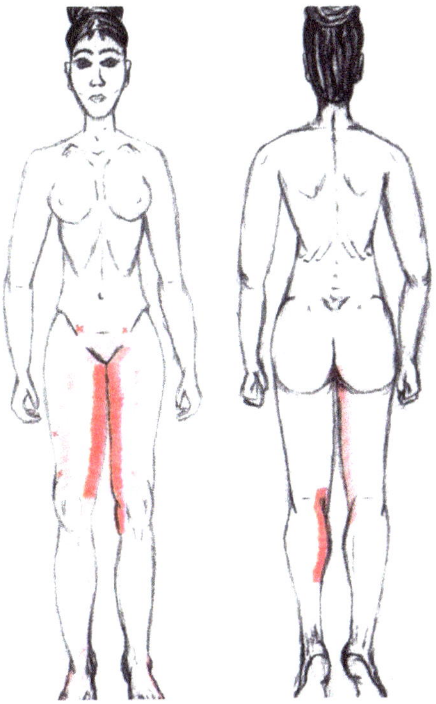

Figure 7. Graphical simulation of referred pain areas of the adductor magnus muscle.

The frequency at the areas of referred adductor magnus muscle pain in the menstrual phase and in the ovulatory phase is shown in Tables 9 and 10, respectively.

3.10. Gluteus Maximus Muscle

No significant results were found in either the menstrual or ovulatory phase in any of the areas of referred pain for the gluteus maximus muscle. Figure 8 shows a graphical simulation of the representation of the referred pain zones, showing with greater intensity of color the zones where it was referred with greater frequency and, with less intensity, those with less frequency.

The frequency at the areas of referred gluteus maximus muscle pain in the menstrual phase and in the ovulatory phase is shown in Tables 9 and 10, respectively.

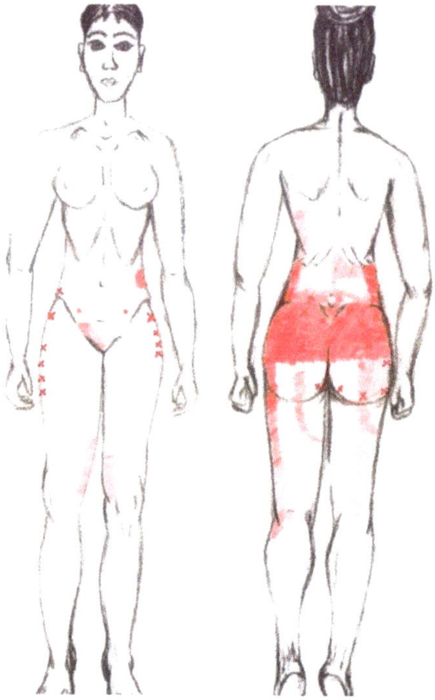

Figure 8. Graphical simulation of referred pain areas of the gluteus maximus muscle.

3.11. Gluteus Medius Muscle

No significant data were found in either the menstrual or ovulatory phase in any of the areas of referred pain for the gluteus medius muscle. Figure 9 shows a graphical simulation of the representation of the referred pain zones, showing with greater intensity of color the zones where it was referred with greater frequency and, with less intensity, those with less frequency.

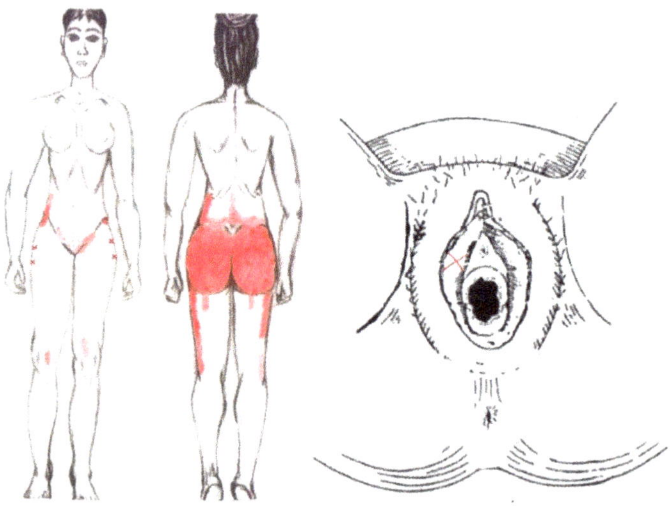

Figure 9. Graphical simulation of referred pain areas of the gluteus medius muscle.

The frequency at the areas of referred gluteus medius muscle pain in the menstrual phase and in the ovulatory phase is shown in Tables 9 and 10, respectively.

3.12. Gluteus Minimus Muscle

No statistically significant results emerged from either the menstrual or ovulatory phase in any of the areas of referred pain for the gluteus minimus muscle. Figure 10 shows a graphical simulation of the representation of the referred pain zones, showing with greater intensity of color the zones where it was referred more frequently and, with less intensity, those with less frequency.

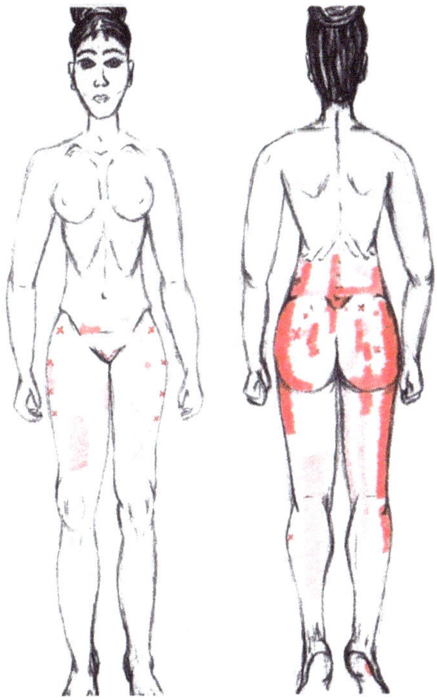

Figure 10. Graphical simulation of referred pain areas of the gluteus minimus muscle.

The frequency at the areas of referred gluteus minimus muscle pain in the menstrual phase and in the ovulatory phase is shown in Tables 9 and 10, respectively.

3.13. Quadratus Lumborum Muscle

No significant results were found in either the menstrual or ovulatory phase in any of the areas of referred pain for the quadratus lumborum muscle. Figure 11 shows a graphical simulation of the representation of the referred pain zones, showing with greater intensity of color the zones where it was referred more frequently and, with less intensity, those with less frequency.

The frequency at the areas of referred quadratus lumborum muscle pain in the menstrual phase and in the ovulatory phase is shown in Tables 9 and 10, respectively.

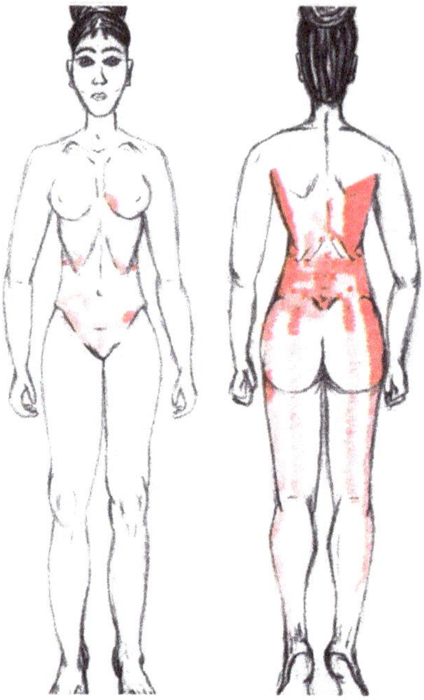

Figure 11. Graphical simulation of referred pain areas of the quadratus lumborum muscle.

3.14. Ischiocavernosus Muscle

No significant findings were found in either the menstrual or ovulatory phase in any of the areas of referred pain for the ischiocavernosus muscle. Figure 12 shows a graphical simulation of the representation of the referred pain zones, showing with greater intensity of color the zones where it was referred with greater frequency and, with less intensity, those with less frequency.

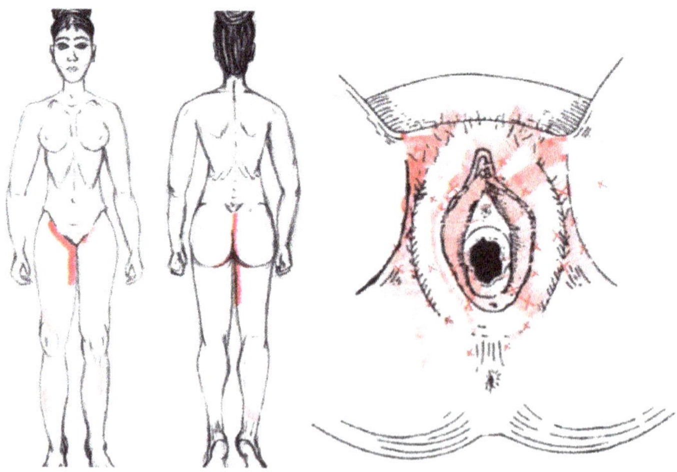

Figure 12. Graphical simulation of referred pain areas of the ischiocavernosus muscle.

The frequency at the areas of referred ischiocavernosus muscle pain in the menstrual phase and in the ovulatory phase is shown in Tables 11 and 12, respectively.

Table 11. Pain reproduced at specific sites after palpation in 84 participants during menstrual phase in the pelvic floor muscles.

	Self-Reported Pain Site																		
Muscles n (%)	**Flank n (%)**	**Iliac Fossa n (%)**	**Hypogastrium n (%)**	**Mesogastrium n (%)**	**Epigastrium n (%)**	**Anterior Part Lower Limb n (%)**	**Posterior Part Lower Limb n (%)**	**Pubis n (%)**	**Groin n (%)**	**Gluteus n (%)**	**Lumbar n (%)**	**Coccyx n (%)**	**Sacrum n (%)**	**Internal Part Lower Limb n (%)**	**Vulva n (%)**	**Vagina n (%)**	**Urethra n (%)**	**Anus n (%)**	**Rectum n (%)**
Ischiocavernosus	0 (0)	0 (0)	2 (2.38)	0 (0)	0 (0)	1 (1.19)	1 (1.19)	1 (1.19)	14 (16.67)	3 (3.57)	1 (1.19)	2 (2.38)	0 (0)	4 (4.76)	55 (65.48)	3 (3.57)	4 (4.76)	0 (0)	0 (0)
Bulbospongiosus	0 (0)	0 (0)	1 (1.19)	0 (0)	0 (0)	0 (0)	0 (0)	0 (0)	1 (1.19)	0 (0)	0 (0)	0 (0)	0 (0)	0 (0)	41 (48.81)	11 (13.10)	6 (7.14)	0 (0)	0 (0)
Transverse Perineal	0 (0)	0 (0)	0 (0)	0 (0)	0 (0)	1 (1.19)	1 (1.19)	0 (0)	1 (1.19)	21 (25.00)	0 (0)	2 (2.38)	0 (0)	2 (2.38)	29 (34.52)	1 (1.19)	0 (0)	9 (10.71)	0 (0)
Puborectalis	0 (0)	1 (1.19)	5 (5.95)	0 (0)	0 (0)	1 (1.19)	0 (0)	9 (10.71)	11 (13.10)	13 (15.48)	0 (0)	6 (7.14)	2 (2.38)	5 (5.95)	41 (48.81)	28 (33.33)	7 (8.33)	19 (22.62)	6 (7.14)
Pubococcygeus	0 (0)	13 (15.48)	23 (27.38)	0 (0)	0 (0)	5 (5.95)	9 (10.71)	14 (16.67)	18 (21.43)	14 (16.67)	4 (4.76)	5 (5.95)	2 (2.38)	6 (7.14)	31 (36.90)	14 (16.67)	4 (4.76)	6 (7.14)	0 (0)
Iliococcygeus	2 (2.38)	18 (21.43)	46 (54.76)	2 (2.38)	0 (0)	4 (4.76)	4 (4.76)	37 (44.05)	23 (27.38)	10 (11.90)	3 (3.57)	4 (4.76)	2 (2.38)	3 (3.57)	37 (44.05)	12 (14.29)	9 (10.71)	5 (5.95)	1 (1.19)
Coccygeus	0 (0)	2 (2.38)	3 (3.57)	0 (0)	0 (0)	0 (0)	2 (2.38)	1 (1.19)	3 (3.57)	20 (23.81)	2 (2.38)	21 (25.00)	5 (5.95)	1 (1.19)	13 (15.48)	2 (2.38)	0 (0)	20 (23.81)	6 (7.14)
External Anal Sphincter	0 (0)	0 (0)	0 (0)	0 (0)	0 (0)	0 (0)	0 (0)	0 (0)	0 (0)	4 (4.76)	0 (0)	1 (1.19)	0 (0)	0 (0)	7 (8.33)	0 (0)	0 (0)	26 (30.95)	0 (0)
Obturator Internus	0 (0)	7 (8.33)	17 (20.24)	0 (0)	0 (0)	9 (10.71)	33 (39.29)	19 (22.62)	19 (22.62)	42 (50.00)	9 (10.71)	8 (9.52)	8 (9.52)	13 (15.48)	35 (41.67)	10 (11.90)	6 (7.14)	25 (29.76)	7 (8.33)

Table 12. Pain reproduced at specific sites after palpation in 84 participants during ovulatory phase in the pelvic floor muscles.

Muscles n (%)	Self-Reported Pain Site																		
	Flank n (%)	Iliac Fossa n (%)	Hypog-astrium n (%)	Mesog-astrium n (%)	Epiga-strium n (%)	Anterior Part Lower Limb n (%)	Pubis n (%)	Groin n (%)	Vulva n (%)	Sacrum n (%)	Lumbar n (%)	Internal Part Lower Limb n (%)	Coccyx n (%)	Posterior Part Lower Limb n (%)	Gluteus n (%)	Vagina n (%)	Urethra n (%)	Anus n (%)	Rectum n (%)
Ischiocaver-nosus	0 (0)	0 (0)	2 (2.38)	0 (0)	0 (0)	2 (2.38)	0 (0)	11 (13.10)	48 (57.14)	0 (0)	0 (0)	2 (2.38)	0 (0)	0 (0)	3 (3.57)	1 (1.19)	0 (0)	0 (0)	0 (0)
Bulbospon-giosus	0 (0)	1 (1.19)	1 (1.19)	0 (0)	0 (0)	2 (2.38)	0 (0)	2 (2.38)	24 (28.57)	0 (0)	0 (0)	1 (1.19)	0 (0)	0 (0)	0 (0)	8 (9.52)	3 (3.57)	0 (0)	0 (0)
Transverse Perineal	0 (0)	0 (0)	0 (0)	0 (0)	0 (0)	1 (1.19)	0 (0)	2 (2.38)	18 (21.43)	1 (1.19)	1 (1.19)	0 (0)	0 (0)	0 (0)	16 (19.04)	2 (2.38)	1 (1.19)	7 (8.33)	0 (0)
Puborectalis	0 (0)	0 (0)	5 (5.95)	1 (1.19)	0 (0)	2 (2.38)	1 (1.19)	6 (7.14)	50 (59.52)	2 (2.38)	2 (2.38)	0 (0)	2 (2.38)	1 (1.19)	11 (13.10)	22 (26.19)	4 (4.76)	20 (23.81)	4 (4.76)
Pubococcy-geus	1 (1.19)	2 (2.38)	22 (26.19)	0 (0)	0 (0)	4 (4.76)	18 (21.43)	16 (19.05)	23 (27.38)	1 (1.19)	2 (2.38)	6 (7.14)	3 (3.57)	5 (5.95)	10 (11.90)	11 (13.10)	6 (7.14)	6 (7.14)	0 (0)
Iliococcygeus	0 (0)	15 (17.86)	42 (50.00)	1 (1.19)	0 (0)	6 (7.14)	22 (26.19)	15 (17.86)	30 (35.71)	2 (2.38)	5 (5.95)	4 (4.76)	1 (1.19)	3 (3.57)	5 (5.95)	9 (10.71)	5 (5.95)	2 (2.38)	0 (0)
Coccygeus	1 (1.19)	2 (2.38)	3 (3.57)	0 (0)	0 (0)	3 (3.57)	3 (3.57)	3 (3.57)	9 (10.71)	4 (4.76)	0 (0)	1 (1.19)	12 (14.29)	0 (0)	13 (15.48)	1 (1.19)	0 (0)	19 (22.62)	5 (5.95)
External Anal Sphincter	0 (0)	0 (0)	0 (0)	0 (0)	0 (0)	0 (0)	0 (0)	0 (0)	3 (3.57)	2 (2.38)	0 (0)	0 (0)	1 (1.19)	0 (0)	4 (4.76)	0 (0)	0 (0)	18 (21.43)	0 (0)
Obturator Internus	2 (2.38)	10 (11.90)	17 (20.24)	1 (1.19)	0 (0)	6 (7.14)	11 (13.10)	14 (16.67)	33 (39.29)	3 (3.57)	4 (4.76)	8 (9.52)	4 (4.76)	23 (27.38)	38 (45.24)	12 (14.29)	4 (4.76)	23 (27.38)	5 (5.95)

3.15. Bulbospongiosus Muscle

No significant results were found in either the menstrual or ovulatory phase in any of the areas of referred pain for the bulbospongiosus muscle. Figure 13 shows a graphical simulation of the representation of the referred pain zones, showing with greater intensity of color the zones where it was referred with greater frequency and, with less intensity, those with less frequency.

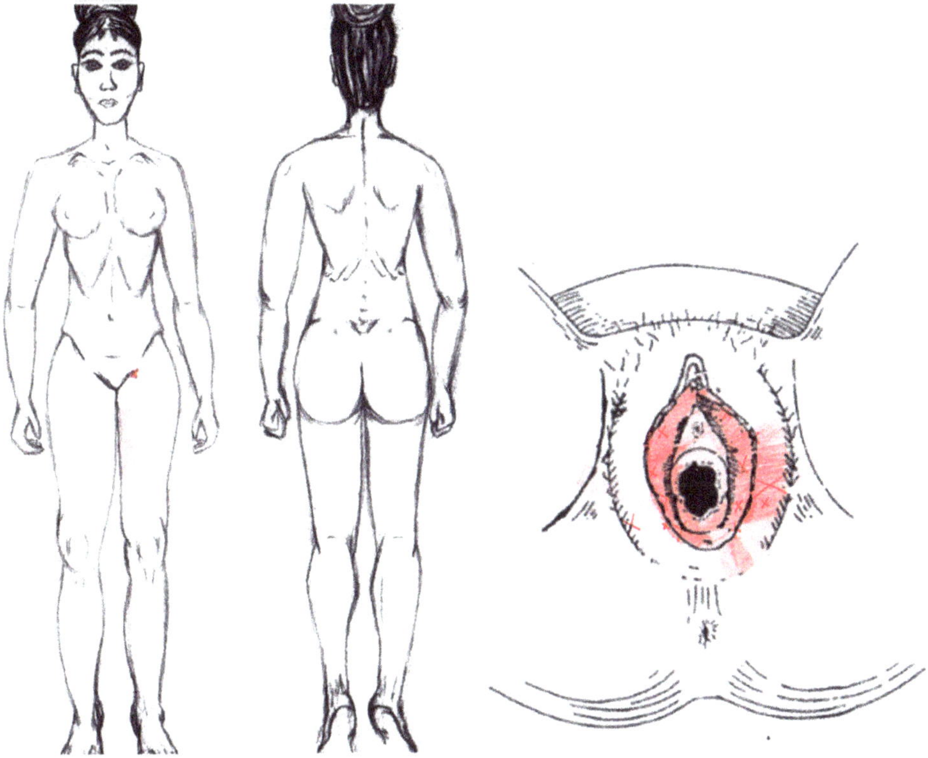

Figure 13. Graphical simulation of referred pain areas of the bulbospongiosus muscle.

The frequency at the areas of referred bulbospongiosus muscle pain in the menstrual phase and in the ovulatory phase is shown in Tables 11 and 12, respectively.

3.16. Transverse Perineal Muscle

No significant results were found in either the menstrual or ovulatory phase in any of the areas of referred pain for the transverse perineal muscle. Figure 14 shows a graphical simulation of the representation of the referred pain zones, showing with greater intensity of color the zones where it was referred more frequently and, with less intensity, those with less frequency.

The frequency at the areas of referred transverse perineal muscle pain in the menstrual phase and in the ovulatory phase is shown in Tables 11 and 12, respectively.

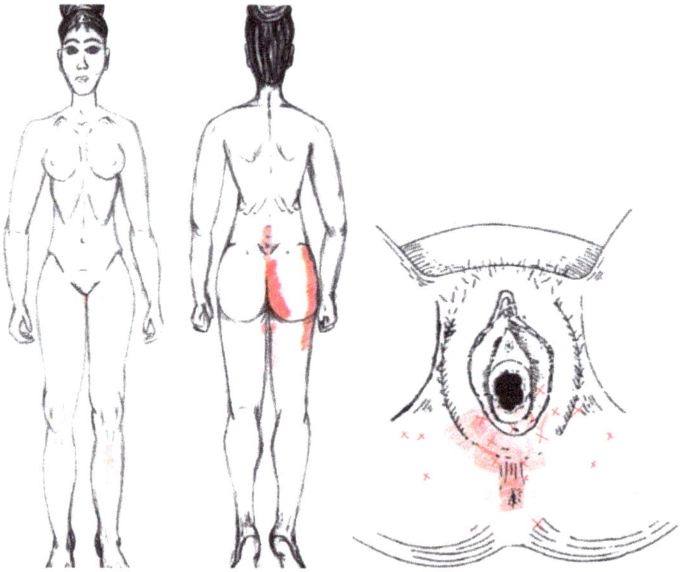

Figure 14. Graphical simulation of referred pain areas of the transverse perineal muscle.

3.17. Puborectalis Muscle

Statistically significant data were found in the ovulatory phase for the areas of referred groin pain, present in the rectum only in 7.14% of the women and felt almost exclusively in the NDNA group. It was identified by 4.76% of women in its entirety in the SDSA group, and it was reported in the anus by 23.81% of respondents, most from the SDSA group. In the rest of the referred pain areas in the ovulatory phase, and in all of referred pain areas in the menstrual phase, no significant results were found for the puborectalis muscle (Figure 15).

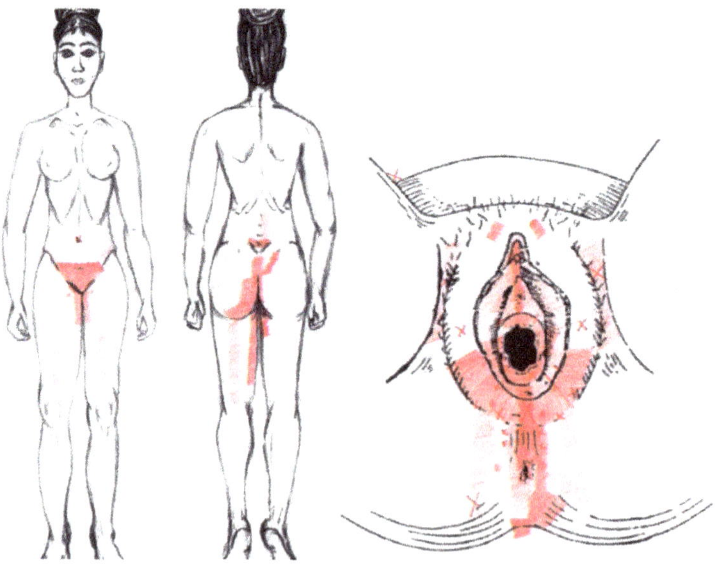

Figure 15. Graphical simulation of referred pain areas of the puborectalis muscle.

The frequency at the areas of referred puborectalis muscle pain in the menstrual phase and in the ovulatory phase is shown in Tables 11 and 12, respectively.

3.18. Pubococcygeus Muscle

No statistically significant results were found in either the menstrual or ovulatory phase in any of the areas of referred pain for the pubococcygeus muscle. Figure 16 shows a graphical simulation of the representation of the referred pain zones, showing with greater intensity of color the zones where it was referred with greater frequency and, with less intensity, those with less frequency.

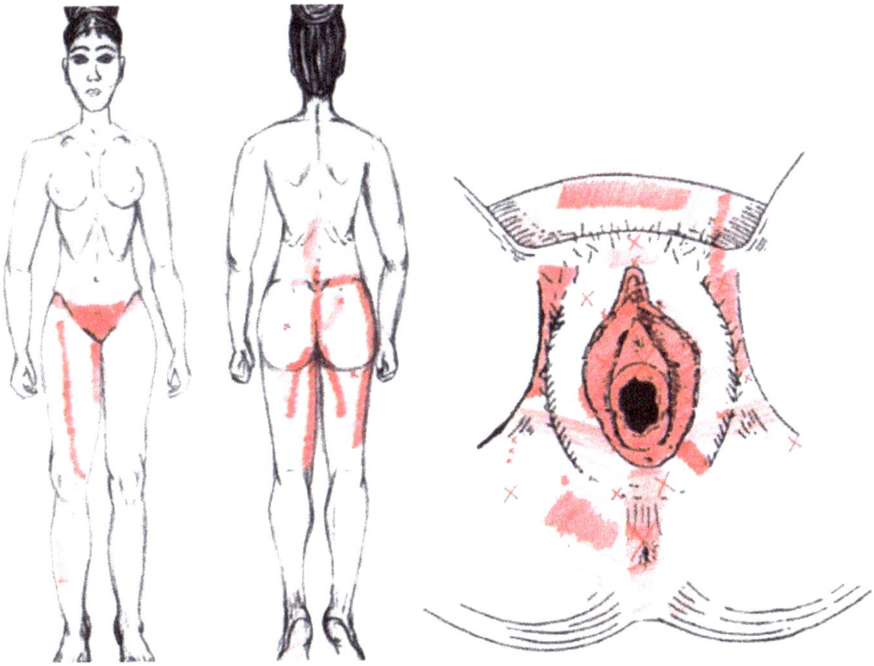

Figure 16. Graphical simulation of referred pain areas of the pubococcygeus muscle.

The frequency at the areas of referred pubococcygeus muscle pain in the menstrual phase and in the ovulatory phase is shown in Tables 11 and 12, respectively.

3.19. Iliococcygeus Muscle

Statistically significant results were found in the ovulatory phase for the area of referred pain from the hypogastrium, which was present in 50% of respondents, most from the SDNA and SDSA groups. In the other referred pain areas in the ovulatory phase, and in all referred pain areas in the menstrual phase, no significant results were found for the iliococcygeus muscle (Figure 17).

The frequency at the areas of referred iliococcygeus muscle pain in the menstrual phase and in the ovulatory phase is shown in Tables 11 and 12, respectively.

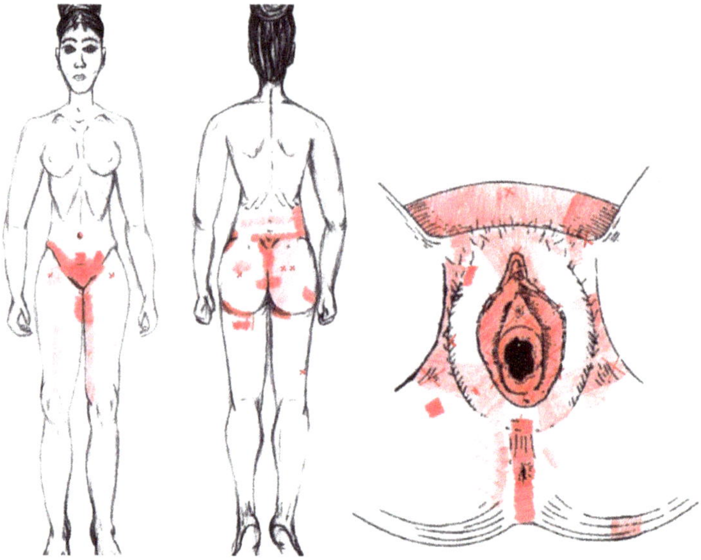

Figure 17. Graphical simulation of referred pain areas of the iliococcygeus muscle.

3.20. Coccygeus Muscle

No significant data were found in either the menstrual or ovulatory phase in any of the areas of referred pain for the coccygeus muscle. Figure 18 shows a graphical simulation of the representation of the referred pain zones, showing with greater intensity of color the zones where it was referred with greater frequency and, with less intensity, those with less frequency.

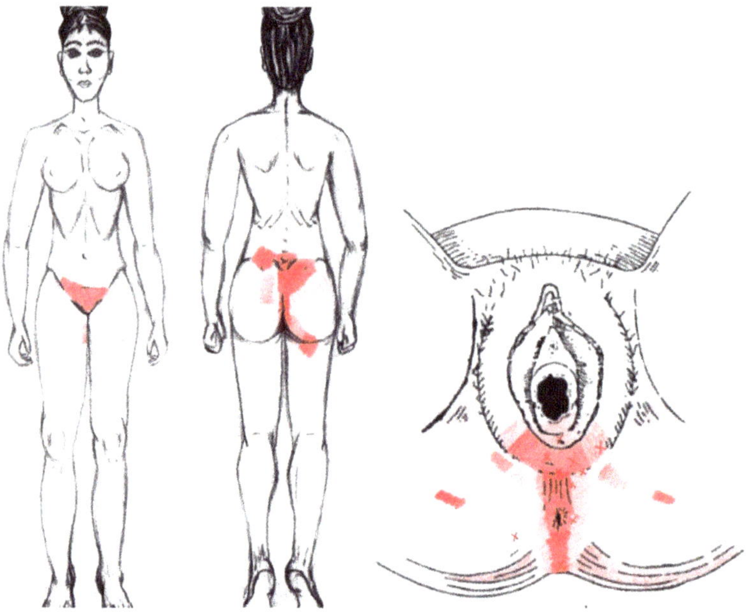

Figure 18. Graphical simulation of referred pain areas of the coccygeus muscle.

The frequency at the areas of referred coccygeus muscle pain in the menstrual phase and in the ovulatory phase is shown in Tables 11 and 12, respectively.

3.21. External Anal Sphincter Muscle

No significant data were found in either the menstrual or ovulatory phase in any of the areas of referred pain for the external anal sphincter muscle. Figure 19 shows a graphical simulation of the representation of the referred pain zones, showing with greater intensity of color the zones where it was referred more frequently and, with less intensity, those with less frequency.

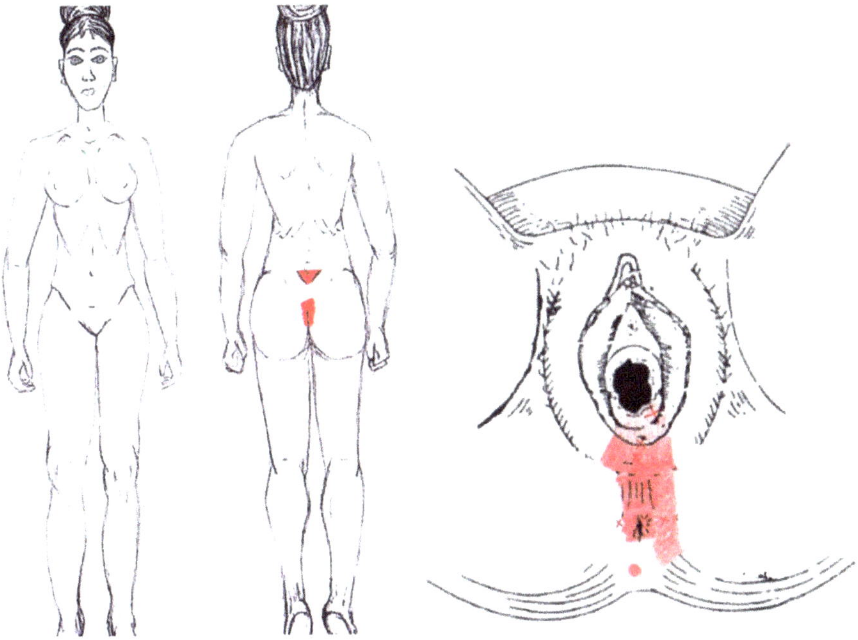

Figure 19. Graphical simulation of referred pain areas of the external anal sphincter muscle.

The frequency at the areas of referred external anal sphincter muscle pain in the menstrual phase and in the ovulatory phase is shown in Tables 11 and 12, respectively.

3.22. Obturator Internus Muscle

Statistically significant data were found in the ovulatory phase for the area of referred pain from the vulva, being present in 39.29% of the women, and its proportion being higher in the SDNA group. In the rest of the referred pain areas in the ovulatory phase, and in all referred pain areas in the menstrual phase, no statistically significant results were found for the obturator internus muscle (Figure 20).

The frequency at the areas of referred obturator internus muscle pain in the menstrual phase and in the ovulatory phase is shown in Tables 11 and 12, respectively.

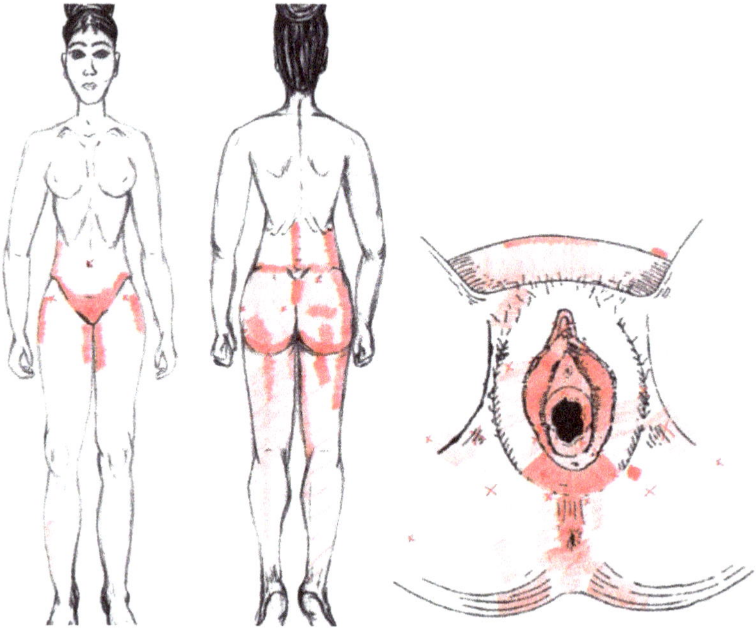

Figure 20. Graphical simulation of referred pain areas of the obturator internus muscle.

3.23. *Piriformis Muscle*

No significant data were found in either the menstrual or ovulatory phase in any of the areas of referred pain for the piriformis muscle. Figure 21 shows a graphical simulation of the representation of the referred pain zones, showing with greater intensity of color the zones where it was referred more frequently and, with less intensity, those with less frequency.

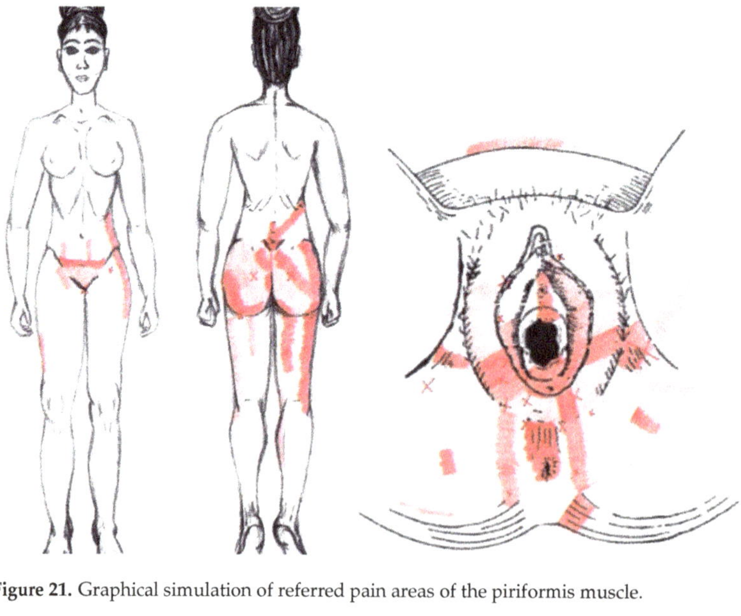

Figure 21. Graphical simulation of referred pain areas of the piriformis muscle.

The frequency at the areas of referred piriformis muscle pain in the menstrual phase and in the ovulatory phase is shown in Tables 9 and 10, respectively.

4. Discussion

Our study sought to provide information on the possible relationship between PD and the presence of MPS, considering not only the existence of both active and latent MTrPs, but also variables such as altered mechanosensitivity to pressure and its relationship with the central sensitization process, and the description of referred pain maps of the study muscles; these factors are usually associated with the presence of MTrPs. The data were obtained from the comparison of women with and without this gynecological disorder and who were or were not receiving contraceptive treatment.

In addition to the clear difference in VAS scores between the groups with and without pain during the menstrual phase, our results indicate that the affective, emotional, and sensory descriptors collected by the McGill Pain Questionnaire yielded higher scores in groups with PD, when they are not receiving contraceptive treatment; lower scores were found in women without PD who were receiving contraceptive treatment. By comparison, there seems to be an impairment in the quality of life in women with PD who were not receiving contraceptive treatment, mainly with respect to physical health.

Despite these differences in pain and quality of life during menstruation in women with PD, these differences were not as clearly reflected in the mechanosensitivity data presented by women in the menstrual phase compared with those with and without menstrual pain. In the mechanosensitivity data, we only found differences in some of the measurement time-points collected between the groups receiving contraceptive treatment. Where we did find greater differences was in the intragroup analysis, which revealed differences between the menstrual phase and the luteal phase. The significant differences that appeared in the PPT in the periovulatory or intermenstrual phase occurred only in the group of women without PD and who were under contraceptive treatment.

The prevalence of MTrPs during menstruation exceeded 80% of the total sample for the deep muscles of the PF, and for muscles such as the rectus abdominis, external oblique, quadratus lumborum, and piriformis; elevated prevalence rates during the periovulatory or intermenstrual phase were found only in the case of the rectus abdominis muscle, with a high prevalence rate of latent MTrPs; and in the case of the iliococcygeus muscle, with a high prevalence rate of active MTrPs, predominantly among the participants with PD.

A record of referred pain areas was made to find a body representation associated with the presence of MTrPs in the different study muscles. The referred pain zones obtained in this study are considerably broader than the patterns previously described for the PF musculature.

4.1. Sociodemographic Factors and Clinical Data

In our study, no significant effects were found in terms of the sociodemographic variables collected, such as age or BMI, nor in the data on the menstrual cycle, such as the length of the cycle, duration of menstruation, and the onset of menstruation (menarche). The available literature continues to investigate the possible risk factors associated with dysmenorrhea, since a lack of consensus remains on some aspects. Although no differences in age groups were observed in our study, the vast majority of extant studies focused on young populations—overwhelmingly university students or those under 25 years of age—with very limited information on older women [19,79]. Data about weight and BMI are also mixed, although several studies focused on the greater predisposition in women with low weight or who have lost or attempted weight loss [19,80]. Latthe et al., found that women with a BMI < 20 kg/m^2 report greater pain intensity [81], which, according to Nalan et al., who obtained similar results, could be due to the fact that low body fat would affect the normal ovulation and the menstrual cycle, causing an excessive release of PGs, which are considered the source of menstrual pain [80].

Regarding the characteristics of the menstrual cycle, other studies relate a greater severity of menstrual pain with longer periods, irregular cycles, or menarche onset before 12 years of age [9,80–82]. In the rest of the clinical variables, we found no significant results in our study, except in the gastrointestinal alterations that women present during the days of menstruation and that are absent outside of menstruation, such as nausea, discomfort, and—mainly—changes in the frequency of passing stool. The data on gastrointestinal disorders, such as constipation and diarrhea, are consistent in most studies, not only on PD, but also on premenstrual syndrome and menstruation in general [20,83,84].

From the data collected on the number of pregnancies and deliveries, and on their subsequent relationship with pain, no significant results were found between the groups. However, it should be noted that only a small percentage of the sample (19%) was under this condition. The most notable was an improvement in menstrual symptoms after childbirth, a condition more commonly described in other investigations [9]. Regarding physical activity and its effects on menstrual symptoms, no significant differences were found in nearly 37% of participants, while improved and worsened symptoms were reported in 27.38% and 10.71% of participants, respectively; these data are similar to those reported in the relevant literature, since the great variety of disciplines and exercise programs used make it difficult to unify criteria that allow clarifying the role of exercise in PD [21]. However, the review by Armor et al., noted that regular physical activity lasting 45–60 min can provide beneficial effects [85].

Almost 65% of the participants in our study required treatment to relieve menstrual symptoms. The most popular treatment were pharmaceuticals, either on their own or combined with thermotherapy (i.e., the application of heat to the affected area). These data are consistent with those reported in the relevant literature [2,9,10,20,68,86–88]. However, one of the treatments most commonly described and used for the treatment of PD is the use of contraceptives, which, in our case, was not included as a form of treatment, since it was part of one of the variables used to classify the participants in our study. Despite being a form of treatment, and helping to improve symptoms, there were women who were recruited in the group of menstrual pain and contraceptive treatment, which indicates that its use does not completely eliminate menstrual pain in all cases. Something that could be assessed in future studies is the type of contraceptive treatment, because even though the vast majority of studies refer to combined oral contraceptives (COCs) for the treatment of PD, not all of the women in our study who were receiving contraceptive treatment were taking COCs; in some cases, they used an intrauterine device (IUD) or vaginal ring. Although the extant literature contends that all three forms of contraceptive treatment cause changes in menstrual flow and pain—and can even affect other symptoms associated with menstruation [2,8–10,20,89–93]—no studies to date have compared contraceptive use with PD. Unlike our research, in the vast majority of reviewed studies on PD, contraceptive treatment was considered an exclusion criterion.

4.2. Menstrual Pain and Severity

In addition to the lack of available data about the perception of physical pain in women with PD, we also found differences in the classification of dysmenorrhea based on the severity of their pain or symptoms, creating a very heterogeneous group in relation to the classification model and clinical criteria. In the case of our sample, the classification was made only using the VAS, considering women with PD who scored 3/10 on the VAS, as described by Huang et al. [23] and Gaubeca et al. [22].

The most subjective data on pain (i.e., the sensory, affective, and evaluative sphere), which we collected through the McGill Pain Questionnaire, revealed higher scores in the groups of women with PD; among this group, the highest scores were higher in the subgroup of women with PD who were not receiving contraceptive treatment. We classified the participants based on these data because, although the McGill Pain Questionnaire has been used in other studies on menstrual pain, it has not to date been used to make a classification based on severity.

4.3. Quality of Life

The results of our study indicate that women with PD and who are not receiving contraceptive treatment suffer from decreased quality of life during the menstrual period, especially with regard to physical function. This finding is in line with those of studies about the effects of menstruation [6,94,95].

4.4. Pain Mechanosensitivity

The main hypothesis of our study was that women with PD would have greater mechanosensitivity than women without PD; however, we did not find significant differences in terms of the decrease in PPT between women with and without dysmenorrhea, except in the measurement made in the right arm, in the luteal phase, between the groups that were under contraceptive treatment with and without PD; and in the left thigh, in the mid-cycle assessment, between the group of women without PD and who were under contraceptive treatment, compared with the two groups that did have PD, both with and without contraceptive treatment. The results differ from those presented in the study by Bajaj et al., who found differences in pressure between dysmenorrheic women and those who were not, even though we used the same anatomical references for our assessment [96]. Unlike our case, in their study, a prior assessment was carried out on all of the participants so that they knew how to indicate the moment of pressure pain. Such training was not carried out in our study, which may have influenced the sensations of perception of the patients. According to Vatine et al., PPT results can be influenced by mood, personality, the interpretation by participants of the instructions, familiarity with the technique, and differences in somatic sensitivity to pain [97]; these may have led to differences between our results and those of Bajaj et al., In addition, their sample comprised nursing and physiotherapy students exclusively, unlike our more heterogeneous sample, and their sample had a higher average age. This mean age of the study patients in the case of Bajaj et al., was 25.5 and 28 years for women with and without PD, respectively [96]. A higher age was found in our study, reaching a mean of 30.71 years for the group of women with PD and 35.47 years for the group of women without PD, who were not under contraceptive treatment. In the study by Bajaj et al., other types of measurements were made at the same points as the PPT, on sensitivity to heat, pressure in a pincer, and tactile stimulation. The assessment of algometry was continuous with that of a pincer in a subcutaneous fold of the same area [96], which could have increased the perception of pain compared with our study. Furthermore, women receiving contraceptive treatment were excluded from their study, but included in ours.

However, our results that coincide with those of Bajaj et al., are from the comparison between the different phases of the menstrual cycle, with the PPT being lower at the menstrual time-point vs. other time-points [96]; however, this was only found in the group of women with PD. In contrast, we found this result within all groups.

By comparison, Amodei and Nelson found no significant differences in pain thresholds and tolerance levels of dysmenorrheic and non-dysmenorrheic women at different phases of the menstrual cycle. They suggest that, although dysmenorrheic women report pain and distress throughout the menstrual and premenstrual phases of their cycles, these symptoms are more intense than those without, and there is no significant difference in their demonstrated ability to tolerate or cope with physical pain [98]. However, Tassorelli et al., suggested, based on their results, that women tended to have a greater susceptibility to the perception of pain symptoms during the luteal phase than during the follicular phase, which is probably the result of complex central and peripheral interactions between specific neurotransmitters, such as serotonin, opiates, and ovarian steroids [99].

We must also highlight that, although in our study three measurements were made on each of the assessment points, which were muscular structures, the measurement areas with algometry have generated discussion. This is because it is considered that the sensitivity to pressure measured with algometry varies according to the muscle and its location. Differences are also shown between the measurement of bone, neural, and muscular structures, with the PPT being less and more unpleasant and painful at the neural and bone level, respectively [100,101]. In addition, a wide diversity in terms of algometry and the number of measurements to establish the PPT can be found, from authors contending that a first measurement can sensitize the measurement point [97,102], to others who affirm that what exists is an accommodation in the successive measurements [103]. Yet others consider that the most accurate measurement is the average between the second and the third measurement [104,105].

One of the striking findings of our study is that in the algometry performed in the lumbar area, no statistically significant differences emerged, either between groups or between groups, despite being one of the main regions described as a zone of referred pain of lower-back menstrual pain. This could be justified by the results of the study by As-Sanie et al., in which the PPT was assessed in women with CPP and endometriosis with and without menstrual pain. They found differences in the perception of pain compared to that of healthy women, but reported a greater sensitivity to pain in locations far from the pelvic area, with the idea that amplification of central pain may play a role in the development of CPP [106].

Moreover, in patients with CPP, Fenton et al., assessed myofascial pain in the abdominal wall using algometry, applying pressure to 14 different points on the abdominal wall and making a second measurement on the same points after infiltrating the MTrPs with a 10 mL solution of 0.5% bupivacaine; they found an improvement of 75% in the PPT after the intervention [107]. However, the study did not have a control group; thus, it can be understood that, since there were so many infiltrated points, and since it involved the infiltration of a local anesthetic, the effects could be similar in the population without CPP.

In the rest of the comparisons regarding the perception of pain between women with and without menstrual pain, we found different ways of measuring and disparate results. Giamberardino et al., compared women with and without dysmenorrhea in different phases of the menstrual cycle; however, we must bear in mind that, in this case, they did so through electrical stimulation of the skin, subcutaneous tissue, and muscle. The measurement zones were also similar to ours, since they were made in the abdomen, deltoids, and quadriceps. The results indicate greater sensitivity in dysmenorrheic women and, in the menstrual phase, in electrical stimulation at the dermal, subcutaneous, and muscular levels in the abdomen and extremities. However, changes were also found in women without dysmenorrhea, in this case only at the muscular and abdominal subcutaneous levels [108]; this showed greater coincidence with our results, since the measurement was in muscular structures. In the study by Granot et al., women with dysmenorrhea had a greater perception of pain compared to women without dysmenorrhea, where the perception of pain was measured through evoked potentials [109].

Costantin et al., also measured pain thresholds via electrical stimulation and performed MTrP treatment at the lumbar level by local anesthetic infiltration. The results of the study show that, in patients with dysmenorrhea plus previous urinary calculosis with residual lumbar MTrPs, whose compression reproduces the typical pattern of urinary pain, viscerovisceral hyperalgesia persists despite not showing new calculosis. In fact, patients continue to experience more menstrual pain/muscle hyperalgesia referred from the uterus than patients with dysmenorrhea alone. Inactivation of lumbar MTrPs through local anesthetic injection results in a significant improvement in menstrual pain and referred muscle hyperalgesia of the uterus, in contrast to no improvement in the same parameters when there was no MTrP treatment [110]. This viscerovisceral hyperalgesia could explain the significant differences obtained in our study in the intragroup PPT measurements between the different phases of the menstrual cycle, since hyperalgesia or changes at the uterine level could affect the perception of pain and variations in mechanosensitivity [110].

Therefore, more in-depth future analysis is warranted, since there are other studies in which measurements have been made to assess sensitivity to pain in other musculoskeletal disorders, but taking into account the menstrual cycle. This was undertaken in the study by Isselee et al., in temporomandibular disorders, where it was observed that the PPTs are lower in the perimenstrual phase, and that they increase significantly and progressively in the follicular and luteal phases [111]. Therefore, these hormonal variations may be important when interpreting the results.

By comparison, the use of exogenous hormones can attenuate the effects of the cycle on experimental pain [112]. Therefore, studies such as ours that include a treatment group receiving contraceptive treatment should report on the type and dosage of that contraceptive [112]. However, a study by Isselee et al., showed that the PPTs of all the muscles evaluated were significantly lower in the perimenstrual phases in women both without contraceptive treatment and those taking COCs [102].

Payne et al., found increased pain sensitivity in adolescent girls and young adult women with PD at all phases of the menstrual cycle, consistent with evidence of central sensitization. However, measures of excitatory and inhibitory pain processing revealed no difference between groups [113]. The presence of generalized sensitivity to pressure pain is considered a manifestation of central sensitization, assuming the assessment areas distant from the area of clinical manifestation are asymptomatic and normal.

Therefore, further studies are required to determine whether women with dysmenorrhea are more susceptible to pain in general and, therefore, more likely to perceive dysmenorrhea; whether dysmenorrhea leads to a general lowering of the pain threshold, so that women who suffer from it are secondarily more susceptible to pain; or whether dysmenorrhea affects all women, because it varies depending on the menstrual cycle and its hormonal variations in the different phases of the cycle.

4.5. Myofascial Trigger Points in Primary Dysmenorrhea

This study found that local and referred pain caused by active MTrPs of the explored musculature of the abdomen, lower back, lower limb, and PF reproduced pain symptoms not only in PD patients, but also caused sensations similar to those felt during menstruation in women who did not have PD.

Despite the lack of previous research assessing the prevalence or relationship of MTrPs with PD, there are studies assessing this relationship with MTrPs of the abdominal muscles, finding that treatment by infiltration with lidocaine or dry needling provides benefits to these women [22–24]. One study included dry needling treatment of the hip muscles and manual therapy for the PF muscles [24]. The present study is the first to identify a direct relationship between MTrPs of the PF musculature in this patient profile.

Although the presence of MTrPs with PD has been little studied, we did find studies of the relationship of abdominal and pelvic MTrPs in women with CPP and with biopsy-confirmed endometriosis, which is relatively common. These studies also indicated that women with MTrPs were more likely to present signs of central sensitization [114].

MTrPs can become a self-sustaining source of pain, even after the visceral injury has resolved [115]. Active MTrPs, in particular, serve as a source of ongoing nociception, and can lower pain thresholds and increase visceral pain, referred pain, and central sensitization [35]. Aredo et al., suggest that, in the case of dysmenorrhea secondary to endometriosis, MTrPs that develop secondarily to the disease can maintain pain and dysfunction despite removal of the endometrial lesion and hormonal management [42]. Some studies promote the effectiveness of these techniques in the treatment of myofascial pelvic pain, such as Pastore et al. [116] and Bedaiwy et al., whose study showed a high prevalence of myofascial pain related to CPP. In their study, improvements were achieved in up to 63% of patients with CPP via physiotherapy treatment of the PF muscles. Improvements have been reported in terms of pain, and in terms of functionality [117], as shown by Espinosa et al., with its treatment in the PD [24].

Our study found a high presence of MTrPs in the abdominal muscles during menstruation, with higher prevalence of active MTrPs in the case of women with dysmenorrhea, and a higher prevalence of latent MTrPs in the case of women without PD for the rectus abdominis muscle, or oblique musculature, in all women. These MTrPs decrease during the periovulatory or intermenstrual phase, with the presence of latent MTrPs becoming greater than that of active MTrPs in the case of women with PD. This relationship with the abdominal muscles is not only present in PD, but also in other pathologies such as CPP, interstitial cystitis, or chronic prostatitis [45,49,50,56]. Montenegro et al., described that, in 15% of cases, CPP is associated with abdominal MPS, which is characterized by deep, intense pain in the abdominal region and generally affects women more than men [44]. In addition, the treatment of MTrPs in the abdominal wall was found to be effective in patients with CPP, although treatment by direct injection with lidocaine provided a clinically superior response to physical therapy in the long term [118].

The highest prevalence in our study of MTrPs related to PD was found in the muscles assessed by intrapelvic examination; a high frequency was found not only in the levator ani muscle, but also in the internal obturator and piriformis muscles. Although present in all exploration groups during menstruation, the rate of active MTrPs was higher in the PD groups, while the rate of latent MTrPs was higher in the non-PD groups. In the periovulatory or intermenstrual assessment, a similar pattern was found as that in the abdominal muscles. The absolute frequency of MTrPs was lower, and the number of active MTrPs was also higher, in proportion, than that of the latent MTrPs. These results align with those of Sedighimehr et al., who found that patients with CPP exhibited more tenderness in the levator ani, piriformis, and internal obturator muscles. They also indicated that more than 70% of the women in their study had dysmenorrhea [119]. Bassaly et al., also found a significant presence of MTrPs in the levator and obturator internus in women with interstitial cystitis, with a higher number of MTrPs in women who had endometriosis. Howard also found that the obturator internus and levator ani are the muscles that most frequently harbor MTrPs, in addition to the coccygeus and external anal sphincter muscles [120]. The data on these last two muscles do not coincide with those of our study. The study of Anderson et al., shows that, despite describing the presence of MTrPs in the coccygeus and anal sphincter muscles in patients with chronic prostatitis, the prevalence rates are much lower than those of the levator ani muscle [45]. In general, more studies support the relationship between PF muscle dysfunction and CPP patients [121–123], in addition to the efficacy of treatment directed at these structures, which provides benefits, relieving pain in patients with CPP after infiltration of lidocaine in the levator ani muscle; for example, the study of Langford et al. [60].

There is a greater number of latent MTrPs during menstruation in muscles that usually have MTrPs within the groups with menstrual pain compared to the groups without pain. This coincides with other studies of myofascial pain in other regions of the body, such as the lateral epicondylalgia [124], plantar fasciitis [125], or chronic lower-back pain [126]. However, we also found opposite data, in which the presence of latent MTrPs is similar in the pain groups compared to the control groups, as is the case of post-menisectomy pain [37] or mechanical neck pain [127]. These results are more consistent with those we found in the comparison between groups in the periovulatory or intermenstrual phase. These discrepancies could be due to the specific areas or muscles explored; in our case, they could be related to hormone levels and visceral referred pain, a hypothesis that we cannot confirm with current data.

Despite the clinical importance described by Shah et al., of active vs. latent MTrPs [128,129], the clinical relevance of latent MTrPs has increased in recent years [130,131], as both alter normal patterns of motor recruitment and movement efficiency, and induce mechanisms of peripheral and central sensitization [36,132,133]. Similar data were obtained by Sedighimehr et al., who found a significant reduction in mean PF muscle strength and endurance in women with CPP compared to those without [119]. This finding led us to consider the possible relevance of these latent MTrPs during the periovulatory or intermenstrual period as precursors of active MTrPs during the menstrual phase. In this way, the importance and additional contribution of MTrPs to the development and perpetuation of PD as a CPP entity could be explained in association with their involvement in peripheral and central sensitization, in addition to their possible bidirectional relationship with central sensitization. Its deactivation could be a relevant aspect to reverse central sensitization and improve associated pain.

In our study, as in the studies described above that found efficacy for PD through the treatment of MTrPs [22–24], the diagnostic criteria for MTrPs used were those established by the expert consensus of the Delphi panel in 2018, which are the presence of a taut band, a tender point, and referred pain [33]. However, other studies, such as the study by Itza et al., which explored the relationship of the CPP with the MTrPs of the PF, showed that gyro-amplitude electromyography is a reliable diagnostic test for detecting MPS of the PF musculature. They estimated the sensitivity (83%), specificity (100%), and positive (95% CI 1.00–1.00) and negative (95% CI 0.77–0.93) predictive values of the test; these findings are important because they support a diagnosis of PF MPS, although they offer insufficient predictive power to constitute it as a diagnostic test in patients with CPP [134]. In this regard, however, Hubbard and Berkoff described a non-specific electrodiagnostic version of MPS, describing electrical activity as a characteristic common to all MTrPs, in which the potentials were characterized by a high-frequency peak [135]. Previously, Simons et al., described low-amplitude motor endplate noise associated with the presence of MTrPs, considering it spontaneous electrical activity [136]. Furthermore, Partanen et al., described that taut bands may be local contraction points in skeletal motor units, which could be caused by a sustained reflex drive in muscle spindles. On electromyography, this can be seen as complex repetitive discharges; therefore, we can deduce that MTrPs are related to increased excitability of muscle spindles [137]. We can only mention this as a future line of research that will help in the earlier detection of the presence of MPS in PF musculature, since there is little evidence available on its presence and the pathology of chronic pelvic pain, including PD.

4.6. Referred Pain Areas

As mentioned above, the presence of MTrPs with PD has been little studied. Less valued, however, is the relationship between the areas of referred pain of MTrPs and menstrual pain, despite the fact that the areas usually described as experiencing menstrual pain are within the referred pain maps of muscles such as the rectus abdominis, external oblique, gluteus, adductor magnus, piriformis, obturator internus, and PF musculature. In this sense, this study is the first to find a relationship between the presence of MTrPs—and their areas of referred pain—with the pain suffered by women with PD. Our study also reproduced the characteristic clinical picture of this pelvic alteration.

The results obtained in our study allow expansion of the referred pain reference maps of the MTrPs of the studied musculature reproduced both at the menstrual moment and in the periovulatory or intermenstrual phase. We found that, although the representation is greater in the women with PD, there was also a similar reality in women without dysmenorrhea. We found that the gluteal musculature extends its referred pain pattern to the abdominal area and anterior pelvic structures such as the pubis, groin, and vulva. In the case of the quadratus lumborum and the abdominal muscles, we found that the abdominal surface in which the referred pain is caused increases with respect to the areas already described by Travell and Simons. The most striking and relevant data that we obtained are the areas of referred pain of the PF muscles and the piriformis and internal obturator muscles. In addition to relating the presence of MTrPs in these muscles within highly restricted areas at the level of the gluteus, sacrum, and coccyx, we can also include as areas of referred pain the abdominal area (mainly suprapubic area and flank); lumbar area; anterior, internal, and posterior parts of the thigh; groin; and genitourinary and vulvar areas. Within the available literature, in the case of the PF muscles, few studies have suggested patterns of referred pain that differed from those described by Travell and Simons [27,39], but not related to PD. In the study by Bassaly et al., an examination of the rectus abdominis, levator ani, and obturator internus muscles was performed in patients with interstitial cystitis. They found that the areas of pain or discomfort caused by MTrPs are projected towards the suprapubic, lumbar, anal, and vulvar regions. These results highlight that a closer relationship was detected with the symptomatology of the study; the MTrPs of the left side of the women were explored, although the relationship was found to be not significant [50]. The study by Anderson et al., had the same objective as ours, regarding the definition of areas of referred pain, but in men with chronic prostatitis [45]. The results coincide with our results and those found by Bassaly et al., highlighting the suprapubic and genital area, with the most prevalent rate of MTrPs being in the levator ani [45,50].

Although this type of exploration was not included in our study, we must consider that visceral structures can also cause referred pain, and their characteristic areas have also not been widely studied. In this regard, Arendt-Nielsen et al., found that women with dysmenorrhea had larger areas of referred pain compared to controls. Pain threshold at first stimulus was significantly higher in patients than that of controls, but significantly decreased when the cervix was repeatedly distended. For prolonged cervical distention, pain ratings increased significantly in women with dysmenorrhea but decreased in control women. This may mean that sensitization to pain by temporary summation (i.e., increased pain during prolonged stimulation) and the facilitation of areas of referred pain can be considered as indicators of changes in the central nervous system in women with dysmenorrhea. Referred pain caused by this cervical distention harbored the usual areas of menstrual pain: the lumbar region, abdominal region, pelvic region, and thighs [138].

4.7. Hormonal Influence of the Menstrual Cycle on the Perception of Pain

There is much controversy in the literature about whether the timing of the menstrual cycle has an effect on pain perception in women. A review by Iacovides et al., reported that most well-controlled studies found that the phase of the menstrual cycle had no effect on pain perception in healthy, pain-free women. However, these results may be surprising considering the fluctuations in reproductive hormones throughout the cycle, and considering that animal studies have shown that progesterone and estradiol influence the response to pain. Some imaging studies show that there are, indeed, differences in patterns of brain activation in regions involved in cognitive modulation of pain in association with hormonal changes in the menstrual cycle, even when behavioral responses to pain have not changed [139]. When other pain conditions are considered, as in the study by LeResche et al., examining temporomandibular disorders, the results obtained suggest that temporomandibular pain in women is higher when estrogen levels are low, although the rapid variation in these levels may also be associated with increased pain [140].

The assessments in our study were made based on the menstrual calendar during menstruation, the periovulatory or intermenstrual phase, and the luteal phase. As with other studies, we assessed differences in hormone levels across these phases [98,108]. However, Sherman et al., suggest that the main limitation of much previous research on the menstrual cycle is that the underlying objective has been to detect relationships between pain and hormones, in the absence of a direct measurement of hormone levels, since the phases of the menstrual cycle have been taken as a reference. Regarding the menstrual cycle, there is significant heterogeneity between the studies when considering the phase and its recognition in the population of women assessed, regardless of the variability in both the length of the menstrual cycle and ovulation, and considering that approximately 20% of cycles may be anovulatory [112].

Bartley et al., assessed differences in perception of mechanical, electrical, and ischemic pain by measuring the tolerance and pain threshold in healthy women in the middle follicular and late luteal phases. They established minimal variations in pain sensitivity and spinal nociceptive processing between the phases, which would imply that the hormonal variation between these two phases has a minimal effect on the response to pain [141].

However, the latest recommendations on the considerations of the menstrual cycle were determined by the type of study and its variables, considering that in cross-sectional studies, the menstrual cycle is not the main variable of interest, although its potential effects should be controlled for the main variables. As is the case in our study, it would not be necessary to make such an exhaustive hormonal registry. The selection of the phase could be adjusted according to the menstrual calendar, regarding women with regular menstrual cycles [142].

MacLean and Hayashi explain that menstrual cycles, which are regulated by complex hormonal mechanisms, repeat and alter the local endometrial environment. Thus, the local hormonal environment cannot be precisely defined in each cycle. They note that some gynecological disorders may be due to disrupted hormone production, progesterone resistance, altered hormone-dependent gene expression, common somatic genetic mutations, and/or side effects of hormonal treatments, and many of these patients suffer from CPP and/or dysmenorrhea, which reduces the quality of life [143].

Pelvic pain is recognized as being driven by hormones, for example, endometriosis; thus, the role of these substances should be considered. In addition, there is considerable overlap between conditions that can cause chronic pelvic pain (endometriosis, interstitial cystitis, and irritable bowel syndrome), making it difficult to definitively assign causality to any one of them [144].

The study by Rezaii et al., showed more effective pain modulation in the ovulatory phase of the menstrual cycle, when estradiol levels are higher and progesterone levels are lower, than in the early follicular phase, when levels of both hormones are low, as measured by pressure tolerance to pain in healthy women. In conclusion, the results of this study showed more effective pain modulation in the ovulatory phase of the menstrual cycle, when estradiol levels are high and progesterone levels are low, than in the early follicular phase, when estradiol and progesterone levels are low [145].

One must ask whether the absolute level or the variation in hormonal levels is more important, and we must consider that most of the studies recorded estrogens levels rather than progestogen levels [144]. According to Christin-Maitre, in the available studies on the menstrual cycle, menstruation, and dysmenorrhea, ample reference can be found to menstruation as a psychosocial phenomenon strongly affected by historical evolution and cultural factors. In many women it is considered an unknown process until the moment of their "suffering"; thus, it can be strongly influenced by the environment, and by external factors such as stress, intense physical activity, and weight extremes, which can alter normal hypothalamic secretion of GnRH [146].

It is tempting to assume that finding an association between an outcome and a particular phase of the cycle implies that concurrent hormonal events drive symptom change. However, at least with respect to premenstrual pain syndrome, studies suggest delayed effects of hormonal change, such that the onset of symptoms occurs at a different phase than the hormonal event [142].

For all these reasons, the phases or moments of measurement should be standardized. Alternatively, hormone tests and more frequent assessments can be conducted to establish a more direct relationship between the different variables with respect to hormone levels. The importance of understanding the hormonal flow and how it affects human physiological and psychosocial factors should be recognized.

4.8. Peripheral and Central Sensitization, and Their Relationship with Menstruation and Primary Dysmenorrhea

One of our study's objectives was to detect a generalized sensitivity of pain to pressure in women with PD. Therefore, we considered it a manifestation of the central sensitization that these women could experience compared with women without menstrual pain. However, the data we obtained on PPT between the different phases of the menstrual cycle led us to consider that there may not be an alteration in sensitivity exclusive to PD but, rather, generalized by the menstrual cycle. According to Greenwald and Shafritz, the lowest PPT found in symptomatic areas, such as the abdomen in our study, would represent primary hyperalgesia due to sensitized polymodal nociceptors within the injured musculoskeletal structures related to peripheral sensitization. In addition, the lower PPT in the extremities in our study implies the presence of secondary hyperalgesia, with generalized hyperexcitability of the central nociceptive pathways related to central sensitization [147].

We must also consider the role of MTrPs in peripheral and central sensitization, and consider the high number of both active and latent MTrPs in some muscles in our research, since their presence may contribute to exacerbating and perpetuating pain in women with PD. In line with our results, Wang et al., concluded that MTrPs were associated with an early manifestation of local and generalized mechanical hyperalgesia that contributes to peripheral and central sensitization, which favors the spatial spread of mechanical pain [148]. Furthermore, MTrPs can be the generators of nociceptive impulses that lead to the process of generalized hyperalgesia and central sensitization [133,149].

Central sensitization, including lower PPT and extension of pain areas, may contribute to increased MTrPs [35], in the same way that active MTrPs may contribute to the spatial spread of pain and/or generalized pain in conditions of musculoskeletal pain [150]. In addition, this hyperalgesia can favor the presence of more active MTrPs in the same muscle [151] or in several functionally related muscles in situations of chronic musculoskeletal pain [118].

The sustained nociceptive stimuli that can cause hyperirritability of the MTrPs of a muscle can cause the secretion of sensitizing substances such as PGs, among others, which lower the activation threshold of the neuron such that they sensitize nociceptors [36,152]. These are PGs, which are also considered the main cause of the etiopathogenesis of menstrual pain [5,9–12,80].

We can also see differences between genders in terms of pain perception; more specifically, we found that a greater sensitivity to pain and risk of clinical pain was more common in women. In addition, although the specific etiology underlying these sex differences is unknown, it is highly likely that multiple biological and psychosocial processes are contributing factors [153]. Pieretti et al., highlight the importance of the interaction of the opioidergic system with sex hormones [154].

There are two aspects of central sensitization that are especially relevant for women with CPP: viscerosomatic convergence and viscerosomatic reflex [42]. Almost all spinal neurons that receive visceral input also receive somatosensory input from muscle and skin through a process known as viscerosomatic convergence [155]. Input convergence makes precise localization and discrimination of sensory information difficult [156]. This is also the basis of referred pain and explains why visceral pathologies are commonly felt as pain in somatic structures—particularly muscles—innervated by the same spinal segment; in addition, since visceral afferent fibers terminate in several spinal segments above and below the entry level of the segment, referred pain may be present in areas remote from the affected visceral organ [42,155]. Therefore, this viscerosomatic convergence would explain how noxious visceral input can sensitize multiple areas of the spinal cord, generating the broad areas of allodynia, hyperalgesia, and referred pain seen with somatic dysfunction [42].

The data provided by Sánchez et al., recently demonstrated that somatovisceral reflexes involving the bladder, urethra, and musculature of PF are sensitive to ovarian hormones, and estrogens play an essential role in these reflexes. Their findings support the notion that alterations in the activity of the pubococcygeus muscle during urination are sensitive to estrogens. This highlights the need to establish a more direct relationship between muscle assessment and hormone levels, which will depend on the moment of the menstrual cycle in which it occurs [157]. Prendergast and Weiss suggest that chronic pain caused by viscerovisceral and somatovisceral reflexes could be an indirect mechanism involved in interstitial cystitis that is accompanied by painful spasms of the PF musculature [158].

Viscerosomatic convergence may not only provide the means for pain referral to somatic structures, but also govern the reflex that induces muscle spasm and eventual MTrP formation. In turn, the MTrPs can serve as an additional source of nociceptive information and become a key component of the CPP. Therefore, its inhibition could reverse central sensitization and improve the pain associated with endometriosis [42].

Visceroviscera hyperalgesia between the uterus and urinary tract may persist after stone passage due to nociceptive inputs of MTrPs into the referred urinary area, since MTrP treatment effectively reverses intensified menstrual symptoms [110].

Central sensitization and myofascial pain secondary to active MTrPs are likely other sources of pain initiation, amplification, and perpetuation. Either could easily spread pain-related symptoms in women, even after surgical and medical/hormonal treatment for endometriosis has been optimized. Unfortunately, both central sensitization and myofascial dysfunction are frequently overlooked in the evaluation, diagnosis, and treatment of CPP associated with endometriosis [42].

Tu et al., noted that excessive excitatory input during menstrual pain can induce a compensatory inhibitory mechanism in several somatic sensorimotor regions [159]. In addition, like Vincent et al., they considered that constant and repeated stimulation of nociceptive pathways, as in the case of menstrual pain, can give rise to functional and structural alterations of the CNS, thereby giving rise to central sensitization [159,160]. In the same regard, Iacovides et al., concluded that limiting cyclical noxious input to the central nervous system in women with severe dysmenorrhea via analgesic treatment could reduce the chances of developing hyperalgesia and possibly other chronic pain conditions, as dysmenorrhea predisposes women to diffuse muscle hyperalgesia and clinically relevant deep muscle pain [161].

It is important to consider CPP associated with dysmenorrhea secondary to endometriosis from a global pain-focused perspective, as MTrPs and central sensitization appear to contribute significantly to clinical manifestations. Although the direct innervation of endometrial lesions may set the stage for visceral nociception and peripheral sensitization, over time central sensitization creates a process for pain maintenance that is independent of the initial pathology and is potentially reversible [115].

Oladosu et al., demonstrated the association of menstrual pain with abnormal autonomic activity and bladder sensitivity, even 2 weeks after menstruation. Both dysmenorrheic and bladder pain syndrome participants reported increased sensitivity to bladder pain compared to controls, with frequent comorbidity [162].

4.9. Future Lines of Research

Due to the large amount of data collected in this study and the controversial results found in existing studies, more research is required to clarify whether the relationship between MPS and PD is clinically relevant. If so, it may offer new therapeutic approaches for women with PD whose quality of life is affected monthly, and who resign themselves to the use of pharmacological treatments on a regular basis.

Our study is observational in nature and relied on a convenience sample. As such, clinical trials with randomized procedures are encouraged, as they may provide additional important data about women with PD.

Furthermore, although there is a high correlation between the summary measures of physical health and mental health between the SF-12 and the SF-36 data, it would have been convenient to use the SF-36 to avoid a loss of precision in the scores given our small sample size.

Our participants were also not classified based on the severity of their dysmenorrhea, which could have helped us determine the relevance of the study variables according to their degree of severity. Moreover, classifications did not consider the type of contraceptive treatment used.

Despite complying with the recommendations on the choice of menstrual phases (according to the menstrual calendar), using hormonal controls through urine or saliva tests could have allowed us to establish a more direct relationship between our results and hormonal levels.

In addition, exploration by palpation of some study muscles may not be completely reliable because the muscles we studied are found in deeper planes, which may undermine the accuracy of our conclusions regarding the direct relationship indicated by the results, or relate these to more superficial muscle planes. Thus, as in the case of the subregions of the levator ani, it is difficult to ensure that the identified referred pain originated exclusively from that portion. Furthermore, despite our awareness of the fact that the most anterior and most posterior fibers do correspond to the so-called bundle, it would be convenient to encompass the referred pain patterns of the puborectalis, pubococcygeus, and iliococcygeus muscles into one pattern.

Finally, despite having made a very detailed and specific percentage record of referred pain areas, validated software used either at the time of recording the pain areas or during analysis would have allowed us to make a real representation of the pain maps instead of creating a graphical illustration based on the data.

5. Conclusions

We conclude that there are few differences in musculoskeletal mechanosensitivity between women with and without PD, except in the luteal phase in women with PD who are under contraceptive treatment compared to those who, while under contraceptive treatment, do not present PD, in dermatomes C7-C8; and in the ovulatory phase in women with PD compared to those who do not have PD, but who are under contraceptive treatment, in dermatomes L2-L3. Furthermore, we conclude that there are bilateral differences in musculoskeletal mechanosensitivity in dermatomes C7-C8, L2-L3, and T10-T12, but there are no differences in dermatomes S2-S4 between the different phases of the menstrual cycle. However, a lower PPT in the menstrual phase was found, which was more pronounced in some locations in women receiving contraceptive treatment.

A higher prevalence of active MTrPs was found in the rectus abdominis, gluteus maximus, ischiocavernosus, and pubococcygeus muscles during the menstrual phase. A higher prevalence of active MTrPs in the iliococcygeus muscle and latent MTrPs in the ischiocavernosus muscle was found in the menstrual, periovulatory, and intermenstrual phases in women with PD. We also highlight that, during the menstrual phase, active MTrPs in the iliococcygeus muscle are common, being present in more than 50% of women in all experimental groups, in more than 70% of women with PD, and in almost all women who were not under contraceptive treatment. The internal obturator muscle presented MTrPs, whether active or latent, during the menstrual phase in all of our participants.

The areas of referred pain in the studied muscles, especially in the PF muscles, were found to be greatly extended relative to previous conceptions, including abdominal areas and the lower extremities. At the time of menstruation, the inguinal area was referred to with the greatest significance by women with PD among the abdominal muscles and the levator ani muscle. Outside of menstruation, the areas in which the pain was significantly referred were the hypogastrium, the vulva and the rectum, and the anus, from the iliococcygeus, obturator internus, and puborectalis muscles, respectively.

Author Contributions: Conceptualization, A.S.-I., D.P.-M., C.C.-M., A.G.-M. and C.C.-L.; methodology, A.S.-I., D.P.-M., C.C.-M., A.G.-M. and C.C.-L.; formal analysis, A.S.-I. and C.C.-L.; investigation, A.S.-I., C.C.-M. and A.G.-M.; data curation, A.S.-I. and C.C.-L.; writing—original draft preparation, A.S.-I., D.P.-M. and C.C.-L.; writing—review and editing, A.S.-I., D.P.-M., C.C.-M., A.G.-M. and C.C.-L.; supervision, D.P.-M. and C.C.-L. All authors have read and agreed to the published version of the manuscript.

Funding: This research did not receive any specific grants from funding agencies in the public, commercial, or non-profit sectors.

Institutional Review Board Statement: This study was approved by the Research Ethics and Animal Experimentation Committee of the University of Alcalá (IEC Code: CEID/HU/2017/01).

Informed Consent Statement: All participants signed the informed consent form before participation in the present study.

Data Availability Statement: Raw data are available upon corresponding author request.

Conflicts of Interest: The authors of this study declare no conflict of interest.

References

1. Hurtado, B.G.; Chillón-Martínez, R.; Roldán, J.R.; Orta-Perez, M. Dismenorrea primaria y fisioterapia. *Fisioterapia* **2005**, *27*, 327–342. [CrossRef]
2. Durain, D. Primary Dysmenorrhea: Assessment and Management Update. *J. Midwifery Women's Health* **2004**, *49*, 520–528. [CrossRef] [PubMed]
3. Latthe, P.; Latthe, M.; Say, L.; Gülmezoglu, A.M.; Khan, K.S. WHO systematic review of prevalence of chronic pelvic pain: A neglected reproductive health morbidity. *BMC Public Health* **2006**, *6*, 177. [CrossRef]
4. Larroy, C.; Crespo, M.; Meseguer, C. Dismenorrea Funcional En La Comunidad Autónoma de Madrid: Estudio de La Prevalencia En Función de La Edad. *Rev. Soc. Esp. Dolor* **2001**, *8*, 11–22.
5. Abarca, L.; Molero, J.M.; Casimiro, C. Dismenorrea. Una revisión multidisciplinaria en el contexto de la medicina basada en la evidencia. *FMC* **2006**, *13*, 550–559. [CrossRef]
6. Chrisler, J.C.; Gorman, J.A. Menstruation. In *Encyclopedia of Mental Health*, 2nd ed.; Academic Press: Cambridge, MA, USA, 2016; pp. 75–81. [CrossRef]
7. Terranova, P. Dysmenorrhea. In *Reference Module in Biomedical Sciences*; Elsevier: Amsterdam, The Netherlands, 2018. [CrossRef]
8. Coco, A.S. Primary Dysmenorrhea. *Am. Fam. Physician* **1999**, *60*, 489.
9. Guimarães, I., Póvoa, A.M. Primary Dysmenorrhea: Assessment and Treatment Dismenorreia Primária: Avaliação e Trata mento. *Rev. Bras. Ginecol. Obstet.* **2020**, *42*, 501–507. [CrossRef]
10. Iacovides, S.; Avidon, I.; Baker, F.C. What we know about primary dysmenorrhea today: A critical review. *Hum. Reprod. Update* **2015**, *21*, 762–778. [CrossRef]
11. Pickles, V.R. Myometrial Responses to the Menstrual Plain Muscle Stimulant. *J. Endocrinol.* **1959**, *19*, 150–157. [CrossRef]
12. Pickles, V.R. A Plain-muscle Stimulant in the Menstruum. *Nature* **1957**, *180*, 1198–1199. [CrossRef]
13. Akman, A.O.; Bozdag, G.; Pehlivantürk-Kizilkan, M.; Akgul, S.; Derman, O.; Kanbur, N. Menstrual Cycle Pain Is Independent of Ovulation in Adolescents with Primary Dysmenorrhea. *J. Pediatr. Adolesc. Gynecol.* **2021**, *34*, 635–642. [CrossRef]
14. Deligeoroglou, E. Dysmenorrhea. *Ann. N. Y. Acad. Sci.* **2006**, *900*, 237–244. [CrossRef]
15. Alfonsín, M.G.; López-Roca, A.; Rodríguez-Pampín, M.; Novo-Domínguez, A. Fisiología femenina II: Ciclo uterino. Ciclo endometrial. Menstruación. Procesos reparativos cervicales. Ciclo endocervical. Ciclo y fisiología de la vagina. Y la vulva. EN: Bajo JM, compilador. In *Fundamentos de Obstetricia (SEGO)*; Grupo ENE Publicidad: Madrid, Spain, 2007; pp. 65–92.
16. Dawood, M.Y. Dysmenorrhoea and Prostaglandins: Pharmacological and Therapeutic Considerations. *Drugs* **1981**, *22*, 42–56. [CrossRef]
17. Sima, R.-M.; Sulea, M.; Radosa, J.C.; Findeklee, S.; Hamoud, B.H.; Popescu, M.; Gorecki, G.P.; Bobircă, A.; Bobirca, F.; Cirstoveanu, C.; et al. The Prevalence, Management and Impact of Dysmenorrhea on Medical Students' Lives—A Multicenter Study. *Healthcare* **2022**, *10*, 157. [CrossRef]
18. Andersch, B.; Milsom, I. An epidemiologic study of young women with dysmenorrhea. *Am. J. Obstet. Gynecol.* **1982**, *144*, 655–660. [CrossRef]
19. Karout, S.; Soubra, L.; Rahme, D.; Karout, L.; Khojah, H.M.J.; Itani, R. Prevalence, risk factors, and management practices of primary dysmenorrhea among young females. *BMC Women's Health* **2021**, *21*, 1–14. [CrossRef]
20. Burnett, M.; Lemyre, M. No. 345-Primary Dysmenorrhea Consensus Guideline. *J. Obstet. Gynaecol. Can.* **2017**, *39*, 585–595. [CrossRef]
21. López-Liria, R.; Torres-Álamo, L.; Vega-Ramírez, F.; García-Luengo, A.; Aguilar-Parra, J.; Trigueros-Ramos, R.; Rocamora-Pérez, P. Efficacy of Physiotherapy Treatment in Primary Dysmenorrhea: A Systematic Review and Meta-Analysis. *Int. J. Environ. Res. Public Health* **2021**, *18*, 7832. [CrossRef]
22. Gaubeca-Gilarranz, A.; Fernández-De-Las-Peñas, C.; Medina-Torres, J.R.; Seoane-Ruiz, J.M.; Company-Palonés, A.; A Cleland, J.; Arias-Buría, J.L. Effectiveness of Dry Needling of Rectus Abdominis Trigger Points for the Treatment of Primary Dysmenorrhoea: A Randomised Parallel-Group Trial. *Acupunct. Med. J. Br. Med. Acupunct. Soc.* **2018**, *36*, 302–310. [CrossRef]
23. Huang, Q.-M.; Liu, L. Wet Needling of Myofascial Trigger Points in Abdominal Muscles for Treatment of Primary Dysmenorrhoea. *Acupunct. Med.* **2014**, *32*, 346–349. [CrossRef]
24. Díaz, M.E.; Cabellos, C.F. Relationship between Dysmenorrhoea and Myofascial Pain Syndrome. A Physiotherapist Perspective. Pilot Randomized Trial. *Fisioterapia* **2020**, *43*, 5–11. [CrossRef]
25. Howard, F.M. Chronic Pelvic Pain in Women. *Am. J. Manag. Care* **2001**, *7*, 1001–1011. [PubMed]
26. Merskey, H.; Bogduk, N. *Classification of Chronic Pain, IASP Task Force on Taxonomy*; International Association for the Study of Pain Press: Seattle, WA, USA, 1994.
27. Simons, D.G.; Travell, J.G.; Simons, L.S. *Myofascial Pain and Dysfunction: The Trigger Point Manual. Volume 1 "Upper Half of Body"*, 2nd ed.; Lippincott Williams & Wilkins: Baltimore, PA, USA, 1999.
28. Cao, Q.-W.; Peng, B.-G.; Wang, L.; Huang, Y.-Q.; Jia, D.-L.; Jiang, H.; Lv, Y.; Liu, X.-G.; Liu, R.-G.; Li, Y.; et al. Expert consensus on the diagnosis and treatment of myofascial pain syndrome. *World J. Clin. Cases* **2021**, *9*, 2077–2089. [CrossRef] [PubMed]
29. Gerwin, R.D. Myofascial Trigger Point Pain Syndromes. *Semin. Neurol.* **2016**, *36*, 469–473. [CrossRef] [PubMed]
30. Giamberardino, M.A.; Tana, C.; Costantini, R. Pain thresholds in women with chronic pelvic pain. *Curr. Opin. Obstet. Gynecol.* **2014**, *26*, 253–259. [CrossRef]

31. Rathbone, A.T.; Grosman-Rimon, L.; Kumbhare, D. Interrater Agreement of Manual Palpation for Identification of Myofascial Trigger Points: A Systematic Review and Meta-Analysis. *Clin. J. Pain* **2017**, *33*, 715–729. [CrossRef]
32. Li, L.; Stoop, R.; Clijsen, R.; Hohenauer, E.; Fernández-De-Las-Peñas, C.; Huang, Q.; Barbero, M. Criteria Used for the Diagnosis of Myofascial Trigger Points in Clinical Trials on Physical Therapy: Updated Systematic Review. *Clin. J. Pain* **2020**, *36*, 955–967. [CrossRef]
33. Fernández-De-Las-Peñas, C.; Dommerholt, J. International Consensus on Diagnostic Criteria and Clinical Considerations of Myofascial Trigger Points: A Delphi Study. *Pain Med.* **2018**, *19*, 142–150. [CrossRef]
34. Saxena, A.; Chansoria, M.; Tomar, G.; Kumar, A. Myofascial Pain Syndrome: An Overview. *J. Pain Palliat. Care Pharmacother.* **2015**, *29*, 16–21. [CrossRef]
35. Gerwin, R.D. Diagnosis of Myofascial Pain Syndrome. *Phys. Med. Rehabil. Clin. N. Am.* **2014**, *25*, 341–355. [CrossRef]
36. Shah, J.P.; Thaker, N.; Heimur, J.; Aredo, J.V.; Sikdar, S.; Gerber, L. Myofascial Trigger Points Then and Now: A Historical and Scientific Perspective. *PM R* **2015**, *7*, 746–761. [CrossRef]
37. Torres-Chica, B.; Núñez-Samper-Pizarroso, C.; Ortega-Santiago, R.; Cleland, J.A.; Salom-Moreno, J.; Laguarta-Val, S.; Fernández-De-Las-Peñas, C. Trigger Points and Pressure Pain Hypersensitivity in People with Postmeniscectomy Pain. *Clin. J. Pain* **2015**, *31*, 265–272. [CrossRef]
38. Lucas, K.R.; Rich, P.A.; Polus, B.I. Muscle activation patterns in the scapular positioning muscles during loaded scapular plane elevation: The effects of Latent Myofascial Trigger Points. *Clin. Biomech.* **2010**, *25*, 765–770. [CrossRef]
39. Travell, J.; Simons, D. *Myofascial Pain and Dysfunction: The Trigger Point Manual*, 1st ed.; Lippincott Williams & Wilkins: Baltimore, PA, USA, 1999; Volume 2.
40. Maddux:Menstruation—Google Académico. Available online: https://scholar.google.com/scholar_lookup?title=Menstruation&author=H.C.Maddux&publication_year=1975 (accessed on 2 March 2022).
41. Abreu-Sánchez, A.; Ruiz-Castillo, J.; Onieva-Zafra, M.D.; Parra-Fernández, M.L.; Fernández-Martínez, E. Interference and Impact of Dysmenorrhea on the Life of Spanish Nursing Students. *Int. J. Environ. Res. Public Health* **2020**, *17*, 6473. [CrossRef]
42. Aredo, J.V.; Heyrana, K.J.; Karp, B.I.; Shah, J.P.; Stratton, P. Relating Chronic Pelvic Pain and Endometriosis to Signs of Sensitization and Myofascial Pain and Dysfunction. *Semin. Reprod. Med.* **2017**, *35*, 088–097. [CrossRef]
43. Itza, F.; Zarza, D.; Serra, L.; Gómez-Sancha, F.; Salinas, J.; Allona-Almagro, A. Myofascial pain syndrome in the pelvic floor: A common urological condition. *Actas Urológicas Españolas* **2010**, *34*, 318–326. [CrossRef]
44. Montenegro, M.L.; Gomide, L.B.; Mateus-Vasconcelos, E.L.; Rosa-E-Silva, J.C.; Candido-Dos-Reis, F.J.; Nogueira, A.A.; Poli-Neto, O.B. Abdominal myofascial pain syndrome must be considered in the differential diagnosis of chronic pelvic pain. *Eur. J. Obstet. Gynecol. Reprod. Biol.* **2009**, *147*, 21–24. [CrossRef]
45. Anderson, R.U.; Sawyer, T.; Wise, D.; Morey, A.; Nathanson, B.H. Painful Myofascial Trigger Points and Pain Sites in Men With Chronic Prostatitis/Chronic Pelvic Pain Syndrome. *J. Urol.* **2009**, *182*, 2753–2758. [CrossRef]
46. Jarrell, J.; Giamberardino, M.A.; Robert, M.; Nasr-Esfahani, M. Bedside Testing for Chronic Pelvic Pain: Discriminating Visceral from Somatic Pain. *Pain Res. Treat.* **2011**, *2011*, 692102. [CrossRef]
47. Oyama, I.A.; Rejba, A.; Lukban, J.C.; Fletcher, E.; Kellogg-Spadt, S.; Holzberg, A.S.; Whitmore, K.E. Modified Thiele massage as therapeutic intervention for female patients with interstitial cystitis and high-tone pelvic floor dysfunction. *Urology* **2004**, *64*, 862–865. [CrossRef]
48. Weiss, J.M. Pelvic Floor Myofascial Trigger Points: Manual Therapy for Interstitial Cystitis and the Urgency-Frequency Syndrome. *J. Urol.* **2001**, *166*, 2226–2231. [CrossRef] [PubMed]
49. Doggweiler-Wiygul, R.; Wiygul, P.J. Interstitial cystitis, pelvic pain, and the relationship to myofascial pain and dysfunction: A report on four patients. *World J. Urol.* **2002**, *20*, 310–314. [CrossRef] [PubMed]
50. Bassaly, R.; Tidwell, N.; Bertolino, S.; Hoyte, L.; Downes, K.; Hart, S. Myofascial pain and pelvic floor dysfunction in patients with interstitial cystitis. *Int. Urogynecology J.* **2010**, *22*, 413–418. [CrossRef] [PubMed]
51. Anderson, R.U.; Wise, D.; Sawyer, T.; Nathanson, B.H.; Smith, J.N. Equal Improvement in Men and Women in the Treatment of Urologic Chronic Pelvic Pain Syndrome Using a Multi-modal Protocol with an Internal Myofascial Trigger Point Wand. *Appl. Psychophysiol. Biofeedback* **2016**, *41*, 215–224. [CrossRef] [PubMed]
52. Fitzgerald, M.P.; Anderson, R.U.; Potts, J.; Payne, C.K.; Peters, K.M.; Clemens, J.Q.; Kotarinos, R.; Fraser, L.; Cosby, A.; Fortman, C.; et al. Randomized Multicenter Feasibility Trial of Myofascial Physical Therapy for the Treatment of Urological Chronic Pelvic Pain Syndromes. *J. Urol.* **2013**, *189*, S75–S85. [CrossRef]
53. Tadros, N.N.; Shah, A.B.; Shoskes, D.A. Utility of trigger point injection as an adjunct to physical therapy in men with chronic prostatitis/chronic pelvic pain syndrome. *Transl. Androl. Urol.* **2017**, *6*, 534–537. [CrossRef]
54. Anderson, R.U. Management of chronic prostatitis–chronic pelvic pain syndrome. *Urol. Clin. N. Am.* **2002**, *29*, 235–239. [CrossRef]
55. Anderson, R.U.; Wise, D.; Sawyer, T.; Chan, C. Integration of Myofascial Trigger Point Release and Paradoxical Relaxation Training Treatment of Chronic Pelvic Pain in Men. *J. Urol.* **2005**, *174*, 155–160. [CrossRef]
56. Anderson, R.U.; Wise, D.; Sawyer, T.; Chan, C.A. Sexual Dysfunction in Men with Chronic Prostatitis/Chronic Pelvic Pain Syndrome: Improvement After Trigger Point Release and Paradoxical Relaxation Training. *J. Urol.* **2006**, *176*, 1534–1539. [CrossRef]
57. Bharucha, A.E.; Lee, T.H. Anorectal and Pelvic Pain. *Mayo Clin. Proc.* **2016**, *91*, 1471–1486. [CrossRef]

58. Ashrafi, A.; Arab, A.M.; Abdi, S.; Nourbakhsh, M.R. The association between myofascial trigger points and the incidence of chronic functional constipation. *J. Bodyw. Mov. Ther.* **2020**, *26*, 201–206. [CrossRef]
59. Yacubovich, Y.; Cohen, N.; Tene, L.; Kalichman, L. The prevalence of primary dysmenorrhea among students and its association with musculoskeletal and myofascial pain. *J. Bodyw. Mov. Ther.* **2019**, *23*, 785–791. [CrossRef]
60. Langford, C.F.; Nagy, S.U.; Ghoniem, G. Levator ani trigger point injections: An underutilized treatment for chronic pelvic pain. *Neurourol. Urodyn.* **2007**, *26*, 59–62. [CrossRef]
61. Hong, C.-Z. Lidocaine Injection versus Dry Needling to Myofascial Trigger Point. The Importance of the Local Twitch Response. *Am. J. Phys. Med. Rehabil.* **1994**, *73*, 256–263. [CrossRef]
62. Venancio, R.D.A.; Alencar, F.G.P.; Zamperini, C. Botulinum Toxin, Lidocaine, and Dry-Needling Injections in Patients with Myofascial Pain and Headaches. *CRANIO®* **2009**, *27*, 46–53. [CrossRef]
63. Bhide, A.A.; Puccini, F.; Khullar, V.; Elneil, S.; Digesu, G.A. Botulinum neurotoxin type A injection of the pelvic floor muscle in pain due to spasticity: A review of the current literature. *Int. Urogynecology J.* **2013**, *24*, 1429–1434. [CrossRef]
64. Von Elm, E.; Altman, D.G.; Egger, M.; Pocock, S.J.; Gøtzsche, P.C.; Vandenbroucke, J.P. The Strengthening the Reporting of Observational Studies in Epidemiology (STROBE) Statement: Guidelines for Reporting Observational Studies. *Ann. Intern. Med.* **2007**, *147*, 573–577. [CrossRef]
65. Reed, B.G.; Carr, B.R. The Normal Menstrual Cycle and the Control of Ovulation. In *Endotext*; MDText.com, Inc.: South Dartmouth, MA, USA, 2018.
66. Macías, A.S.A.; de Miranda, M.L.A.; Díaz, A.Q. La Mujer, El Ciclo Menstrual y La Actividad Física The Woman, the Menstrual Cycle, and the Physical Activity. *Rev. Arch. Médico De Camagüey* **2017**, *21*, 294–307.
67. Úbeda-D'Ocasar, E.; Valera-Calero, J.; Hervás-Pérez, J.; Caballero-Corella, M.; Ojedo-Martín, C.; Gallego-Sendarrubias, G. Pain Intensity and Sensory Perception of Tender Points in Female Patients with Fibromyalgia: A Pilot Study. *Int. J. Environ. Res. Public Health* **2021**, *18*, 1461. [CrossRef]
68. American College of Obstetricians and Gynecologists. ACOG Committee Opinion No. 760: Dysmenorrhea and Endometriosis in the Adolescent. *Obstet. Gynecol.* **2018**, *132*, e249–e258. [CrossRef]
69. Gandek, B.; Ware, J.E.; Aaronson, N.K.; Apolone, G.; Bjorner, J.B.; Brazier, J.E.; Bullinger, M.; Kaasa, S.; Leplege, A.; Prieto, L.; et al. Cross-validation of item selection and scoring for the sf-12 health survey in nine countries: Results from the iqola project. International quality of life assessment. *J. Clin. Epidemiol.* **1998**, *51*, 1171–1178. [CrossRef]
70. Melzack, R. The McGill Pain Questionnaire: Major properties and scoring methods. *Pain* **1975**, *1*, 277–299. [CrossRef] [PubMed]
71. The Development of a Spanish Questionnaire for Assessing Pain: Preliminary Data Concerning Reliability and Validity—PsycNET. Available online: https://psycnet.apa.org/record/1995-11922-001 (accessed on 6 February 2022).
72. Masedo, A.I.; Esteve, R. Some empirical evidence regarding the validity of the Spanish Version of the McGill Pain Questionnaire (MPQ-SV). *Pain* **2000**, *85*, 451–456. [CrossRef]
73. Kahl, C.; Cleland, J.A. Visual analogue scale, numeric pain rating scale and the McGill pain Questionnaire: An overview of psychometric properties. *Phys. Ther. Rev.* **2005**, *10*, 123–128. [CrossRef]
74. Blanca, M.J.; Alarcón, R.; Arnau, J.; Bono, R.; Bendayan, R. Non-Normal Data: Is ANOVA still a Valid Option? *Psicothema* **2017**, *29*, 552–557. [CrossRef] [PubMed]
75. Haverkamp, N.; Beauducel, A. Violation of the Sphericity Assumption and Its Effect on Type-I Error Rates in Repeated Measures ANOVA and Multi-Level Linear Models (MLM). *Front. Psychol.* **2017**, *8*, 1841. [CrossRef]
76. Cohen, J. Eta-Squared and Partial Eta-Squared in Fixed Factor Anova Designs. *Educ. Psychol. Meas.* **1973**, *33*, 107–112. [CrossRef]
77. Kelley, K.; Preacher, K.J. On effect size. *Psychol. Methods* **2012**, *17*, 137–152. [CrossRef]
78. Hazra, A.; Gogtay, N. Biostatistics series module 4: Comparing groups—Categorical variables. *Indian J. Dermatol.* **2016**, *61*, 385–392. [CrossRef]
79. Maity, S.; Wray, J.; Coffin, T.; Nath, R.; Nauhria, S.; Sah, R.; Waechter, R.; Ramdass, P.; Nauhria, S. Academic and Social Impact of Menstrual Disturbances in Female Medical Students: A Systematic Review and Meta-Analysis. *Front. Med.* **2022**, *9*, 821908. [CrossRef]
80. Çinar, G.N.; Akbayrak, T.; Gürşen, C.; Baran, E.; Üzelpasacı, E.; Nakip, G.; Bozdağ, G.; Beksaç, M.S.; Özgül, S. Factors Related to Primary Dysmenorrhea in Turkish Women: A Multiple Multinomial Logistic Regression Analysis. *Reprod. Sci.* **2020**, *28*, 381–392. [CrossRef]
81. Latthe, P.; Mignini, L.; Gray, R.; Hills, R.; Khan, K. Factors predisposing women to chronic pelvic pain: Systematic review. *BMJ* **2006**, *332*, 749–755. [CrossRef]
82. Hu, Z.; Tang, L.; Chen, L.; Kaminga, A.C.; Xu, H. Prevalence and Risk Factors Associated with Primary Dysmenorrhea among Chinese Female University Students: A Cross-sectional Study. *J. Pediatr. Adolesc. Gynecol.* **2020**, *33*, 15–22. [CrossRef]
83. Gudipally, P.R.; Sharma, G.K. *Premenstrual Syndrome*; StatPearls Publishing: Treasure Island, FL, USA, 2022.
84. Bouchoucha, M.; Devroede, G.; Rompteaux, P.; Mary, F.; Bejou, B.; Benamouzig, R. Clinical, Physiological, and Psychological Correlates of the Improvement of Defecation during Menses in Women with Functional Gastrointestinal Disorders. *Visc. Med.* **2020**, *36*, 487–493. [CrossRef]
85. Armour, M.; Ee, C.C.; Naidoo, D.; Ayati, Z.; Chalmers, K.J.; A Steel, K.; de Manincor, M.; Delshad, E. Exercise for dysmenorrhoea. *Cochrane Database Syst. Rev.* **2019**, *2019*, CD004142. [CrossRef]
86. French, L. Dysmenorrhea. *Am. Fam. Physician* **2005**, *71*, 285–292. [CrossRef]

87. Dawood, M.Y. Ibuprofen and Dysmenorrhea. *Am. J. Med.* **1984**, *77*, 87–94. [CrossRef]
88. Lefebvre, G.; Pinsonneault, O.; Antao, V.; Black, A.; Burnett, M.; Feldman, K.; Lea, R.; Robert, M. Sogc Primary Dysmenorrhea Consensus Guideline. *J. Obstet. Gynaecol. Can.* **2005**, *27*, 1117–1130. [CrossRef]
89. Sachedina, A.; Todd, N. Dysmenorrhea, Endometriosis and Chronic Pelvic Pain in Adolescents. *J. Clin. Res. Pediatr. Endocrinol.* **2020**, *12*, 7–17. [CrossRef]
90. Wildemeersch, D.; Jandi, S.; Pett, A.; Hasskamp, T. Management of primary dysmenorrhea in young women with frameless LNG-IUS. *Open Access J. Contracept.* **2014**, *5*, 23–28. [CrossRef]
91. Lindh, I.; Milsom, I. The influence of intrauterine contraception on the prevalence and severity of dysmenorrhea: A longitudinal population study. *Hum. Reprod.* **2013**, *28*, 1953–1960. [CrossRef] [PubMed]
92. Fox, M.C.; Klipping, C.; Nguyen, A.M.; Frenkl, T.L.; Cruz, S.M.; Wang, Y.; Korver, T. A phase 2b multicenter, randomized, double-blind, placebo-controlled clinical trial to evaluate the efficacy and safety of vaginal rings containing nomegestrol acetate or etonogestrel and 17β-estradiol in the treatment of women with primary dysmenorrhea. *Contraception* **2019**, *99*, 125–130. [CrossRef] [PubMed]
93. Gupta, D.R.; Prabhakar, B.; Wairkar, S. Non-oral routes, novel formulations and devices of contraceptives: An update. *J. Control. Release* **2022**, *345*, 798–810. [CrossRef]
94. dos Santos, L.B.; Ferreira, C.W.S.; Gonçalves, C.G.; Xavier, M.A.D.O.; Dantas, J.H.; Barbosa, I.R.; da Câmara, S.M.A.; Dantas, D. Association among dysmenorrhea and activity limitation and participation restrictions in adult women: A cross-sectional study, Brazil-2017. *Arch. Public Health* **2021**, *79*, 1–7. [CrossRef] [PubMed]
95. Fraser, I.S.; Critchley, H.; Munro, M.; Broder, M. Can we achieve international agreement on terminologies and definitions used to describe abnormalities of menstrual bleeding? *Hum. Reprod.* **2007**, *22*, 635–643. [CrossRef]
96. Bajaj, P.; Bajaj, P.; Madsen, H.; Arendt-Nielsen, L. A Comparison of Modality-Specific Somatosensory Changes During Menstruation in Dysmenorrheic and Nondysmenorrheic Women. *Clin. J. Pain* **2002**, *18*, 180–190. [CrossRef]
97. Vatine, J.-J.; Shapira, S.C.; Magora, F.; Adler, D.; Magora, A. Electronic pressure algometry of deep pain in healthy volunteers. *Arch. Phys. Med. Rehabil.* **1993**, *74*, 526–530. [CrossRef]
98. Amodei, N.; Nelson-Gray, R.O. Reactions of dysmenorrheic and nondysmenorrheic women to experimentally induced pain throughout the menstrual cycle. *J. Behav. Med.* **1989**, *12*, 373–385. [CrossRef]
99. Tassorelli, C.; Sandrini, G.; Proietti Cecchini, A.; Nappi, R.E.; Sances, G.; Martignoni, E. Changes in Nociceptive Flexion Reflex Threshold Across the Menstrual Cycle in Healthy Women. *Psychosom. Med.* **2002**, *64*, 621–626. [CrossRef]
100. Fischer, A.A. Pressure algometry over normal muscles. Standard values, validity and reproducibility of pressure threshold. *Pain* **1987**, *30*, 115–126. [CrossRef]
101. Kosek, E.; Ekholm, J.; Hansson, P. Pressure Pain Thresholds in Different Tissues in One Body Region. The Influence of Skin Sensitivity in Pressure Algometry. *Scand. J. Rehabil. Med.* **1999**, *31*, 89–93. [CrossRef]
102. Isselée, H.; Laat, A.; Bogaerts, K.; Lysens, R. Long-term fluctuations of pressure pain thresholds in healthy men, normally menstruating women and oral contraceptive users. *Eur. J. Pain* **2001**, *5*, 27–37. [CrossRef]
103. Chesterton, L.S.; Sim, J.; Wright, C.C.; Foster, N.E. Interrater Reliability of Algometry in Measuring Pressure Pain Thresholds in Healthy Humans, Using Multiple Raters. *Clin. J. Pain* **2007**, *23*, 760–766. [CrossRef]
104. Isselée, H.; Laat, A.; Lesaffre, E.; Lysens, R. Short-term reproducibility of pressure pain thresholds in masseter and temporalis muscles of symptom-free subjects. *Eur. J. Oral Sci.* **1997**, *105*, 583–587. [CrossRef]
105. Nussbaum, E.L.; Downes, L. Reliability of Clinical Pressure-Pain Algometric Measurements Obtained on Consecutive Days. *Phys. Ther.* **1998**, *78*, 160–169. [CrossRef]
106. As-Sanie, S.; Harris, R.E.; Harte, S.E.; Tu, F.F.; Neshewat, G.; Clauw, D.J. Increased Pressure Pain Sensitivity in Women With Chronic Pelvic Pain. *Obstet. Gynecol.* **2013**, *122*, 1047–1055. [CrossRef]
107. Fenton, B.W.; Palmieri, P.A.; Durner, C.; Fanning, J. Quantification of Abdominal Wall Pain Using Pain Pressure Threshold Algometry in Patients with Chronic Pelvic Pain. *Clin. J. Pain* **2009**, *25*, 500–505. [CrossRef]
108. Giamberardino, M.A.; Berkley, K.J.; Iezzi, S.; de Bigontina, P.; Vecchiet, L. Pain threshold variations in somatic wall tissues as a function of menstrual cycle, segmental site and tissue depth in non-dysmenorrheic women, dysmenorrheic women and men. *Pain* **1997**, *71*, 187–197. [CrossRef]
109. Granot, M.; Yarnitsky, D.; Itskovitz-Eldor, J.; Granovsky, Y.; Peer, E.; Zimmer, E.Z. Pain perception in women with dysmenorrhea. *Obstet. Gynecol.* **2001**, *98*, 407–411. [CrossRef]
110. Costantini, R.; Affaitati, G.; Fiordaliso, M.; Giamberardino, M.A. Viscero-visceral hyperalgesia in dysmenorrhoea plus previous urinary calculosis: Role of myofascial trigger points and their injection treatment in the referred area. *Eur. J. Pain* **2020**, *24*, 933–944. [CrossRef]
111. Isselée, H.; de Laat, A.; de Mot, B.; Lysens, R. Pressure-pain threshold variation in temporomandibular disorder myalgia over the course of the menstrual cycle. *J. Orofac. Pain* **2002**, *16*, 105–117. [PubMed]
112. Sherman, J.J.; LeResche, L. Does experimental pain response vary across the menstrual cycle? A methodological review. *Am. J. Physiol. Regul. Integr. Comp. Physiol.* **2006**, *291*, R245–R256. [CrossRef] [PubMed]
113. Payne, L.A.; Seidman, L.C.; Sim, M.-S.; Rapkin, A.J.; Naliboff, B.D.; Zeltzer, L.K. Experimental evaluation of central pain processes in young women with primary dysmenorrhea. *Pain* **2019**, *160*, 1421–1430. [CrossRef] [PubMed]

114. Stratton, P.; Khachikyan, I.; Sinaii, N.; Ortiz, R.; Shah, J. Association of Chronic Pelvic Pain and Endometriosis With Signs of Sensitization and Myofascial Pain. *Obstet. Gynecol.* **2015**, *125*, 719–728. [CrossRef] [PubMed]
115. Woolf, C.J. Central sensitization: Implications for the diagnosis and treatment of pain. *Pain* **2011**, *152*, S2–S15. [CrossRef]
116. Pastore, E.A.; Katzman, W.B. Recognizing Myofascial Pelvic Pain in the Female Patient with Chronic Pelvic Pain. *J. Obstet. Gynecol. Neonatal Nurs.* **2012**, *41*, 680–691. [CrossRef]
117. Bedaiwy, M.; Patterson, B.; Mahajan, S. Prevalence of myofascial chronic pelvic pain and the effectiveness of pelvic floor physical therapy. *J. Reprod. Med.* **2013**, *58*, 504–510.
118. Montenegro, M.L.L.S.; Braz, C.A.; Rosa-E-Silva, J.C.; Candido-Dos-Reis, F.J.; Nogueira, A.A.; Poli-Neto, O.B. Anaesthetic injection versus ischemic compression for the pain relief of abdominal wall trigger points in women with chronic pelvic pain. *BMC Anesthesiol.* **2015**, *15*, 1–8. [CrossRef]
119. Sedighimehr, N.; Manshadi, F.D.; Shokouhi, N.; Baghban, A.A. Pelvic musculoskeletal dysfunctions in women with and without chronic pelvic pain. *J. Bodyw. Mov. Ther.* **2018**, *22*, 92–96. [CrossRef]
120. Howard, F. *Pelvic Pain: Diagnosis and Management*; Lippincott Williams & Wilkins: Baltimore, PA, USA, 2000.
121. Tu, F.; Kane, J.; Hellman, K. Noninvasive experimental bladder pain assessment in painful bladder syndrome. *BJOG Int. J. Obstet. Gynaecol.* **2016**, *124*, 283–291. [CrossRef]
122. Hetrick, D.C.; Ciol, M.; Rothman, I.; Turner, J.A.; Frest, M.; Berger, R.E. Musculoskeletal Dysfunction in Men with Chronic Pelvic Pain Syndrome Type III: A Case-control Study. *J. Urol.* **2003**, *170*, 828–831. [CrossRef]
123. Montenegro, M.L.L.D.S.; Mateus-Vasconcelos, E.C.L.; Silva, J.C.R.E.; Nogueira, A.A.; Dos Reis, F.J.C.; Neto, O.B.P. Importance of Pelvic Muscle Tenderness Evaluation in Women with Chronic Pelvic Pain. *Pain Med.* **2010**, *11*, 224–228. [CrossRef]
124. Fernández-Carnero, J.; Fernández-De-Las-Peñas, C.; de la Llave-Rincón, A.I.; Ge, H.-Y.; Arendt-Nielsen, L. Prevalence of and Referred Pain from Myofascial Trigger Points in the Forearm Muscles in Patients with Lateral Epicondylalgia. *Clin. J. Pain* **2007**, *23*, 353–360. [CrossRef]
125. Ríos-León, M.; Ortega-Santiago, R.; Madeleine, P.; Fernández-De-Las-Peñas, C.; Plaza-Manzano, G. Topographical Pressure Pain Sensitivity Maps of the Feet Reveal Bilateral Pain Sensitivity in Patients with Unilateral Plantar Heel Pain. *J. Orthop. Sports Phys. Ther.* **2019**, *49*, 640–646. [CrossRef]
126. Iglesias-González, J.J.; Muñoz-García, M.T.; Rodrigues-De-Souza, D.P.; Alburquerque-Sendín, F.; Fernández-De-Las-Peñas, C. Myofascial Trigger Points, Pain, Disability, and Sleep Quality in Patients with Chronic Nonspecific Low Back Pain. *Pain Med.* **2013**, *14*, 1964–1970. [CrossRef]
127. Muñoz-Muñoz, S.; Muñoz-García, M.T.; Alburquerque-Sendín, F.; Arroyo-Morales, M.; Fernández-De-Las-Peñas, C. Myofascial Trigger Points, Pain, Disability, and Sleep Quality in Individuals with Mechanical Neck Pain. *J. Manip. Physiol. Ther.* **2012**, *35*, 608–613. [CrossRef]
128. Shah, J.P.; Phillips, T.M.; Danoff, J.V.; Gerber, L. An in vivo microanalytical technique for measuring the local biochemical milieu of human skeletal muscle. *J. Appl. Physiol.* **2005**, *99*, 1977–1984. [CrossRef]
129. Shah, J.P.; Danoff, J.V.; Desai, M.J.; Parikh, S.; Nakamura, L.Y.; Phillips, T.M.; Gerber, L. Biochemicals Associated with Pain and Inflammation are Elevated in Sites Near to and Remote From Active Myofascial Trigger Points. *Arch. Phys. Med. Rehabil.* **2008**, *89*, 16–23. [CrossRef]
130. Ge, H.-Y.; Monterde, S.; Graven-Nielsen, T.; Arendt-Nielsen, L. Latent Myofascial Trigger Points Are Associated with an Increased Intramuscular Electromyographic Activity During Synergistic Muscle Activation. *J. Pain* **2014**, *15*, 181–187. [CrossRef]
131. Quesada, S.A.; Arias-Buría, J.L.; Courtney, C.A.; Arendt-Nielsen, L.; Fernández-De-Las-Peñas, C. Exploration of Quantitative Sensory Testing in Latent Trigger Points and Referred Pain Areas. *Clin. J. Pain* **2018**, *34*, 409–414. [CrossRef]
132. Kimura, Y.; Ge, H.-Y.; Zhang, Y.; Kimura, M.; Sumikura, H.; Arendt-Nielsen, L. Evaluation of sympathetic vasoconstrictor response following nociceptive stimulation of latent myofascial trigger points in humans. *Acta Physiol.* **2009**, *196*, 411–417. [CrossRef]
133. Ibarra, J.M.; Ge, H.-Y.; Wang, C.; Vizcaino, V.M.; Graven-Nielsen, T.; Arendt-Nielsen, L. Latent Myofascial Trigger Points are Associated with an Increased Antagonistic Muscle Activity During Agonist Muscle Contraction. *J. Pain* **2011**, *12*, 1282–1288. [CrossRef] [PubMed]
134. Itza, F.; Zarza, D.; Salinas, J.; Teba, F.; Ximenez, C. Turn-amplitude analysis as a diagnostic test for myofascial syndrome in patients with chronic pelvic pain. *Pain Res. Manag.* **2015**, *20*, 96–100. [CrossRef] [PubMed]
135. Hubbard, D.R.; Berkoff, G.M. Myofascial Trigger Points Show Spontaneous Needle EMG Activity. *Spine* **1993**, *18*, 1803–1807. [CrossRef] [PubMed]
136. Simons, D.G.; Hong, C.-Z.; Simons, L.S. Endplate Potentials Are Common to Midfiber Myofacial Trigger Points. *Am. J. Phys. Med. Rehabilitation* **2002**, *81*, 212–222. [CrossRef]
137. Partanen, J.V.; Ojala, T.A.; Arokoski, J.P. Myofascial syndrome and pain: A neurophysiological approach. *Pathophysiology* **2010**, *17*, 19–28. [CrossRef]
138. Arendt-Nielsen, L.; Madsen, H.; Jarrell, J.; Gregersen, H.; Drewes, A.M. Pain evoked by distension of the uterine cervix in women with dysmenorrhea: Evidence for central sensitization. *Acta Obstet. Et Gynecol. Scand.* **2014**, *93*, 741–748. [CrossRef]
139. Iacovides, S.; Avidon, I.; Baker, F. Does pain vary across the menstrual cycle? A review. *Eur. J. Pain* **2015**, *19*, 1389–1405. [CrossRef]
140. LeResche, L.; Mancl, L.; Sherman, J.J.; Gandara, B.; Dworkin, S.F. Changes in temporomandibular pain and other symptoms across the menstrual cycle. *Pain* **2003**, *106*, 253–261. [CrossRef]

141. Bartley, E.J.; Rhudy, J.L. Comparing Pain Sensitivity and the Nociceptive Flexion Reflex Threshold Across the Mid-follicular and Late-luteal Menstrual Phases in Healthy Women. *Clin. J. Pain* **2013**, *29*, 154–161. [CrossRef]
142. Schmalenberger, K.M.; Tauseef, H.A.; Barone, J.C.; Owens, S.A.; Lieberman, L.; Jarczok, M.N.; Girdler, S.S.; Kiesner, J.; Ditzen, B.; Eisenlohr-Moul, T.A. How to Study the Menstrual Cycle: Practical Tools and Recommendations. *Psychoneuroendocrinology* **2021**, *123*, 104895. [CrossRef]
143. MacLean, J.A.; Hayashi, K. Progesterone Actions and Resistance in Gynecological Disorders. *Cells* **2022**, *11*, 647. [CrossRef]
144. Hassan, S.; Muere, A.; Einstein, G. Ovarian hormones and chronic pain: A comprehensive review. *Pain* **2014**, *155*, 2448–2460. [CrossRef]
145. Rezaii, T.; Hirschberg, A.L.; Carlström, K.; Ernberg, M. The Influence of Menstrual Phases on Pain Modulation in Healthy Women. *J. Pain* **2012**, *13*, 646–655. [CrossRef]
146. Christin-Maitre, S. Human Menstrual Cycle. In *Encyclopedia of Endocrine Diseases*; Academic Press: Cambridge, MA, USA, 2018; pp. 399–403. [CrossRef]
147. Greenwald, J.D.; Shafritz, K.M. An Integrative Neuroscience Framework for the Treatment of Chronic Pain: From Cellular Alterations to Behavior. *Front. Integr. Neurosci.* **2018**, *12*, 18. [CrossRef]
148. Wang, C.; Ge, H.-Y.; Ibarra, J.M.; Yue, S.-W.; Madeleine, P.; Arendt-Nielsen, L. Spatial Pain Propagation Over Time Following Painful Glutamate Activation of Latent Myofascial Trigger Points in Humans. *J. Pain* **2012**, *13*, 537–545. [CrossRef]
149. Fernández-De-Las-Peñas, C.; Dommerholt, J. Myofascial Trigger Points: Peripheral or Central Phenomenon? *Curr. Rheumatol. Rep.* **2014**, *16*, 1–6. [CrossRef]
150. Ge, H.-Y.; Fernández-De-Las-Peñas, C.; Yue, S.-W. Myofascial trigger points: Spontaneous electrical activity and its consequences for pain induction and propagation. *Chin. Med.* **2011**, *6*, 13. [CrossRef]
151. Ge, H.-Y.; Nie, H.; Madeleine, P.; Danneskiold-Samsøe, B.; Graven-Nielsen, T.; Arendt-Nielsen, L. Contribution of the local and referred pain from active myofascial trigger points in fibromyalgia syndrome. *Pain* **2009**, *147*, 233–240. [CrossRef]
152. McPartland, J.M.; Simons, D.G. Myofascial Trigger Points: Translating Molecular Theory into Manual Therapy. *J. Man. Manip. Ther.* **2006**, *14*, 232–239. [CrossRef]
153. Bartley, E.J.; Fillingim, R.B. Sex differences in pain: A brief review of clinical and experimental findings. *Br. J. Anaesth.* **2013**, *111*, 52–58. [CrossRef] [PubMed]
154. Pieretti, S.; Di Giannuario, A.; Di Giovannandrea, R.; Marzoli, F.; Piccaro, G.; Minosi, P.; Aloisi, A.M. Gender differences in pain and its relief. *Ann. Dell'istituto Super. Di Sanita* **2016**, *52*, 184–189. [CrossRef]
155. Schwartz, E.S.; Gebhart, G.F. Visceral Pain. *Curr. Top Behav. Neurosci.* **2014**, *20*, 171–197. [CrossRef] [PubMed]
156. Rogers, R.M. Basic neuroanatomy for understanding pelvic pain. *J. Am. Assoc. Gynecol. Laparosc.* **1999**, *6*, 15–29. [CrossRef]
157. Sánchez-García, O.; López-Juárez, R.; Corona-Quintanilla, D.L.; Ruiz, C.; Martínez-Gómez, M.; Cuevas-Romero, E.; Castelán, F. Estrogens influence differentially on the pelvic floor muscles activation at somatovisceral reflexes involved in micturition of rabbits. *Menopause* **2021**, *28*, 1287–1295. [CrossRef] [PubMed]
158. Prendergast, S.A.; Weiss, J.M. Screening for Musculoskeletal Causes of Pelvic Pain. *Clin. Obstet. Gynecol.* **2003**, *46*, 773–782. [CrossRef]
159. Tu, C.-H.; Niddam, D.M.; Chao, H.-T.; Liu, R.-S.; Hwang, R.-J.; Yeh, T.-C.; Hsieh, J.-C. Abnormal cerebral metabolism during menstrual pain in primary dysmenorrhea. *NeuroImage* **2009**, *47*, 28–35. [CrossRef]
160. Vincent, K.; Warnaby, C.; Stagg, C.; Moore, J.; Kennedy, S.; Tracey, I. Dysmenorrhoea is associated with central changes in otherwise healthy women. *Pain* **2011**, *152*, 1966–1975. [CrossRef]
161. Iacovides, S.; Baker, F.C.; Avidon, I.; Bentley, A. Women with Dysmenorrhea Are Hypersensitive to Experimental Deep Muscle Pain Across the Menstrual Cycle. *J. Pain* **2013**, *14*, 1066–1076. [CrossRef]
162. Oladosu, F.A.; Hellman, K.M.; Ham, P.J.; Kochlefl, L.E.; Datta, A.; Garrison, E.F.; Steiner, N.D.; Roth, G.E.; Tu, F.F. Persistent autonomic dysfunction and bladder sensitivity in primary dysmenorrhea. *Sci. Rep.* **2019**, *9*, 1–10. [CrossRef]

diagnostics

MDPI

Article

Screening Clinical Changes for the Diagnosis of Early Knee Osteoarthritis: A Cross-Sectional Observational Study

Ana Alabajos-Cea [1], Luz Herrero-Manley [1], Luis Suso-Martí [2,*], Núria Sempere-Rubio [3], Ferran Cuenca-Martínez [2,*], Vicente Muñoz-Alarcos [2], Juan Alonso Pérez-Barquero [1], Enrique Viosca-Herrero [1] and Isabel Vázquez-Arce [1]

[1] Servicio de Medicina Física y Rehabilitación, Hospital La Fe, 46026 Valencia, Spain
[2] Exercise Intervention for Health Research Group (EXINH-RG), Department of Physiotherapy, University of Valencia, 46010 Valencia, Spain
[3] UBIC, Department of Physiotherapy, Faculty of Physiotherapy, Universitat de Valencia, 46010 Valencia, Spain
[*] Correspondence: luis.suso@uv.es (L.S.-M.); [illegible]@gmail.com (F.C.-M.); Tel.: +34-963-983-855

Abstract: Background: The main objective was to evaluate differences in the clinical, motor, or functional variables in patients with Early Osteoarthritis (EOA) and individuals at risk of developing osteoarthritis (OA). **Methods:** A cross-sectional study was performed. All the participants were divided into two groups: EOA patients and healthy subjects (HS) at risk of developing OA. The main outcomes were clinical tests, such as those of knee morphology, instability, or proprioception; motor and functional variables, such as knee strength, range of motion, walking speed, and the sit-to-stand test; pain and disability, assessed through the Western Ontario McMaster Universities Osteoarthritis Index (WOMAC) and Knee injury and Osteoarthritis Outcome Score (KOOS) scales; and knee alignment and leg length inequality, assessed via X-ray images. **Results:** A total of 97 participants were included (54 EOA and 43 HS). Patients with EOA showed a greater presence of knee pain ($p < 0.01$). In addition, more EOA patients showed instability both in the left ($p < 0.01$) and right legs ($p < 0.05$). Regarding the knee alignment variable, significant differences were found ($p < 0.04$), with more patients with EOA diagnosed as possessing a varus alignment. In addition, EOA patients showed lower knee strength, since statistically significant differences were found regarding flexion and extension strength in the left leg (Mean Difference (MD): 12.92; $p = 0.03$; $d = -0.46$ and MD:7.81; $p = 0.04$; $d = -0.39$). Differences were found for the sit-to-stand test scores, showing lower results for the EOA group (MD: −1.91; $p < 0.01$; $d = 0.54$). **Conclusions:** The results of this research show statistically significant differences between patients with EOA and HS at risk of developing OA with respect to pain, disability, instability, knee strength, and the sit-to-stand test. Our results suggest that the evaluation of clinical, motor, and functional features could contribute to an early management of knee OA.

Keywords: osteoarthritis; knee osteoarthritis; early osteoarthritis; musculoskeletal disorders; risk factors

1. Introduction

Osteoarthritis (OA) is a common joint disease that causes disability and a reduction in patients' quality of life. It is a leading cause of chronic pain and health-care utilization [1]. OA is characterized by cartilage loss, subchondral bone changes, synovial inflammation, and meniscus degeneration [2]. Basic research approaches have allowed for the identification of pathophysiological factors that determine the existence of OA. However, the main part of this research is performed in the late stage of OA, and the pathological processes involved in the early stages of joint disease are not well understood [3].

Previous studies suggest that many of the structural findings grounded in X-ray evidence in persons with knee OA are late phenomena, which occur after a considerable progression of the pathology [4,5]. In this regard, it has been suggested that the limited

A)

B)

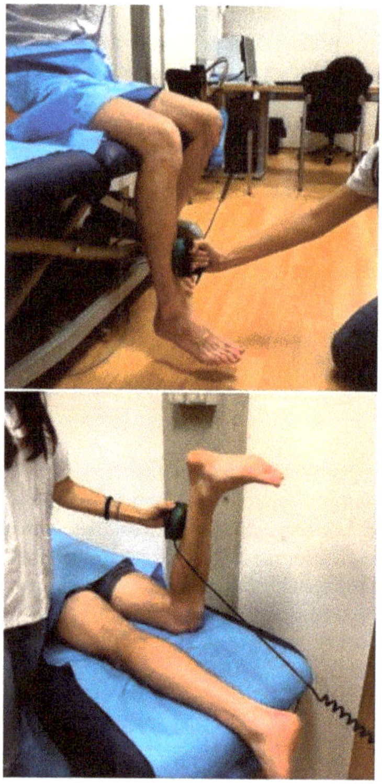

Figure 1. Knee strength measurement: (**A**) extension movement; (**B**) flexion movement.

Knee Range of Motion

To obtain knees' range of motion (ROM) measurements, particular care was taken to align the goniometer to the femur by palpating the greater trochanter and then aligning the proximal arm of the goniometer close to the femur. The distal arm of the goniometer was parallel to the tibia [19].

Sit-to-Stand

To assess functional capacity, the sit-to-stand test was employed. The test was performed as follows: with the patient seated with their back against the back of the chair, the clinician counted each standing movement aloud so that the patient remained oriented. The clinician stopped the test when the patient achieved the standing position on the 5th repetition [20].

Walking Speed

Subject walked without assistance 10 m (32.8 feet) and the time was measured for the intermediate 6 m (19.7 feet). Assistive devices could be used but had to be kept consistent and documented from test to test. Test was performed at the fastest speed possible. There were three trials collected and the average of the three trials was calculated for the measurement [21,22].

2.3.4. Pain and Disability Variables

Pain Intensity

Visual Analogue Scale (VAS) was used to measure pain intensity. The VAS is a 100 mm line with two endpoints representing the extreme states "no pain" and "the maximal pain imaginable". It has been shown to have good re-test reliability (r = 0.94, $p < 0.001$) and a minimal detectable change of 15.0 mm [23,24]. Pain intensity was measured both at rest and while walking.

Pain Type

Pain was also assessed with National Health and Nutrition Examination Survey (NHANES)-type pain questions, wherein duration of pain is indicated as 'most days in a month' (NHANES A and NHANES C), following published recommendations [25].

Western Ontario and McMaster Universities Osteoarthritis Index (WOMAC)

This instrument is the most extensively used for the functional and symptomatic assessment of patients with osteoarthritis. The WOMAC questionnaire is self-administered and is used to assess patients who progress with hip and/or knee osteoarthritis. The questionnaire is a multidimensional scale composed of 24 items divided into 3 aspects: functional pain (consisting of 5 items), stiffness (2 items), and activities of daily life difficulties (17 items). Higher values mean poorer WOMAC subscales scores of pain and physical function. The Spanish version of the WOMAC questionnaire has adequate psychometric properties, presenting an index of internal consistency (a) of 0.82 for pain and 0.93 for physical function subscales [26].

Knee Injury and Osteoarthritis Outcome Score (KOOS)

The KOOS is a knee-specific instrument, developed to assess a patient's opinion about their knee and associated problems. The KOOS evaluates both short-term and long-term consequences of knee injury. It holds 42 items in 5 separately scored subscales: Pain, other Symptoms, Function in daily living (ADL), Function in Sport and Recreation (Sport/Rec), and knee-related Quality of Life (QOL). The psychometric properties and the ICC of the Spanish version have shown acceptable properties for both the total score and the subscales [27].

2.3.5. Image Variables

Knee Alignment

Knee alignment was measured based on bilateral standard anterior–posterior weight-bearing radiographs as the angle formed by the intersection of the mechanical axes of the femur (the line from femoral head center to femoral intercondylar notch center) and the tibia (the line from ankle talus center to the center of the tibial spine tips). A knee was defined as varus when alignment was more than 0° in the varus direction, valgus when it was more than 0° in the valgus direction, and neutral when alignment was 0° (the angle made by the femur and tibia on a knee X-ray does not consider the proximal femur, femoral or tibial shafts, or ankle, so it is highly variable as opposed to full-limb measurements) [15].

Leg-Length Inequality (LLI)

We measured LLI in a bilateral standard anterior–posterior weight-bearing radiograph. We drew a line from the top of the femoral head that was lower than the other one. In addition, we then measured the distance between that line and the highest point of the other femoral head.

2.4. Procedures

An information sheet with an explanation of the procedure and an informed consent form were given to all the participants. Once the subjects had read the information from the study, they were allowed to ask any questions about its nature. The subjects that agreed to participate proceeded to fill in the sociodemographic questionnaire. Self-reported measures of disability, pain, and disability variables were then assessed. Finally, the physical examination was performed, including physical tests and motor and functional tests. The study protocol lasted approximately one hour. In order to avoid the influence of fatigue on the physical tests, an interval of 3 min between tests was maintained. This procedure was identical for both groups.

2.5. Statistical Analysis

The sociodemographic and clinical variables of the participants were analyzed. The data were summarized using frequency counts, descriptive statistics, summary tables, and figures. The data analysis was performed using the Statistics Package for the Social Sciences (SPSS 24, IBM Inc., Chicago, IL, USA). The categorical variables are shown as frequencies and percentages. The quantitative results are represented by descriptive statistics (confidence interval, mean, and standard deviation). For all variables, the z-score was assumed to follow a normal distribution based on the central limit theorem because all the groups had more than 30 participants [28,29]. Student's *t*-test was used for group comparisons. Cohen's *d* effect sizes were calculated for multiple comparisons of the outcome variables. According to Cohen's method, the magnitude of the effect was classified as small (0.20–0.49), medium (0.50–0.79), or large (0.80).

The relationships between pain and disability measures and between physical measurements were examined using Pearson's correlation coefficients. A Pearson's correlation coefficient greater than 0.60 indicated a strong correlation, a coefficient between 0.30 and 0.60 indicated a moderate correlation, and a coefficient below 0.30 indicated a low or very low correlation [30].

3. Results

A total of 97 participants were included in the study, with a mean age of 51.51 ± 5.89 (36 men and 61 women). A total of 54 of the participants met the criteria to be classified as EOA while 43 were classified as HS. All the physical tests established in the protocol were performed on all the participants included in the study; no abandonment of any study participant was recorded. No adverse effects were reported during the assessments. There were no statistically significant differences between the groups in terms of the descriptive, demographic, and control variables (Table 1).

Table 1. Descriptive, demographic data and control variables.

	EOA (*n* = 54)	HS (*n* = 43)	*p* Value
Age (years)	51.81 ± 5.65	51.05 ± 6.21	0.44
BMI (kg/m^2)	27.28 ± 4.08	28.01 ± 2.96	0.59
KL Grade			
0	19 (35)	23 (54)	0.67
1	35 (65)	20 (46)	
Gender			
Men	22 (40.8)	14 (32.5)	0.78
Women	32 (59.2)	21 (67.5)	
Hormonal status			
Pre-menopausal	12 (37.5)	14 (66.6)	0.19
Post-menopausal	20 (62.5)	7 (33.3)	
Smoking			
Yes	9 (16.6)	4 (9.3)	
No	21 (38.9)	19 (44.2)	0.55
Ex	24 (44.5)	20 (46.5)	

Table 1. *Cont.*

	EOA (*n* = 54)	HS (*n* = 43)	*p* Value
Alcohol			0.66
Never	6 (11.1)	4 (9.3)	
Seldom	14 (25.9)	12 (27.9)	
1–2 times/month	13 (24.1)	11 (25.6)	
1–2 times/week	17 (31.5)	13 (30.3)	
1 time per day	3 (5.5)	2 (4.6)	
More than 1 a day	1 (1.9)	1 (2.3)	
Previous Injuries Left			0.35
No	42 (77.3)	27 (62.8)	
Yes	12 (22.2)	16 (37.2)	
Meniscus	8	3	
Ligament	0	4	
Bone	0	2	
Cartilage	1	2	
Unspecific	3	5	
Previous Injuries Right			0.47
No	40 (74.1)	25 (58.2)	
Yes	14 (25.9)	18 (41.8)	
Meniscus	4	7	
Ligament	5	2	
Bone	1	1	
Cartilage	1	2	
Unspecific	3	6	
Knee morphology			0.89
Normal	52 (96.3)	43 (100)	
Altered	2 (3.7)	0 (0)	
Occupational risk			0.68
Never	16 (29.6)	10 (23.3)	
Seldom	12 (22.2)	11 (25.6)	
1–2 times/month	3 (5.6)	5 (11.6)	
1–2 times/week	6 (11.1)	1 (2.3)	
1 a day	9 (16.7)	9 (20.9)	
Always	8 (14.8)	7 (16.3)	
Family history			0.56
Yes	38 (70.4)	32 (74.4)	
No	16 (29.6)	11 (25.6)	
OA Hand history			0.25
Yes	11 (20.4)	6 (14.0)	
No	43 (79.6)	37 (86.0)	

Table 1. *Cont.*

	EOA (*n* = 54)	HS (*n* = 43)	*p* Value
OA Hip history			0.66
Yes	8 (14.8)	7 (16.3)	
No	46 (85.2)	36 (83.7)	
Sport			0.54
Yes	24 (45.5)	27 (62.8)	
No	30 (55.5)	16 (37.2)	
Education level			
Primary	9 (16.6)	6 (13.9)	0.92
Secondary	19 (35.2)	15 (34.9)	
College	26 (48.2)	22 (51.2)	
Marital status			
Single	6 (11.1)	7 (16.2)	0.22
Married	36 (66.7)	32 (74.4)	
Divorced	10 (18.5)	2 (4.7)	
Widow	2 (3.7)	2 (4.7)	

The categorical variables are shown as frequencies and percentages. The quantitative results are represented by descriptive statistics (confidence interval, mean, and standard deviation). BMI: Body Mass index; EOA: Early Osteoarthritis; HS: Healthy subjects; KL: Kellgren-Laurence.

3.1. Clinical and Image Variables

Regarding differences in the clinical and image variables, the patients with EOA presented more knee pain ($p < 0.01$). In addition, more EOA patients showed instability both in the left ($p < 0.01$) and the right leg ($p < 0.05$). Significant differences were found with respect to the knee alignment variable ($p < 0.04$), wherein more patients with EOA diagnosed as possessing varus alignment. Detailed results are presented in Table 2.

Table 2. Clinical and image variable results.

	EOA (*n* = 54)	HS (*n* = 43)	*p* Value
Pain			
Yes	**45 (83.3)**	**16 (37.2)**	**<0.01**
No	**9 (16.6)**	**27 (62.8)**	
Pain side			
Left	7 (15.6)	3 (18.8)	0.55
Right	14 (31.1)	4 (25)	
Both	24 (53.3)	9 (56.2)	
NHANES Pain Left			0.67
No pain	34 (63.0)	29 (67.5)	
A	10 (18.5)	9 (20.9)	
C	10 (18.5)	5 (11.6)	
NHANES Pain Right			0.2
No pain	30 (55.6)	29 (67.4)	
A	14 (25.9)	5 (11.6)	
C	10 (18.5)	9 (20.9)	
Crepitus Left			0.65
Yes	39 (72.2)	33 (76.7)	
No	15 (27.8)	10 (23.3)	

Table 2. *Cont.*

	EOA (n = 54)	HS (n = 43)	p Value
Crepitus Right			0.66
Yes	34 (62.9)	29 (67.4)	
No	20 (37.1)	14 (32.6)	
Instability Left Yes No	 18 (33.3) 36 (66.6)	 5 (11.6) 38 (88.4)	0.01
Instability Right Yes No	 26 (48.1) 28 (51.9)	 12 (27.9) 31 (72.1)	0.05
Deformity Left			0.69
Yes	16 (29.6)	13 (30.2)	
No	38 (70.4)	30 (69.8)	
Deformity Right			0.86
Yes	16 (29.6)	12 (27.9)	
No	38 (70.4)	31 (72.1)	
Knee alignment Left			0.04
Neutral	6 (11.1)	11 (25.6)	
Varus	32 (59.3)	16 (37.2)	
Valgus	16 (29.6)	16 (37.2)	
Knee alignment Right			0.47
Neutral	7 (12.9)	5 (11.6)	
Varus	32 (57.4)	21 (48.8)	
Valgus	15 (27.8)	17 (39.6)	
Leg length inequality			0.13
Yes	18 (33.3)	8 (18.6)	
No	36 (66.7)	35 (81.4)	
Leg circumference			0.32
Yes	42 (77.7)	34 (79.1)	
No	12 (22.3)	9 (20.9)	
Proprioception Left			0.88
Altered	44 (81.5)	32 (74.4)	
Normal	10 (18.5)	11 (25.6)	
Proprioception Right			0.33
Altered	35 (64.8)	31 (72.1)	
Normal	19 (35.2)	12 (27.9)	

The categorical variables are shown as frequencies and percentages. The quantitative results are represented by descriptive statistics (confidence interval, mean, and standard deviation). EOA: Early Osteoarthritis; HS: Healthy subjects.

3.2. Motor and Functional Variables

Regarding the differences between the groups, the patients with EOA showed higher levels of pain intensity at rest with a medium effect size (Mean Difference (MD): −2.35; $p = 0.01$; d = 0.5) and walking with a large effect size (MD: −2.21; $p < 0.01$; d = 0.88) (Figure 2).

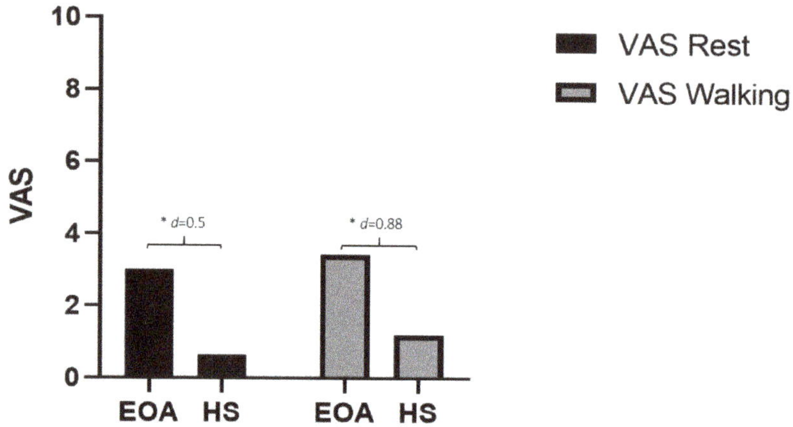

Figure 2. Differences in pain variable. * $p < 0.05$; *d*: Effect size; VAS: Visual Analogue Scale.

In addition, the EOA patients showed lower knee strength, since statistically significant differences were found for flexion and extension strength in the left leg with a small effect size (MD: 12.92; $p = 0.03$; $d = -0.46$ and MD:7.81; $p = 0.04$; $d = -0.39$). In the right leg, similar significant differences were found between groups, but only regarding flexion movement, with a medium effect size (MD: 13.06; $p = 0.01$; $d = 0.55$) (Figure 3). No differences were found for the knee ROM values between groups.

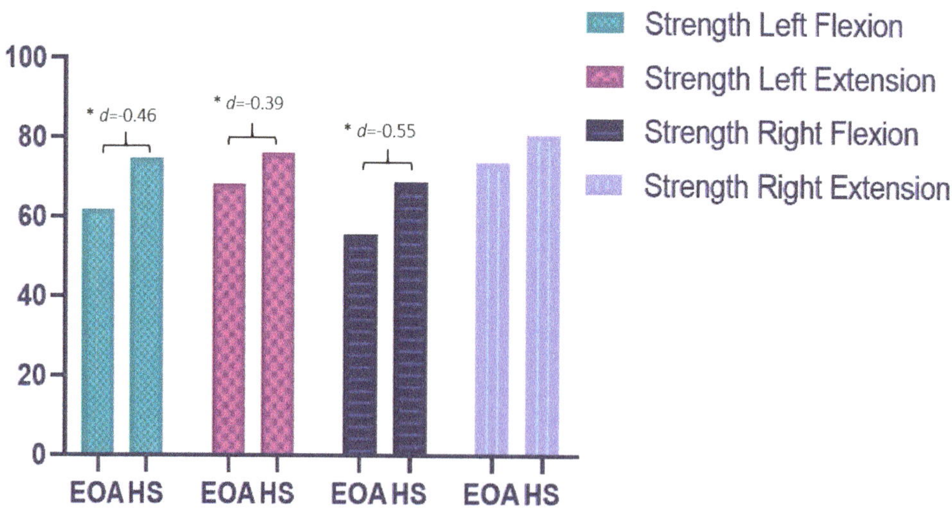

Figure 3. Differences in strength variable. * $p < 0.05$; *d*: Effect size.

Regarding the functional variables, statistically significant differences were found for the sit-to-stand test, showing more time expended for the EOA group, with a medium effect size (MD: −1.91; $p < 0.01$; $d = 0.54$) (Table 3).

Table 3. Between-group comparisons regarding pain, disability, motor, and functional variables.

Measures	EOA (n = 54)	HS (n = 43)	Mean Difference (95% CI)	Effect Size (d)
VAS Rest	3.0 ± 6.44	0.65 ± 1.53	−2.35 * (−4.35 to −0.35)	0.5
VAS Walking	3.42 ± 2.75	1.21 ± 2.23	−2.21 * (−3.24 to −1.18)	0.88
WOMAC	0.25 ± 0.13	0.12 ± 0.13	−0.13 ** (−0.19 to −0.7)	1.01
KOOS				
Pain	73.5 ± 13.79	89.29 ± 14.56	15.79 ** (10.01 to 21.56)	−1.11
Symptoms	77.87 ± 12.66	90.79 ± 12.76	12.91 ** (7.73 to 18.1)	−1.01
ADL	77.7 ± 15.94	90.83 ± 10.56	13.13 ** (7.47 to 18.79)	−0.97
QQL	52.63 ± 24.86	76.17 ± 23.96	23.54 ** (13.58 to 33.49)	−0.96
Strength Left (Kg)				
Flexion	61.91 ± 21.57	74.83 ± 33.00	12.92 * (0.45 to 25.39)	−0.46
Extension	68.24 ± 21.47	76.05 ± 17.81	7.81 * (1.26 to 16.88)	−0.39
Strength Right (Kg)				
Flexion	55.71 ± 16.52	68.77 ± 28.85	13.06 * (2.59 to 23.52)	−0.55
Extension	73.89 ± 22.98	80.86 ± 22.21	6.97 (−3.34 to 17.29)	−0.31
ROM Left Leg (°)	132.39 ± 9.61	132.43 ± 12.75	0.04 (−4.91 to 5.00)	−0.01
ROM Right Leg (°)	132.61 ± 8.11	131.84 ± 12.19	−0.78 (−5.29 to 3.74)	0.07
Sit to stand (sec)	13.18 ± 4.27	11.26 ± 2.61	−1.91 * (−3.52 to −0.31)	0.54
Walking speed (sec)	3.54 ± 0.89	3.36 ± 0.63	−0.17 (−0.53 to 0.18)	0.23

Note: ** $p < 0.01$; * $p < 0.05$; CI: confidence interval; EOA: Early osteoarthritis; HS: Healthy subjects.

3.3. Correlation Analysis

The strongest correlations were found in the EOA group between the left leg flexion strength, left knee ROM, and walking speed with walking VAS. These correlations were low (r = −0.33, r = −0.41 and r = 0.44; $p < 0.05$), and we also found the same trend for the right side, although it was not statistically significant. Correlations were also found between pain intensity at rest and ROM in both groups. Finally, correlations were found between the BMI and the ROM for left and right sides in the EOA patients (r = −0.66 and −0.55; $p < 0.01$) (Table 4).

Table 4. Correlation analysis.

Variable	Group	VAS Rest	VAS Walking	Strength Left F	Strength Left E	Strength Right F	Strength Right E	ROM Left	ROM Right	Sit-to-Stand	Walking Speed
VAS Rest	EOA	1	0.28 *	−0.01	0.15	−0.1	−0.05	−0.14	−0.32 *	0.02	0.04
	HS	1	0.69 **	−0.09	0.05	−0.16	−0.09	−0.62 **	−0.62 *	0.35*	0.4 *
VAS Walking	EOA	0.28 *	1	−0.33 *	−0.20	−0.13	−0.24	−0.41 **	−0.24	0.31 *	0.44 **
	HS	0.69 **	1	−0.13	−0.22	−0.22	−0.13	−0.28	−0.24	0.14	0.32
BMI	EOA	0.09	0.24	0.14	0.13	0.09	0.01	−0.66 **	−0.55 **	0.11	0.32 *
	HS	0.01	−0.03	0.27	0.28	0.25	−0.18	−0.31	−0.34	0.26	0.05
WOMAC	EOA	0.15	0.56 **	−0.12	−0.05	0.11	−0.15	−0.17	−0.27	0.27	0.19
	HS	0.52 **	0.63 **	−0.24	−0.17	−0.27	0.06	−0.08	−0.09	0.25	0.59 **

Note: ** $p < 0.01$; * $p < 0.05$; EOA: Early osteoarthritis; HS: Healthy subject.

4. Discussion

The main objective of this study was to evaluate which clinical, motor, or functional variables could be related to the appearance of EOA. Our study highlights some relevant data in relation to the early diagnosis of OA. In recent years, many efforts have been made to diagnose and classify these patients. However, this remains a challenge in such a heterogeneous disease, and our data provide new information about the risk factors and mechanisms involved in EOA [31]. Firstly, some of the risk factors (gender, personal history, or daily habits) previously identified in the scientific literature have not been found in our population with OAE. However, some other related physical or functional features have been associated with OA in this population, suggesting the importance of these factors in the diagnosis and prevention of OA.

First, it is believed that non-modifiable factors such as age, gender, familial OA, and hormonal status could have an important role in the development of OA. Women have consistently been shown to be at higher risk of hip, knee, and hand OA, and whether this increase in risk is constant with age and changes in relation to endogenous estrogen production and menopause has been studied [32]. However, we found no differences in these variables. In addition, personal OA histories have been studied, with controversial results. Some studies have found the hand and/or hip OA history as one of the main factors that is consistently associated with knee OA [32], while other authors found it to be insignificant [8]. Our results follow the line of the latter authors, as we found no differences in the personal history of OA between subjects with EOA and HS.

On the other hand, some modifiable factors such as overweight and obesity (usually quantified using BMI), occupational risk, knee extensor muscle weakness, leg-length inequalities, or lifestyle habits could also significantly contribute to the onset of the pathology. A higher BMI was associated with greater knee pain accounting for OA severity in persons with or at a high risk for knee OA in the Osteoarthritis Initiative [33]. However, in our population, correlations were found between BMI and ROM in the subjects with EOA, but not with respect to pain intensity. Regarding lifestyle habits, drinking alcohol and smoking have been found to be statistically insignificant as either risk or protective factors [8,32]. Our data are in accordance with this statement, since no significant differences were found between the groups. The association of occupational activities with the development of knee OA has also been studied, finding an increased risk in floor-layers or in frequent occupational kneeling and lifting [34]. These differences were not found in our data, but it should be considered that our sample represented a small number of people with an occupational risk. Perhaps a larger sample of people with a high occupational risk would be necessary to detect differences in this aspect.

Regarding physical activity, a Cochrane Library's review concluded that people are confused about the cause of their pain, and without adequate information from healthcare professionals, they avoid activity for fear of causing harm [35]. In addition, sport activities, defined as regular leisure activities, have been found to predict the progression of knee OA [34]. Being less sedentary was associated with better function in the Osteoarthritis Initiative, independent of moderate–vigorous physical activity minutes [36,37]. A greater degree of walking was associated with a lower risk of incident function limitation in persons with or at higher risk for knee OA in the Multicenter Osteoarthritis Study [38]. In our population, there seems to be a trend toward a greater sedentary lifestyle in the EOA group, but the differences were not significant.

The association of risk factors with the onset of knee pain has also been studied, establishing knee pain not as a predictor, but part of outcome measures for knee OA [8,25,32]. In our population, we combined radiographic and clinical criteria to classify patients into HS or EOA, as suggested by Luyten [11], and we found that the subjects with EOA showed higher levels of disability in terms of WOMAC and pain through VAS both at rest and during walking. In addition, our results show that higher levels of pain may be related to lower levels of ROM in both EOA and HS.

A systematic review and meta-analysis showed that knee extensor muscle weakness was associated with an increased risk of developing symptomatic knee OA [7]. Ruhdorfer et al., analyzing data from the Osteoarthritis Initiative, found that the reduction in thigh muscle strength in knee OA is related to pain but not to the structural (radiographic) disease status [39]. In this regard, our results showed that motor variables such as strength, or functional variables such as functional capacity, are significantly altered in patients with EOA compared to HS at risk of developing OA. In this regard, we also found differences between the right and left leg with respect to variables such as strength or ROM. The reasons for this may be varied, given that more subjects in both groups had pain or instability in the right leg due to a greater dominance of this leg with respect to the left.

Knee alignment, both static and dynamic, has important implications for load distribution within the knee. There is insufficient evidence to draw a conclusion regarding the effects of alignment on incident OA. It is possible that malalignment may be a reflection of the severity of the disease, with joint space loss due to cartilage and meniscal abnormalities, and bone contour alterations occurring as part of the OA disease process contributing to malalignment. In middle-aged, overweight women without knee OA in the Prevention of Knee Osteoarthritis in Overweight Females study, varus alignment was associated with incident radiographic OA; the association for valgus was borderline [40]. Similarly, LLI is an easily modifiable abnormality that can also affect lower extremity biomechanics. An LLI of at least 2 cm has been shown to be almost twice as likely to correspond to prevalent radiographic knee OA, but no such association was noted for incident knee OA [34]. Our data showed a predominance of varus alignment in the EOA group, suggesting its relevance in the development of EOA, but no significant differences were found with respect to LLI in our sample.

Previous studies suggest a relationship between instability and the onset and development of OA [41]. Our results are in line with these findings, as we found higher rates of subjects with ligamentous instability in the group of patients with EOA compared to healthy subjects. In this regard, it has also been suggested that previous knee injuries may contribute to the development of OA [8,34]. Although our results do not show significant differences between the groups, a higher percentage of injuries in the EOA group has been observed.

In addition, previous studies have shown that patients with higher levels of knee strength have higher levels of functional stability [42]. Our results show lower levels of strength in patients with EOA, suggesting that stability may also be dependent on this factor, and not just on ligamentous status. We hypothesize that these lower strength levels may lead to greater joint instability, which may play a role in the development of EOA, although future studies are needed to establish a cause–effect relationship.

Limitations

This research study has several limitations that should be considered when interpreting the results. First, the cross-sectional nature of this study makes it impossible to establish causality. In this sense, we did not find significant differences in many of the variables that have previously been identified as risk factors. This may be due to the fact that these variables (i.e., knee morphology, sports practice, or knee deformity) are not risk factors for the development of OA but rather consequences of the establishment of this pathology. This could entail that our sample would not present these alterations because we are dealing with an 'early' OA. Secondly, the lack of consensus and clear definition of EOA makes it difficult to draw clear conclusions about the differences between these groups of individuals. In this regard, several classifications have been proposed for EOA, and further research into the validity of these classifications is needed [43,44]. Third, in our sample, we have found a low percentage of patients presenting occupational risk, previous injuries, or toxic life habits, which have been previously related to the onset of OA. Studies with a larger sample size or in another type of population may be necessary to obtain relevant data in this regard. Finally, it would have been interesting to collect more information on physical activity in order to explore the implication of its intensity on the onset of EOA.

5. Conclusions

The results of this research show statistically significant differences between patients with EOA and HS at risk of developing OA with respect to pain, disability, instability, knee strength, sit-to-stand test scores, and walking speed. Our results suggest that the evaluation of clinical, motor, and functional features could contribute to an early management of knee OA. However, further longitudinal research is needed to clarify the role of these variables in the onset and development of OA.

Author Contributions: Conceptualization, A.A.-C., L.H.-M., J.A.P.-B., E.V.-H. and I.V.-A.; methodology, A.A.-C., L.H.-M., J.A.P.-B., E.V.-H. and I.V.-A.; formal analysis, L.S.-M., N.S.-R. and F.C.-M.; investigation, A.A.-C., L.H.-M., J.A.P.-B., E.V.-H. and I.V.-A.; data curation, L.S.-M., N.S.-R., F.C.-M. and V.M.-A.; writing—original draft preparation, All authors; writing—review and editing, L.S.-M., N.S.-R. and F.C.-M.; visualization, L.S.-M. and V.M.-A.; supervision, A.A.-C., L.H.-M., J.A.P.-B., E.V.-H. and I.V.-A.; project administration, A.A.-C., L.H.-M., J.A.P.-B., E.V.-H. and I.V.-A.; funding acquisition, A.A.-C., L.H.-M., J.A.P.-B., E.V.-H. and I.V.-A. All authors have read and agreed to the published version of the manuscript.

Funding: This research was funded by the European Union's Horizon 2020 research and innovation programme under grant agreement No 777159.

Institutional Review Board Statement: The study was conducted in accordance with the Declaration of Helsinki and approved by the Institutional Review Board of Hospital La Fe (CEIm La Fe 2017/0147; Valencia, Spain).

Informed Consent Statement: Informed consent was obtained from all subjects involved in the study.

Data Availability Statement: Not applicable.

Acknowledgments: The authors would like to thank the participants of this study.

Conflicts of Interest: The authors declare no conflict of interest.

References

1. Emery, C.A.; Whittaker, J.L.; Mahmoudian, A.; Lohmander, L.S.; Roos, E.M.; Bennell, K.L.; Toomey, C.M.; Reimer, R.A.; Thompson, D.; Ronsky, J.L.; et al. Establishing outcome measures in early knee osteoarthritis. *Nat. Rev. Rheumatol.* **2019**, *15*, 438–448. [CrossRef] [PubMed]
2. Loeser, R.F.; Goldring, S.R.; Scanzello, C.R.; Goldring, M.B. Osteoarthritis: A disease of the joint as an organ. *Arthritis Rheum.* **2012**, *64*, 1697–1707. [CrossRef] [PubMed]
3. Favero, M.; Ramonda, R.; Goldring, M.B.; Goldring, S.R.; Punzi, L. Early knee osteoarthritis. *RMD Open* **2015**, *1*, e000062. [CrossRef] [PubMed]
4. Felson, D.T.; Hodgson, R. Identifying and treating preclinical and early osteoarthritis. *Rheum. Dis. Clin. N. Am.* **2014**, *40*, 699–710. [CrossRef]
5. Neogi, T.; Bowes, M.A.; Niu, J.; De Souza, K.M.; Vincent, G.R.; Goggins, J.; Zhang, Y.; Felson, D.T. Magnetic resonance imaging-based three-dimensional bone shape of the knee predicts onset of knee osteoarthritis: Data from the osteoarthritis initiative. *Arthritis Rheum.* **2013**, *65*, 2048–2058. [CrossRef] [PubMed]
6. Madry, H.; Kon, E.; Condello, V.; Peretti, G.M.; Steinwachs, M.; Seil, R.; Berruto, M.; Engebretsen, L.; Filardo, G.; Angele, P. Early osteoarthritis of the knee. *Knee Surg. Sports Traumatol. Arthrosc.* **2016**, *24*, 1753–1762. [CrossRef] [PubMed]
7. Øiestad, B.E.; Juhl, C.B.; Eitzen, I.; Thorlund, J.B. Knee extensor muscle weakness is a risk factor for development of knee osteoarthritis. A systematic review and meta-analysis. *Osteoarthr. Cartil.* **2015**, *23*, 171–177. [CrossRef]
8. Silverwood, V.; Blagojevic-Bucknall, M.; Jinks, C.; Jordan, J.L.; Protheroe, J.; Jordan, K.P. Current evidence on risk factors for knee osteoarthritis in older adults: A systematic review and meta-analysis. *Osteoarthr. Cartil.* **2015**, *23*, 507–515. [CrossRef]
9. Von Elm, E.; Altman, D.G.; Egger, M.; Pocock, S.J.; Gøtzsche, P.C.; Vandenbroucke, J.P. STROBE Initiative the Strengthening the Reporting of Observational Studies in Epidemiology (STROBE) statement: Guidelines for reporting observational studies. *J. Clin. Epidemiol.* **2008**, *61*, 344–349. [CrossRef]
10. Mahmoudian, A.; Lohmander, L.S.; Jafari, H.; Luyten, F.P. Towards classification criteria for early-stage knee osteoarthritis: A population-based study to enrich for progressors. *Semin. Arthritis Rheum.* **2021**, *51*, 285–291. [CrossRef]
11. Luyten, F.P.; Denti, M.; Filardo, G.; Kon, E.; Engebretsen, L. Definition and classification of early osteoarthritis of the knee. *Knee Surg. Sports Traumatol. Arthrosc.* **2012**, *20*, 401–406. [CrossRef] [PubMed]

12. Zhang, W.; McWilliams, D.F.; Ingham, S.L.; Doherty, S.A.; Muthuri, S.; Muir, K.R.; Doherty, M. Nottingham knee osteoarthritis risk prediction models. *Ann. Rheum. Dis.* **2011**, *70*, 1599–1604. [CrossRef] [PubMed]
13. Deep, K.; Nunag, P.; Willcox, N.; Deakin, A.H.; Picard, F. A Comparison of Three Different Methods of Measurement of Knee Deformity in Osteoarthritis. *J. Orthop. Rheumatol. Sports Med.* **2016**, *1*, 107. [CrossRef]
14. Bakar, Y.; Özdemir, Ö.; Sevim, S.; Duygu, E.; Tuğral, A.; Sürmeli, M. Intra-observer and inter-observer reliability of leg circumference measurement among six observers: A single blinded randomized trial. *J. Med. Life* **2017**, *10*, 176–181. [PubMed]
15. Malanga, G.A.; Andrus, S.; Nadler, S.F.; McLean, J. Physical examination of the knee: A review of the original test description and scientific validity of common orthopedic tests. *Arch. Phys. Med. Rehabil.* **2003**, *84*, 592–603. [CrossRef] [PubMed]
16. Lokhande, M.V.; Shetye, J.; Mehta, A.; Deo, M.V. Assessment of Knee Joint Proprioception in Weight Bearing and in Non-Weight Bearing Positions in Normal Subjects. *J. Krishna Inst. Med. Sci. Univ.* **2013**, *2*, 94–101.
17. Ruhdorfer, A.; Wirth, W.; Eckstein, F. Longitudinal Change in Thigh Muscle Strength Prior to and Concurrent with Minimum Clinically Important Worsening or Improvement in Knee Function: Data from the Osteoarthritis Initiative. *Arthritis Rheumatol.* **2016**, *68*, 826–836. [CrossRef]
18. Bohannon, R.W.; Bubela, D.J.; Magasi, S.R.; Gershon, R.C. Relative reliability of three objective tests of limb muscle strength. *Isokinet. Exerc. Sci.* **2011**, *19*, 77–81. [CrossRef]
19. Bhave, A.; Shabtai, L.; Woelber, E.; Apelyan, A.; Paley, D.; Herzenberg, J.E. Muscle strength and knee range of motion after femoral lengthening: 2- to 5-year follow-up. *Acta Orthop.* **2017**, *88*, 179–184. [CrossRef]
20. Paul, S.S.; Canning, C.G. Five-repetition sit-to-stand. *J. Physiother.* **2014**, *60*, 168. [CrossRef]
21. Bohannon, R.W.; Andrews, A.W.; Thomas, M.W. Walking speed: Reference values and correlates for older adults. *J. Orthop. Sports Phys. Ther.* **1996**, *24*, 86–90. [CrossRef] [PubMed]
22. Bohannon, R.W. Comfortable and maximum walking speed of adults aged 20–79 years: Reference values and determinants. *Age Ageing* **1997**, *26*, 15–19. [CrossRef] [PubMed]
23. Bijur, P.E.; Silver, W.; Gallagher, E.J. Reliability of the visual analog scale for measurement of acute pain. *Acad. Emerg. Med.* **2001**, *8*, 1153–1157. [CrossRef] [PubMed]
24. Ostelo, R.W.J.G.; Deyo, R.A.; Stratford, P.; Waddell, G.; Croft, P.; Von Korff, M.; Bouter, L.M.; de Vet, H.C. Interpreting Change Scores for Pain and Functional Status in Low Back Pain. *Spine* **2008**, *33*, 90–94. [CrossRef]
25. Leyland, K.M.; Gates, L.S.; Nevitt, M.; Felson, D.; Bierma-Zeinstra, S.M.; Conaghan, P.G.; Engebretsen, L.; Hochberg, M.; Hunter, D.J.; Jones, G.; et al. Harmonising measures of knee and hip osteoarthritis in population-based cohort studies: An international study. *Osteoarthr. Cartil.* **2018**, *26*, 872–879. [CrossRef]
26. Escobar, A.; Quintana, J.M.; Bilbao, A.; Azkárte, J.; Güenaga, L.I. Validation of the Spanish version of the WOMAC questionaire for patients with hip or knee osteoarthritis. *Clin. Rheumatol.* **2002**, *21*, 466–471. [CrossRef]
27. Vaquero, J.; Longo, U.G.; Forriol, F.; Martinelli, N.; Vethencourt, R.; Denaro, V. Reliability, validity and responsiveness of the Spanish version of the Knee Injury and Osteoarthritis Outcome Score (KOOS) in patients with chondral lesion of the knee. *Knee Surg. Sports Traumatol. Arthrosc.* **2014**, *22*, 104–108. [CrossRef]
28. Mouri, H. Log-normal distribution from a process that is not multiplicative but is additive. *Phys. Rev. E* **2013**, *88*, 42124. [CrossRef]
29. Nixon, R.M.; Wonderling, D.; Grieve, R.D. Non-parametric methods for cost-effectiveness analysis: The central limit theorem and the bootstrap compared. *Health Econ.* **2010**, *19*, 316–333. [CrossRef]
30. Hinkle, D.E.; Wiersma, W.; Jurs, S.G. Applied Statistics for the Behavioral Sciences. *Source J. Educ. Stat.* **1990**, *15*, 84–87.
31. Mahmoudian, A.; Lohmander, L.S.; Mobasheri, A.; Englund, M.; Luyten, F.P. Early-stage symptomatic osteoarthritis of the knee—Time for action. *Nat. Rev. Rheumatol.* **2021**, *17*, 621–632. [CrossRef] [PubMed]
32. Prieto-Alhambra, D.; Judge, A.; Javaid, M.K.; Cooper, C.; Diez-Perez, A.; Arden, N.K. Incidence and risk factors for clinically diagnosed knee, hip and hand osteoarthritis: Influences of age, gender and osteoarthritis affecting other joints. *Ann. Rheum. Dis.* **2014**, *73*, 1659–1664. [CrossRef] [PubMed]
33. Weiss, E. Knee osteoarthritis, body mass index and pain: Data from the osteoarthritis initiative. *Rheumatoogy* **2014**, *53*, 2095–2099. [CrossRef] [PubMed]
34. Neogi, T.; Zhang, Y. Osteoarthritis prevention. *Curr. Opin. Rheumatol.* **2011**, *23*, 185–191. [CrossRef]
35. Hurley, M.; Dickson, K.; Hallett, R.; Grant, R.; Hauari, H.; Walsh, N.; Stansfield, C.; Oliver, S. Exercise interventions and patient beliefs for people with hip, knee or hip and knee osteoarthritis: A mixed methods review. *Cochrane Database Syst. Rev.* **2018**, *4*, CD010842. [CrossRef]
36. Lee, J.; Chang, R.W.; Ehrlich-Jones, L.; Kwoh, C.K.; Nevitt, M.; Semanik, P.A.; Sharma, L.; Sohn, M.W.; Song, J.; Dunlop, D.D. Sedentary behavior and physical function: Objective evidence from the osteoarthritis initiative. *Arthritis Care Res.* **2015**, *67*, 366–373. [CrossRef]
37. Sharma, L. Osteoarthritis year in review 2015: Clinical. *Osteoarthr. Cartil.* **2016**, *24*, 36–48. [CrossRef]
38. White, D.K.; Tudor-Locke, C.; Zhang, Y.; Fielding, R.; Lavalley, M.; Felson, D.T.; Gross, K.D.; Nevitt, M.C.; Lewis, C.E.; Torner, J.; et al. Daily walking and the risk of incident functional limitation in knee osteoarthritis: An observational study. *Arthritis Care Res.* **2014**, *66*, 1328–1336. [CrossRef]
39. Ruhdorfer, A.; Wirth, W.; Hitzl, W.; Nevitt, M.; Eckstein, F. Association of Thigh Muscle Strength with Knee Symptoms and Radiographic Disease Stage of Osteoarthritis: Data from the Osteoarthritis Initiative. *Arthritis Care Res.* **2014**, *66*, 1344–1353. [CrossRef]

40. Runhaar, J.; van Middelkoop, M.; Reijman, M.; Vroegindeweij, D.; Oei, E.H.G.; Bierma-Zeinstra, S.M.A. Malalignment: A possible target for prevention of incident knee osteoarthritis in overweight and obese women. *Rheumatology* **2014**, *53*, 1618–1624. [CrossRef]
41. Marks, P.H.; Donaldson, M.L.C. Inflammatory cytokine profiles associated with chondral damage in the anterior cruciate ligament-deficient knee. *Arthrosc.—J. Arthrosc. Relat. Surg.* **2005**, *21*, 1342–1347. [CrossRef] [PubMed]
42. Keays, S.L.; Bullock-Saxton, J.E.; Newcombe, P.; Keays, A.C. The relationship between knee strength and functional stability before and after anterior cruciate ligament reconstruction. *J. Orthop. Res.* **2003**, *21*, 231–237. [CrossRef]
43. Greif, D.N.; Kouroupis, D.; Murdock, C.J.; Griswold, A.J.; Kaplan, L.D.; Best, T.M.; Correa, D. Infrapatellar Fat Pad/Synovium Complex in Early-Stage Knee Osteoarthritis: Potential New Target and Source of Therapeutic Mesenchymal Stem/Stromal Cells. *Front. Bioeng. Biotechnol.* **2020**, *8*, 860. [CrossRef] [PubMed]
44. Roman-Blas, J.A.; Mendoza-Torres, L.A.; Largo, R.; Herrero-Beaumont, G. Setting up distinctive outcome measures for each osteoarthritis phenotype. *Ther. Adv. Musculoskelet. Dis.* **2020**, *12*. [CrossRef] [PubMed]

diagnostics

MDPI

Article

Network Analysis Reveals That Headache-Related, Psychological and Psycho–Physical Outcomes Represent Different Aspects in Women with Migraine

César Fernández-de-las-Peñas [1,*], Lidiane L. Florencio [1], Umut Varol [2], Juan A. Pareja [3], Carlos Ordás-Bandera [4] and Juan A. Valera-Calero [2,5,*]

1 Department of Physical Therapy, Occupational Therapy, Rehabilitation and Physical Medicine, Universidad Rey Juan Carlos, 28922 Alcorcón, Spain
2 VALTRADOFI Research Group, Department of Physiotherapy, Faculty of Health, Camilo Jose Cela University, 28692 Villafranca del Castillo, Spain
3 Department of Neurology, Hospital Quirón Pozuelo, 28223 Madrid, Spain
4 Department of Neurology, Hospital Rey Juan Carlos, 28933 Móstoles, Spain
5 Department of Physiotherapy, Faculty of Health, Camilo José Cela University, 28692 Villafranca del Castillo, Spain
* Correspondence: cesar.fernandez@urjc.es (C.F.-d.-l.-P.); javalera@ucjc.edu (J.A.V.-C.)

Abstract: Evidence supports that migraine is a complex pain condition with different underlying mechanisms. We aimed to quantify potential associations between demographic, migraine-related, and psychophysical and psychophysical variables in women with migraine. Demographic (age, height, and weight), migraine-related (intensity, frequency, and duration), related-disability (Migraine Disability Assessment Scale, Headache Disability Inventory), psychological (Hospital Anxiety and Depression Scale), and psycho–physical (pressure pain thresholds -PPTs-) variables were collected from a sample of 74 women suffering from migraine. We calculated adjusted correlations between the variables by using a network analysis. Additionally, we also calculated centrality indices to identify the connectivity among the variables within the network and the relevance of each variable in the network. Multiple positive correlations (ρ) between PPTs were observed ranging from 0.1654 (C5-C6 and tibialis anterior) to 0.40 (hand and temporalis muscle). The strongest associations within the network were those between migraine attack frequency and diagnosis of chronic migraine (ρ = 0.634) and between the HDI-E and HDI-P (ρ = 0.545). The node with the highest strength and betweenness centrality was PPT at the second metacarpal, whereas the node with the highest harmonic centrality was PPT at the tibialis anterior muscle. This is the first study applying a network analysis to understand the underlying mechanisms in migraine. The identified network revealed that a model where each subgroup of migraine-related, psychological, and psycho–physical variables showed no interaction between each variable. Current findings could have clinical implications for developing multimodal treatments targeting the identified mechanisms.

Keywords: migraine; pressure pain; disability; network analysis

1. Introduction

Primary headaches are the pain disorders most commonly attended by neurologists in clinical practice and are ranked among the top ten disabling conditions worldwide in individuals under the age of 50 years [1,2]. The global prevalence of migraine is estimated to be up to 11.6% (13.8% in females, 6.9% in males) [3].

Current theories support the presence of complex mechanisms for underlying pathogenesis of migraine [4]. Although the main hypothesis associate migraine to an abnormal neuronal excitability with cortical spreading depression and to a hyperexcitability of trigeminovascular pathways [4], other factors such as pressure pain hyperalgesia [5], emotional–psychological factors [6], sleep disorders [7], or genetics [8] are also involved in migraine pathogenesis in a complex matrix. Previous studies investigating the potential associations between different aspects of migraine have commonly used Pearson Product-Moment Correlations or linear regressions. However, it should be noted that these analyses ignore the potential associations to arise from their interaction with another variable, as it is the case of Pearson Product-Moment Correlations, or ignore the possibility of bidirectional relationships between the variables, as it is the case of linear regression [9]. These potential limitations can be addressed using network analysis [10].

Network analysis provides a statistical method to identify the most important variables in the identified network, which could be used to potentially design better therapeutic strategies [11]. In fact, network analysis is starting to be used to better understand the complexity of chronic pain conditions such as tension-type headaches [12], fibromyalgia syndrome [13], carpal tunnel syndrome [14], or post-COVID pain [15]. From a network perspective, migraine represents a chronic pain condition sustained by multivariate interactions between migraine-related, emotional/psychological, and physiological systems. Since no previous study has used network analysis in individuals with migraine, we applied network analysis to better understand those potential interactions between migraine-related, emotional/psychological, and psychophysical variables. Therefore, the aim of this study was to describe a network including demographic, migraine-related, and emotional/psychophysical or psychophysical variables in women with migraine to illustrate its potential use for a better understanding of underlying mechanisms of migraine.

2. Methods

2.1. Participants

Consecutive women with migraine recruited from a headache unit located in a tertiary university-based hospital were screened for eligibility criteria between January 2017 and December 2018. Migraine diagnosis was conducted according to the third edition criteria of the International Classification of Headache Disorders (ICHD-III), the beta [16] or final [17] version by neurologists with more than 20 years of experience. Participants were excluded if they presented: 1, other concomitant headache; 2, neck or head trauma; 3, cervical herniated disk; 4, comorbid underlying medical disease; 5, fibromyalgia; 6, had changed medication intake within the previous 6 months; 7, had received any treatment including anesthetic blocks, botulinum toxin or physical therapy the previous 6 months; or, 8, pregnancy. The study was properly revised and approved by the Local Human Ethical Committee of Hospital Rey Juan Carlos (HRJ 07/14). All participants read and signed a written consent form prior to their participation in the study.

Participants were examined when they were headache-free or, in those with chronic migraine, when the intensity of the migraine attack the day of the evaluation was $\leq$3 points on the numerical pain rate scale (NPRS). Patients were asked to avoid taking any analgesic or muscle relaxant 24 h before their examination.

2.2. Migraine-Related Variables

Participants registered in a 4-week headache diary their number of days per week with a migraine attack, the duration of the attack (hours/day), and the pain intensity of each migraine attack on an 11-points NPRS (0: no pain; 10: the worst unimaginable pain) [18].

2.3. Disability-Related Variables

Since migraine is a highly disabling condition, we used two general questionnaires of headache and one specific for migraine.

The Headache Disability Inventory (HDI) is a 25-item questionnaire focusing on the impact of headache on emotional functioning and daily activities [19] with good test-retest reliability [20] and therefore was used for assessing the headache-related disability. Thirteen items evaluate the emotional burden (HDI-E, score from 0 to 52), and 12 items the physical burden (HDI-P, score from 0 to 48) of headache. A greater score suggests a greater headache-related burden. The Headache Impact Test (HIT-6) was the second headache-related general variables used for assessing a headache's impact [21]. The final score varies between 36 and 78 and higher scores suggest a more severe impact.

The Migraine Disability Assessment Scale (MIDAS) is a specific-disease questionnaire used to assess the degree of migraine-related disability in daily activities (work or school, family, and social) [22]. The MIDAS includes 5 questions related to days of partial or total loss within the last 3 months on: 1, paid work or school; 2, household chores; 3, family, social and leisure activities. The final score comes from the sum of the missed days regarding the 3 three activities. In the current study, we used the Spanish version of the MIDAS questionnaire which has proved to be a valid and reliable tool [23].

2.4. Emotional/Psychological Variables

For assessing the presence of anxiety and depression, we used The Hospital Anxiety and Depression Scale (HADS). This self-reported questionnaire consists of seven items assessing the presence or absence of anxiety (HADS-A) and seven analyzing depressive symptoms (HADS-D) [24]. Scores of each item range from 0 to 3 in a 4-point Likert scale (where higher scores indicate a worse health status), providing a maximum of 21 points for each subscale and 42 points in total. This scale was selected as it demonstrated good internal consistency in people with headaches [25].

2.5. Psycho–Physical Variables

An electronic pressure algometer (Somedic® Algometer, Sollentuna, Sweden) was used to calculate pressure pain thresholds (PPTs). We assessed PPT bilaterally over the temporalis muscle (a trigeminal point), C5-C6 joint (an extra-trigeminal point), as well as second metacarpal and tibialis anterior muscles (two remote pain-free points), as these sites have been found to exhibit pressure pain hyperalgesia in migraine sufferers [26]. A training session for familiarization with the procedure was conducted. The mean of 3 trials on each point, with a 30s resting period, was calculated and used in the analysis. The order of assessment was randomized between points on each participant. Since no side-to-side differences were observed (Student's *t*-test), the mean of both sides for each point was used in the network.

2.6. Statistical Analysis

2.6.1. Software and Packages

Data analyses were conducted on R software v.4.1.1 for Windows 10. Several packages were used for different purposes: qgraph (v.1.6.9) and glasso (v.1.11) for network estimation, igraph (v.1.2.6) for community detection, huge (v.1.3.5) for variable transformation, bootnet (v.1.4.3) for stability analysis, CINNA (v.1.1.54) for harmonic centrality measurement and mgm (v. 1.2-12) for estimating k-order mixed graphical models [27–29].

2.6.2. Exploratory Analysis

After conducting an exploratory data analysis on the dataset, 1 missing value was found for the MIDAS score. Since the removal of this missing value would result in loss of 1.35% of the data (73 records), this record was dropped from the dataset.

2.6.3. Network Estimation

The procedure of network analyses has been extensively described in previous papers by our research group [12–15]. We will briefly describe some important points here. Networks represent the variables as nodes and the associations between the variables as edges. The current network included 16 nodes, 15 continuous variables (age, psycho–physical, psychological, headache and health related variables), and one categorical variable (type of migraine).

We used the least absolute shrinkage and selection operator (LASSO, $\ell 1$-regularization) for including as few false positives as possible [27]. LASSO utilizes a tuning parameter λ (the strength of the penalty) for controlling the sparsity level that directly penalizes the likelihood function for the sum of absolute parameter values [27], and for creating a network structure that minimizes the number of spurious edges while maximizing the number of true edges [11].

2.6.4. Node Centrality

Centrality indices provide an estimation of the relevance of each node in the network. We calculated strength, harmonic, and betweenness centrality [30–33].

Node strength considers the total involvement of a particular node in a network for identifying the most relevant node. The node with a higher strength centrality may involve changes to the other nodes [33]. However, strength centrality does not consider the mediating role of other nodes and the number of connections with other nodes. Accordingly, using other centrality indicators is important to derive accurate conclusions [34].

Harmonic centrality was calculated instead of closeness centrality for the unconnected nodes found in the current network [35]. A node with high harmonic centrality could be easily affected by changes in another node's value directly or through changes in other nodes [33].

Finally, a node with a high betweenness centrality acts as an intermediary in the transmission of information or resources between other nodes or even clusters of nodes in the network [31].

2.6.5. Network Edge and Node Centrality Variability

Edge weights and centrality indices variability were assessed by using 1000 iterations to bootstrap 95% confidence intervals (CIs) of edge weights [31]. Wide confidence intervals would entangle the interpretation of the edge strength, yet not the presence, since model selection is already performed by LASSO.

For assessing the variability of the centrality indices (CS-coefficient), participant-dropping subset bootstrap was used [31]. This approach drops a percentage of participants, re-estimates the network, and relates three centrality indices. The CS-coefficient (correlation stability) reflects the maximum proportion of data that can be dropped (ideally >0.25 [11,31]) to retain a correlation > 0.7 with the original centrality indices (95% certainty) [11].

3. Results

Table 1 summarizes the descriptive data of the sample before and after missing value imputation. The network identified in our sample of 74 women with migraine is showed in Figure 1. Up to 18 correlations were seen between and within the variables. The network identified multiple positive correlations between PPTs among the different locations (nodes 13 to 16), with correlations (ρ) ranging from 0.165 (C5-C6 and tibialis anterior) to 0.409 (hand and temporalis). The strongest associations in the network were between migraine attack frequency and diagnosis of chronic migraine (ρ = 0.634) and between the HDI-E and HDI-P (ρ = 0.545). The rest of correlations ranged from 0.171 to 0.409 (Figure 1).

Edge weights variability is shown in Figure S1. The non-overlap of the 95% CI of the edge between PPTs at the neck and tibialis anterior locations (nodes 13 and 16) with the 95% CI of the edge between physical and emotional burden because of headache disability (nodes 7 and 8) indicates that the strength of former is significantly greater than the latter.

As shown in Figure 2, the node with the highest strength and betweenness centrality was PPT at the second metacarpal (hand), followed by emotional burden because of migraine (HDI-E).

Table 1. Values (mean ± standard deviation= of baseline characteristics of the total sample (n = 74).

Variable	Baseline Scores	Missing Values (n; %)
Age (years)	42.3 ± 12.1	0; 0
Migraine Type (n; %)		
Episodic (1)	56; 75.6	0; 0
Chronic (2)	18; 24.4	0; 0
Years with Migraine (years)	19.6 ± 13.9	0; 0
Migraine Intensity (0–10)	8.1 ± 2.0	0; 0
Migraine Frequency (n/month)	9.9 ± 8.1	0; 0
Migraine Duration (hours/episode)	24.2 ± 20.6	0; 0
HDI-E (0–52)	27.0 ± 13.4	0; 0
HDI-P (0–48)	34.7 ± 11.5	0; 0
HADS-A (0–21)	12.3 ± 2.5	0; 0
HADS-D (0–21)	10.5 ± 3.0	0; 0
HIT6 (36–78)	63.0 ± 7.3	0; 0
MIDAS (days missed work)	46.3 ± 69.3	1; 1.35
PPT Neck (kPa)	135.4 ± 46.5	0; 0
PPT Temporalis (kPa)	156.7 ± 61.6	0; 0
PPT Hand (kPa)	194.5 ± 64.1	0; 0
PPT Tibialis Anterior (kPa)	327.0 ± 114.2	0; 0

HADS: Hospital Anxiety and Depression Scale; HDI: Headache Disability Index; HIT: Headache Impact Test; MIDAS: Migraine Disability Assessment Scale; PPT: Pressure Pain Thresholds.

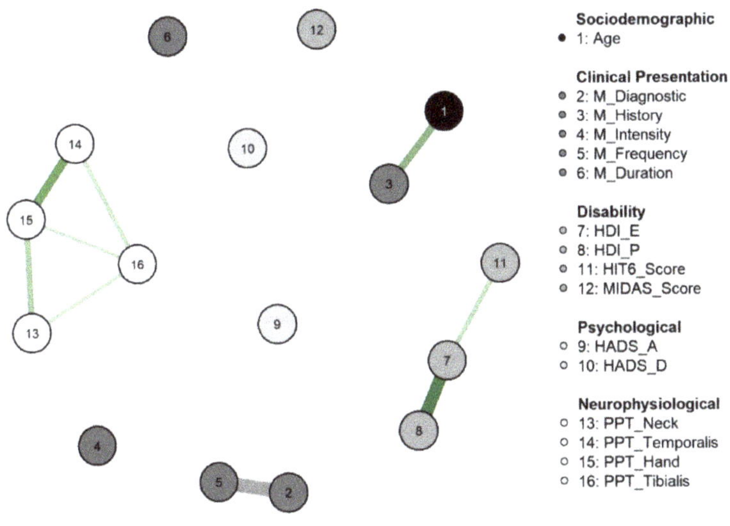

Figure 1. Network analysis of the association between demographic, migraine-related, psychological, and psycho–physical/neuro-physiological measures. Edges represent connections between two nodes and adjusted for the remaining nodes. Direction of the partial correlations were expressed as the color green for positive associations. The color Grey represents the association for categorical variables which no sign is defined. The thickness and color saturation of an edge denotes its weight (the strength of the association between two nodes).

The node with the highest harmonic centrality was PPT at the tibialis anterior, followed by PPT at the cervical spine (Figure 3).

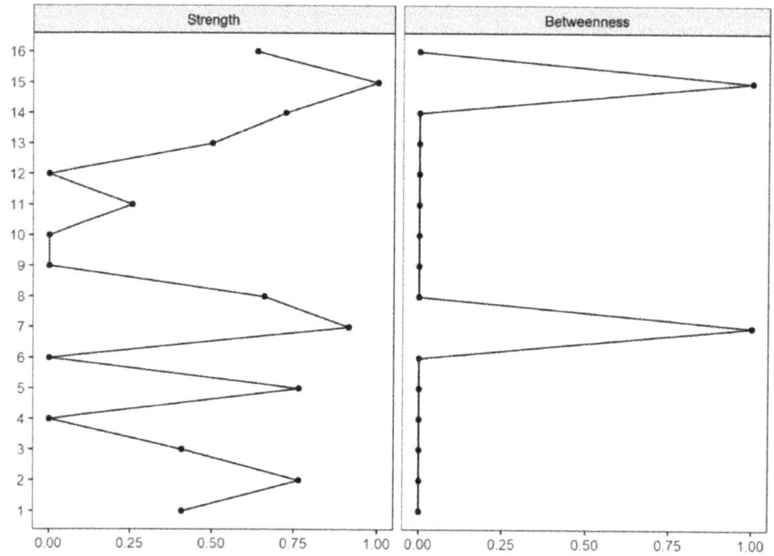

Figure 2. Centrality values (1: maximal importance; 0: no importance) of Strength and Betweenness of each node in the network.

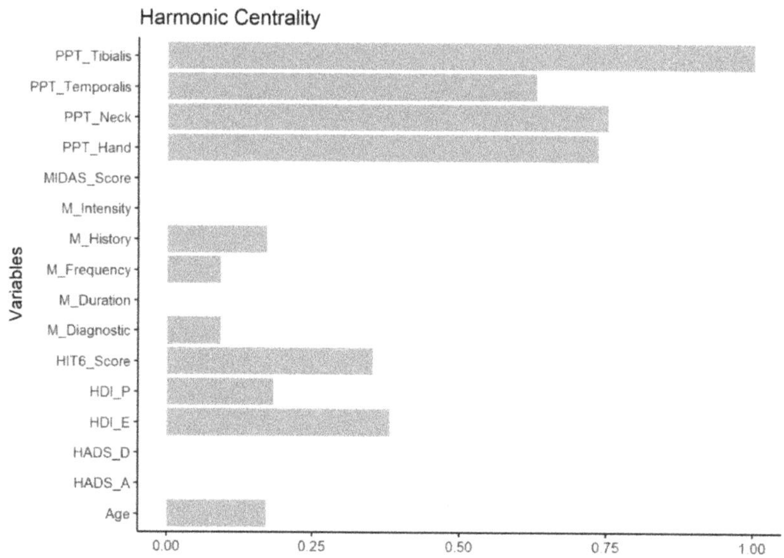

Figure 3. Harmonic Centrality measure (1: maximal importance; 0: no importance) of each node in the network.

The betweenness and strength measures of the network were extremely unstable at $CS_{cor=0.7} = 0.000$ and $CS_{cor=0.7} = 0.287$, respectively. The closeness centrality measure could not be assessed with bootstrapping since the resulting networks were unconnected (Figure 4).

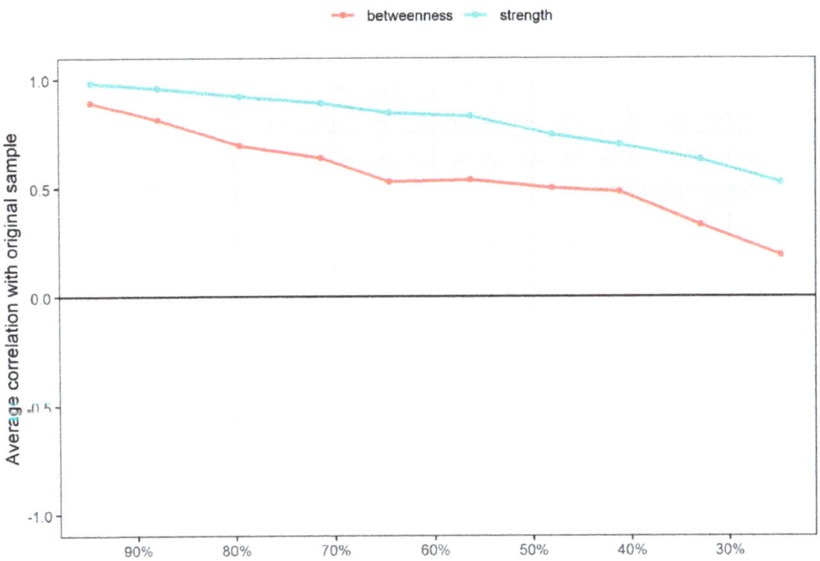

Figure 4. Average correlations between centrality indices of networks sampled with persons dropped and networks built on the entire input dataset, at all follow-up time points. Lines indicate the means and areas indicate the range from the 2.5th quantile to the 97.5th quantile.

4. Discussion

Current evidence supports the influence of multiple biopsychosocial mechanisms contributing to the pathogenesis of migraine [4]. This study used a network analysis for better understanding the multivariate interactions between migraine-related, emotional/psychological, or psychophysical variables in women with migraine. The identified network revealed a model where each subgroup of variables (e.g., migraine-related, psychological, and psycho–physical) showed no interaction between each variable.

The identified network identified different clusters grouping each subtype of variables, but without association between them. These results support the multidimensional complexity of migraine. For instance, psycho–physical variables, i.e., widespread PPTs, were grouped in the same cluster. The topic of pressure hyperalgesia in migraine sufferers has been extensively discussed in headache literature [5]. In fact, PPTs in distant pain-free areas, i.e., the second metacarpal and tibialis anterior, exhibited the strongest centrality values. In such a scenario, current results suggest that if clinicians want to influence other migraine-related variables, e.g., migraine pain or disability, included in the identified network, the best variable to focus treatment on would be PPTs, highlighting the relevance of widespread pressure pain hypersensitivity, as a manifestation of sensitization processes in migraine sufferers. This hypothesis would support current assumptions for applying therapeutic interventions such as aerobic exercise or pain neuroscience education for the treatment of migraine [36,37], since these interventions induce centrally mediated hypoalgesia effects. Accordingly, management of the trigeminal area would be also needed to reduce sensitivity of the trigeminocervical nucleus caudalis, the structure responsible for the triggering of migraine attacks and the sensitization process of the nervous system. Further, it should be noted that the network did not identify significant associations of widespread pressure hypersensitivity with migraine clinical parameters. In agreement with these results, previous data suggested no associations between PPTs and clinical outcomes, such as pain and related disability in chronic spinal pain [38]. It is plausible that pressure pain sensitivity reflects the neurophysiological mechanism, whereas headache clinical variables represent a clinical manifestation of pain pathways, hence representing two different aspects of nociception. Nevertheless, it has been found that higher pressure pain sensitivity as expressed by lower PPTs predict future pain and disability in musculoskeletal pain [39]; accordingly, early management of individuals with migraine could help to reduce the possibility of developing higher degree of sensitization.

The network identified that psychological and migraine-related disability variables did not exhibit significant associations with other variables. A recent meta-analysis has found that depressive and anxiety disorders are the most frequently addressed comorbidities in individuals with migraine and that their prevalence rates seem to be higher than expected [40]. The presence of emotional/psychological disorders support why interventions such as cognitive behavioural therapy have been found to be effective for the management of migraine [41,42]. In fact, psychological interventions are not effective just for improving emotional/cognitive outcomes, but are also effective for reducing headache frequency [43]. In fact, migraine frequency was an independent variable in the identified network, suggesting that it could represent a relevant variable to be addressed in clinical practice. Headache frequency is used to classify patients on episodic or chronic migraine [16,17]. Our sample mostly included women with episodic migraine (75%). The fact that migraine frequency and, accordingly, migraine diagnosis, were independent variables in our network would suggest that identified associations should be similar in either group, episodic or chronic migraine; however, we were unable to conduct separate analyses by group because of the sample size. Future studies should investigate if the identified network is similar (or different) between women with episodic or chronic migraine.

Similarly, management of migraine-related disability should be the focus of specific therapeutic approaches. In such a scenario, [44] it should be observed that manual therapy interventions could be effective for reducing migraine-related disability as assessed with the HIT-6 scale at short and mid-term, although the level of evidence was very low. In fact, specific manual therapy, e.g., spinal manipulation, has been found to be effective for the reduction in migraine days and pain intensity [45]. The results from this network further reinforce the proposal of applying multimodal therapeutic approaches targeting migraine-related pain and disability (i.e., manual therapy), psychological aspects (i.e., cognitive behavior, and relaxation approaches), health-related (i.e., exercise programs), and also nociceptive mechanisms (i.e., neuroscience pain education programs) [46].

Despite the positive aspects of using a network approach in people with migraine, some limitations are also present. First, the edge weights identified in the network cannot be a source of confirmatory causal inference but may provide indicative potential causal pathways [11]. In other words, biological plausibility between the connected variables is needed from a clinical point of view to determine the viability of the analysis. The current network did not report local associations between the subgroups of variables. Second, we recruited women with migraine from a single university-based headache center; therefore, it may be not representative of general population of migraine sufferers. Additionally, since all individuals were women, accordingly, extrapolation to men with migraine would be not appropriate.

5. Conclusions

The application of network analysis in a sample of women with migraine revealed that a model where each subgroup of variables, i.e., migraine-related, psychological, and psycho–physical, showed no interaction between each variable. The network showed that PPTs exhibited the highest centrality measures, supporting a relevant role of pressure pain sensitivity and sensitization in the model. The complex interactions identified in the current network support the contention that migraine treatment should include multimodal therapeutic approaches targeting all these aspects.

Supplementary Materials: The following supporting information can be downloaded at: https://www.mdpi.com/article/10.3390/diagnostics12102318/s1, Figure S1: Bootstrapped 95% quantile confidence interval of the estimated edge weights of the network. "Bootstrap mean" reflects the average magnitude of edge weights across the bootstrapped samples. "Sample" reflects the magnitude of edge weights of the original network built on the entire input dataset.

Author Contributions: Conceptualization, J.A.V.-C.; methodology, all authors; software, U.V.; validation, all authors; formal analysis, J.A.V.-C.; investigation, all authors; resources, C.F.-d.-l.-P.; data curation, U.V.; writing—original draft preparation, J.A.V.-C. and C.F.-d.-l.-P.; writing-review and editing, all authors; visualization, all authors; supervision, J.A.V.-C. and C.F.-d.-l.-P.; project administration, C.F.-d.-l.-P. All authors have read and agreed to the published version of the manuscript.

Funding: This research received no external funding.

Institutional Review Board Statement: The study was conducted according to the guidelines of the Declaration of Helsinki and approved by the Institutional Review Board of Universidad Rey Juan Carlos and Hospital Rey Juan Carlos (URJC 23/2081, HRJ 07/18).

Informed Consent Statement: Informed consent was obtained from all subjects involved in the study.

Data Availability Statement: All data derived from this study are presented in the text.

Conflicts of Interest: The authors declare no conflict of interest.

References

1. GBD 2019 Diseases and Injuries Collaborators. Global burden of 369 diseases and injuries in 204 countries and territories, 1990–2019: A systematic analysis for the Global Burden of Disease Study 2019. *Lancet* **2020**, *396*, 1204–1222. [CrossRef]
2. Steiner, T.J.; Stovner, L.J.; Vos, T. GBD 2015: Migraine is the third cause of disability in under 50s. *J. Headache Pain* **2016**, *17*, 104. [CrossRef] [PubMed]
3. Woldeamanuel, Y.W.; Cowan, R.P. Migraine affects 1 in 10 people worldwide featuring recent rise: A systematic review and meta-analysis of community-based studies involving 6 million participants. *J. Neurol. Sci.* **2017**, *372*, 307–315. [CrossRef] [PubMed]
4. Ashina, M. Migraine. *N. Engl. J. Med.* **2020**, *383*, 1866–1876. [CrossRef]
5. Nahman-Averbuch, H.; Shefi, T.; Schneider, V.J., 2nd; Li, D.; Ding, L.; King, C.D.; Coghill, R.C. Quantitative sensory testing in patients with migraine: A systemic review and meta-analysis. *Pain* **2018**, *159*, 1202–1223. [CrossRef]
6. Garramone, F.; Baiano, C.; Russo, A.; D'Iorio, A.; Tedeschi, G.; Trojano, L.; Santangelo, G. Personality profile and depression in migraine: A meta-analysis. *Neurol. Sci.* **2020**, *41*, 543–554. [CrossRef]
7. Fernández-de-las-Peñas, C.; Fernández-Muñoz, J.J.; Palacios-Ceña, M.; Parás-Bravo, P.; Cigarán-Méndez, M.; Navarro-Pardo, E. Sleep disturbances in tension-type headache and migraine. *Ther. Adv. Neurol. Dis.* **2018**, *11*, 1756285617745444. [CrossRef]
8. Zhao, Y.; Zhu, R.; Xiao, T.; Liu, X. Genetic variants in migraine: A field synopsis and systematic re-analysis of meta-analyses. *J. Headache Pain* **2020**, *21*, 13. [CrossRef]
9. Epskamp, S.; Fried, E.I. A tutorial on regularized partial correlation networks. *Psychol. Methods* **2018**, *23*, 617–634. [CrossRef]
10. Schmittmann, V.D.; Cramer, A.O.J.; Waldorp, L.J.; Epskamp, S.; Kievit, R.A.; Borsboom, D. Deconstructing the construct: A network perspective on psychological phenomena. *New Ideas Psychol.* **2013**, *31*, 43–53. [CrossRef]
11. Valente, T.W. Network Interventions. *Science* **2012**, *337*, 49. [CrossRef] [PubMed]
12. Fernández-de-las-Peñas, C.; Palacios-Ceña, M.; Valera-Calero, J.A.; Cuadrado, M.L.; Guerrero-Peral, A.; Pareja, J.A.; Arendt-Nielsen, L.; Varol, U. Understanding the interaction between clinical, emotional and psychophysical outcomes underlying tension-type headache: A network analysis approach. *J. Neurol.* **2022**, *269*, 4525–4534. [CrossRef] [PubMed]
13. Valera-Calero, J.A.; Arendt-Nielsen, L.; Cigarán-Méndez, M.; Fernández-de-las-Peñas, C.; Varol, U. Network analysis for better understanding the complex psycho-biological mechanisms behind fibromyalgia syndrome. *Diagnostics* **2022**, *12*, 1845. [CrossRef]
14. Liew, B.X.W.; de-la-Llave-Rincón, A.I.; Arias-Buría, J.L.; Ortega-Santiago, R.; Fernández-de-las-Peñas, C. Understanding the psychophysiological mechanisms related to widespread pressure pain hyperalgesia underpinning carpal tunnel syndrome: A network analysis approach. *Pain Med.* **2021**, *22*, 2708–2717. [CrossRef] [PubMed]
15. Fernández-de-las-Peñas, C.; Herrero-Montes, M.; Cancela-Cilleruelo, I.; Rodríguez-Jiménez, J.; Parás-Bravo, P.; Varol, U.; Del-Valle-Loarte, P.; Flox-Benítez, G.; Arendt-Nielsen, L.; Valera-Calero, J.A. Understanding sensitization, cognitive and neuropathic associated mechanisms behind post-COVID Pain: A network analysis. *Diagnostics* **2022**, *12*, 1538. [CrossRef]
16. Headache Classification Committee of the International Headache Society (IHS). The International Classification of Headache Disorders, 3rd edition (beta version). *Cephalalgia* **2013**, *33*, 629–808. [CrossRef]
17. Headache Classification Committee of the International Headache Society (IHS). The International Classification of Headache Disorders, 3rd edition. *Cephalalgia* **2018**, *38*, 1–211. [CrossRef]

18. Phillip, D.; Lyngberg, A.; Jensen, R. Assessment of headache diagnosis. A comparative population study of a clinical interview with a diagnostic headache diary. *Cephalalgia* **2007**, *27*, 1–8. [CrossRef]
19. Jacobson, G.P.; Ramadan, N.M.; Aggarwal, S.K.; Newman, C.W. The Henry Ford Hospital Headache Disability Inventory (HDI). *Neurology* **1994**, *44*, 837–842. [CrossRef]
20. Jacobson, G.P.; Ramadan, N.M.; Norris, L.; Newman, C.W. Headache disability inventory (HDI): Short-term test-retest reliability and spouse perceptions. *Headache* **1995**, *35*, 534–539. [CrossRef]
21. Kosinski, M.; Bayliss, M.S.; Bjorner, J.B.; Ware, J.E.; Garber, W.H.; Batenhorst, A.; Cady, R.; Dahlöf, C.G.H.; Dowson, A.; Tepper, S. A six-item short-form survey for measuring headache impact: The HIT-6TM. *Qual. Life Res.* **2003**, *12*, 963–974. [CrossRef] [PubMed]
22. Stewart, W.F.; Lipton, R.B.; Kolodner, K.; Sawyer, J.; Lee, C.; Liberman, J.N. Validity of the Migraine Disability Assessment (MIDAS) score in comparison to a diary-based measure in a population sample of migraine sufferers. *Pain* **2000**, *88*, 41–52. [CrossRef]
23. Rodríguez-Almagro, D.; Achalandabaso, A.; Rus, A.; Obrero-Gaitán, E.; Zagalaz-Anula, N.; Lomas-Vega, R. Validation of the Spanish version of the migraine disability assessment questionnaire (MIDAS) in university students with migraine. *BMC Neurol.* **2020**, *20*, 67. [CrossRef]
24. Zigmond, A.S.; Snaith, R.P. The hospital anxiety and depression scale. *Acta Psychiatr. Scand.* **1983**, *67*, 361–370. [CrossRef] [PubMed]
25. Juang, K.D.; Wang, S.J.; Lin, C.H.; Fuh, J.L. Use of the hospital anxiety and depression scale as a screening tool for patients with headache. *Zhonghua Yi Xue Za Zhi* **1999**, *62*, 749–755. [PubMed]
26. Palacios-Ceña, M.; Lima Florencio, L.; Natália Ferracini, G.; Barón, J.; Guerrero, Á.L.; Ordás-Bandera, C.; Arendt-Nielsen, L.; Fernández-de-las-Peñas, C. Women with chronic and episodic migraine exhibit similar widespread pressure pain sensitivity. *Pain Med.* **2016**, *17*, 2127–2133. [CrossRef] [PubMed]
27. Friedman, J.; Hastie, T.; Tibshirani, R. Glasso: Graphical Lasso Estimation of Gaussian Graphical Models. R Package Version 20141. Available online: http://www-stat.stanford.edu/~{}tibs/glasso (accessed on 1 March 2022).
28. Stekhoven, D.J.; Bühlmann, P. MissForest: Non-parametric missing value imputation for mixed-type data. *Bioinformatics* **2012**, *28*, 112–118. [CrossRef]
29. Lauritzen, S.L.; Wermuth, N. Graphical models for associations between variables, some of which are qualitative and some quantitative. *Ann. Stat.* **1989**, *17*, 31–57. [CrossRef]
30. Haslbeck, J.M.B.; Waldorp, L.J. How well do network models predict observations? On the importance of predictability in network models. *Behav. Res. Methods* **2018**, *50*, 853–861. [CrossRef]
31. Bloch, F.; Jackson, M.O.; Tebaldi, P. Centrality Measures in Networks. 1 June 2019. Available online: https://papers.ssrn.com/sol3/papers.cfm?abstract_id=2749124 (accessed on 1 March 2022).
32. Freeman, L.C. Centrality in social networks conceptual clarification. *Soc. Netw.* **1978**, *1*, 215–239. [CrossRef]
33. Newman, M.E.J. Analysis of weighted networks. *Phys. Rev. E* **2004**, *70*, 056131. [CrossRef] [PubMed]
34. Opsahl, T.; Agneessens, F.; Skvoretz, J. Node centrality in weighted networks: Generalizing degree and shortest paths. *Soc. Netw.* **2010**, *32*, 245–251. [CrossRef]
35. Rochat, Y. Closeness centrality extended to unconnected graphs: The harmonic centrality index. In Proceedings of the ASNA 2009, Zurich, Switzerland, 27–28 August 2009. Application of Social Network Analysis Conference.
36. Kindelan-Calvo, P.; Gil-Martínez, A.; Paris-Alemany, A.; Pardo-Montero, J.; Muñoz-García, D.; Angulo-Díaz-Parreño, S.; La Touche, R. Effectiveness of therapeutic patient education for adults with migraine. A systematic review and meta-analysis of randomized controlled trials. *Pain Med.* **2014**, *15*, 1619–1636. [CrossRef] [PubMed]
37. La Touche, R.; Fernández Pérez, J.J.; Proy Acosta, A.; González Campodónico, L.; Martínez García, S.; Adraos Juárez, D.; Serrano García, B.; Angulo-Díaz-Parreño, S.; Cuenca-Martínez, F.; Suso-Martí, L.; et al. Is aerobic exercise helpful in patients with migraine? A systematic review and meta-analysis. *Scand. J. Med. Sci. Sports* **2020**, *30*, 965–982. [CrossRef]
38. Hübscher, M.; Moloney, N.; Leaver, A.; Rebbeck, T.; McAuley, J.H.; Refshauge, K.M. Relationship between quantitative sensory testing and pain or disability in people with spinal pain-a systematic review and meta-analysis. *Pain* **2013**, *154*, 1497–1504. [CrossRef]
39. Georgopoulos, V.; Akin-Akinyosoye, K.; Zhang, W.; McWilliams, D.F.; Hendrick, P.; Walsh, D.A. Quantitative sensory testing and predicting outcomes for musculoskeletal pain, disability, and negative affect: A systematic review and meta-analysis. *Pain* **2019**, *160*, 1920–1932. [CrossRef]
40. Caponnetto, V.; Deodato, M.; Robotti, M.; Koutsokera, M.; Pozzilli, V.; Galati, C.; Nocera, G.; De Matteis, E.; De Vanna, G.; Fellini, E.; et al. Comorbidities of primary headache disorders: A literature review with meta-analysis. *J. Headache Pain* **2021**, *22*, 71. [CrossRef]
41. Probyn, K.; Bowers, H.; Mistry, D.; Caldwell, F.; Underwood, M.; Patel, S.; Sandhu, H.K.; Matharu, M.; Pincus, T.; CHESS Team. Non-pharmacological self-management for people living with migraine or tension-type headache: A systematic review including analysis of intervention components. *BMJ Open* **2017**, *7*, e016670. [CrossRef]
42. Perlini, C.; Donisi, V.; Del Piccolo, L. From research to clinical practice: A systematic review of the implementation of psychological interventions for chronic headache in adults. *BMC Health Serv. Res.* **2020**, *20*, 459. [CrossRef]

43. Lee, H.J.; Lee, J.H.; Cho, E.Y.; Kim, S.M.; Yoon, S. Efficacy of psychological treatment for headache disorder: A systematic review and meta-analysis. *J. Headache Pain* **2019**, *20*, 17. [CrossRef]
44. Falsiroli Maistrello, L.; Rafanelli, M.; Turolla, A. Manual therapy and quality of life in people with headache: Systematic review and meta-analysis of randomized controlled trials. *Curr. Pain Headache Rep.* **2019**, *23*, 78. [CrossRef] [PubMed]
45. Rist, P.M.; Hernandez, A.; Bernstein, C.; Kowalski, M.; Osypiuk, K.; Vining, R.; Long, C.R.; Goertz, C.; Song, R.; Wayne, P.M. The impact of spinal manipulation on migraine pain and disability: A systematic review and meta-analysis. *Headache* **2019**, *59*, 532–542. [CrossRef] [PubMed]
46. Fernández-de-las-Peñas, C.; Florencio, L.L.; Plaza-Manzano, G.; Arias-Buría, J.L. Clinical reasoning behind non-pharmacological interventions for the management of headaches: A narrative literature review. *Int. J. Environ. Res. Public Health* **2020**, *17*, 4126. [CrossRef] [PubMed]

diagnostics

MDPI

Review

Clinical Diagnosis and Treatment of Chronic Pain

Sadiq Rahman, Ali Kidwai, Emiliya Rakhamimova, Murad Elias, William Caldwell and Sergio D. Bergese *

Department of Anesthesiology, Stony Brook University Hospital, Stony Brook, NY 11794, USA; sadiq.rahman@stonybrookmedicine.edu (S.R.); ali.kidwai@stonybrookmedicine.edu (A.K.); emiliya.rakhamimova@stonybrookmedicine.edu (E.R.); murad.elias@stonybrookmedicine.edu (M.E.); william.caldwell@stonybrookmedicine.edu (W.C.)

* Correspondence: sergio.bergese@stonybrookmedicine.edu

Abstract: More than 600 million people globally are estimated to be living with chronic pain. It is one of the most common complaints seen in an outpatient setting, with over half of patients complaining of pain during a visit. Failure to properly diagnose and manage chronic pain is associated with substantial morbidity and mortality, especially when opioids are involved. Furthermore, it is a tremendous financial strain on the healthcare system, as over USD 100 billion is spent yearly in the United States on healthcare costs related to pain management and opioids. This exceeds the costs of diabetes, heart disease, and cancer-related care combined. Being able to properly diagnose, manage, and treat chronic pain conditions can substantially lower morbidity, mortality, and healthcare costs in the United States. This review will outline the current definitions, biopsychosocial model, subclassifications, somatosensory assessments, imaging, clinical prediction models, and treatment modalities associated with chronic pain.

Keywords: chronic pain; pain diagnostics; pain classification; pain approach; biopsychosocial

1. Introduction

Chronic pain has become a ubiquitous condition encountered by many patients seeking medical care. Pain is a subjective experience and one of the leading causes of patient suffering and disability [1]. The Global Burden of Disease (GBD) Study highlighted the high prominence of pain as a global cause of disability in both developed and developing nations. The study also highlighted how this assessment of burden is also an underestimate. Chronic lower back pain, for example, was noted to be the single greatest cause of years lived with disability (YLD) around the world [2]. Lower back pain remains the leading cause of disability globally, impacting 619 million individuals globally in 2020, and it is anticipated to increase to 843 million in the next three decades [3].

Many forms of chronic pain, like lower back pain, come without a diagnosable underlying pathology and are often categorized as "non-specific" [4]. This has led to calls for research efforts to better understand the underlying pathophysiology of various chronic pain conditions. Other conditions of perceived pain, like central pain amplification, cannot currently be explained through somatic or neuropathic processes and are instead due to alterations in pain modulatory pathways [5].

"Non-specific" forms of chronic pain can lead to the pooling of heterogenous disease processes and consequently less specific pain management modalities. For optimized management of chronic pain, proper diagnosis and classification is highly recommended. This review will also discuss the recent somatosensory assessments, imaging, and clinical prediction models used for chronic pain conditions. The biopsychosocial treatment of chronic pain is also complex and multifaceted, including pharmacological interventions, physical rehabilitation, and interventional procedures [6–8].

2. Defining Chronic Pain

The most common symptom reported to health care providers is pain. Chronic pain is often used as an umbrella term for a wide range of painful conditions from nonspecific lower back pain to fibromyalgia to complex regional pain syndrome (CRPS). While acute pain may serve an adaptive role, chronic pain has been widely considered to be clinically maladaptive, that "neither protects nor supports healing and repair" [9]. Chronic pain was previously defined as pain persisting past a normal healing time and lacking the advantage of acute pain's warning function [10].

It is often defined as pain that persists longer than "normal healing" and widely agreed to be at least three months in duration. Chronic pain also has been used as a label for a patient's condition when underlying causes of pain are unclear or have been unidentified. This reinforces the need for more precise and updated methods of diagnosis and treatment for the many patients who encounter chronic pain.

The International Association for the Study of Pain (IASP) characterizes pain as an unpleasant sensory and emotional experience associated with, or resembling, actual or potential tissue damage [11]. The IASP definition of chronic pain has become widely adopted by health care professionals and academic researchers and even adopted by professional organizations such as the World Health Organization (WHO).

The need for adequate revision for chronic pain diagnoses in the International Classification of Diseases (ICD) system has also been expressed as it is crucial for not only improvements in treatment but also for launching relevant research programs. Current iterations and classifications of chronic pain conditions are sometimes poorly defined and arbitrarily distributed in the ICD system [12]. As recently as the release of the ICD-10, chronic postsurgical and posttraumatic pain was not being represented; it was only defined as of 2022 within the ICD-11 [13].

Thoughts, emotions, and stress also affect the perception of pain, so a biopsychosocial assessment of pain helps provide a more complete definition and overview of conditions associated with chronic pain [14]. Neuroscience research indicates pain pathways in the central nervous system (CNS) often work in conjunction with emotions. Pain pathways can also be stimulated by peripheral tissues and traumatic experiences [15].

The biopsychosocial model views illness as a complex interaction between psychological, social, and biological factors [16]. This has also led to the development of an interdisciplinary pain management approach. Conceptualizing, assessing, and treating chronic pain would be incomplete without a sophisticated understanding of the emotional states and processes linked with the condition [17].

3. Burdens of Chronic Pain

Chronic pain does not come without significant personal and economic burden across the globe; affecting more than thirty percent of the world population [18]. Prevalence in the United States has been noted to vary between 11% and 40% with the US Centers for Disease Control and Prevention (CDC) estimating point prevalence at 20.4% (approximately 50 million), with higher prevalence rates associated with women and adults living in poverty and from lower socioeconomic backgrounds and rural areas [19]. Furthermore, the CDC estimates that 8% of U.S. adults (20 million) suffer high-impact chronic pain (i.e., interfering with work or life most days or every day).

In one cohort study [20], 61.4% of adults with chronic pain in 2019 had their condition continue in 2020 and estimated a higher incidence of chronic pain (52.4 cases per 1000 PY) compared to diabetes (7.1 cases per 1000 PY), depression (15.9 cases per 1000 PY), and hypertension (45.3 cases per 1000 PY). A strong example of the prevalence of chronic pain can be seen with lower back pain as it is a very common symptom experienced by patients of all ages [21–23].

Furthermore, chronic pain affects more than 50% of the older population and up to 80% of nursing homes residents [24]. Hyperalgesia and delayed recovery from pain secondary to nerve injury was also observed in this population [25]. Another novel finding in chronic pain research found high comorbidities with insomnia. Approximately 50% of chronic patients experience clinically significant sleep disturbances [26]. A lack of restorative sleep can further exacerbate and continue a cycle of chronic pain related symptoms.

Indicators of socioeconomic status including poverty, education, and health insurance coverage are associated with the presence of specific health conditions like chronic pain. It is estimated that chronic pain has an economic impact estimated to be USD 560 billion in direct medical costs, lost productivity, and disability [27]. Chronic pain also has a functional impact as one study found patients with chronic pain had increased difficulty with activities of daily living (21.5% vs. 4.9%), social engagement (25.4% vs. 5.7%), and work limitations (48.8% vs. 15%), leading to an estimated USD 79.9 billion in lost wages [28]. Effective diagnosis and treatment of chronic pain can help alleviate some of the financial impact chronic pain has on many households and communities.

4. Diagnosing Chronic Pain

Properly diagnosing chronic pain is crucial to the successful management of the condition. In the field of headache research, strict criteria for headaches such as migraines help dictate diagnosis and treatment and facilitate additional inquiry. As previously discussed, chronic pain is currently defined as pain that persists or recurs for more than 3 months, consistent with temporal cutoffs associated with other chronic diseases [29]. The 3-month criterion is a common temporal cutoff for chronic conditions. This allows chronic pain diagnoses to remain consistent with criteria of many other chronic health conditions, which facilitates a uniform measure across clinical practice, health statistics, and academia.

Reaching a timely, accurate diagnosis for chronic pain is important to avoid progression towards a chronic disease. One study examining 180 patients with complex regional pain syndrome (CRPS) found that a long a time between onset and diagnosis was predictive for late recovery and the progression of symptoms [30]. Similarly, data from a cross-sectional study found a median diagnostic delay of eight years for spondyloarthritis, and delayed diagnosis was also associated with worse outcomes and poor treatment responses [31]. Another complex disorder, fibromyalgia, is a challenge for healthcare providers as one study found a mean time to diagnosis as long as 6.42 years, with older patients diagnosed at a slower rate [32].

There have been recent initiatives to develop a more personalized and precision-based approach to chronic pain diagnosis and treatment. For example, one study examined a diagnostic approach that would address specific mechanisms behind "non-specific" chronic low back pain to personalize treatment [33]. Described as a "pain diagnostic ladder", this approach encourages a classification of chronic low back pain based on its anatomical, pathological, and mechanistic base [34–36].

To localize pain anatomically, a proper musculoskeletal (MSK) physical exam and local anesthetic injections may be utilized as diagnostic tools. However, the MSK physical exam has limited localizing value, and local anesthetic injections are an invasive means of deriving diagnostic information. It is valuable to monitor for changes in the quality of the patient's pain that may suggest persistent changes in central nervous system (CNS) nociceptors, which may decrease the relevancy of identifying a precipitating peripheral cause of pain.

The authors of this study additionally suggest increasing the characterization for pathological "degenerative low back pain", advocating for distinctions between pathologies that are nociceptive [37], inflammatory [38], neuropathic, or centralized/dysfunctional [39]. Finally, the mechanistic component of pain refers to its cellular mechanisms, which may be utilized to narrow down pharmacological interventions. Examples include utilization of NMDA-antagonists such as ketamine or dual amine uptake inhibitors for allodynia [40]. Chronic pain diagnoses that follow a "pain diagnostic ladder" or similar schematic may allow greater personalization of treatment plans and targeting of patients' distinct pain etiologies.

5. Pain Subclassifications

The classification of pain is vital for the proper treatment of patients, health care policies, statistics, and reimbursement. Neuropathic pain is one example of a condition that has been brought up numerous times as a major epidemiological problem needing systematic classification [41]. In 2018, the World Health Organization (WHO) released the first ever systematic classification of chronic pain diagnoses as part of the ICD-11. Given the high global prevalence of chronic pain, affecting over 30% of the world population [18], the development of a systematic classification for chronic pain facilitates the collection of thorough epidemiological data. These subclassifications have been used to report health care statistics from January 2022 and onwards. The classification system discussed below is intended to apply to specialized pain management and primary care alike.

When diagnosing chronic pain, it is important to distinguish chronic primary pain from chronic secondary pain syndromes (Table 1). Chronic primary pain is defined by the IASP as pain in one or more anatomical regions that is characterized by significant emotional distress or functional disability, and which is not better explained by an alternative chronic pain subclass [42]. Chronic primary pain syndromes include fibromyalgia, complex regional pain syndrome, chronic primary headache, chronic primary visceral pain such as irritable bowel syndrome, and chronic nonspecific low-back pain. These conditions are precluded by chronic pain that can be characterized as a standalone primary diagnosis.

Table 1. Chronic primary pain syndromes vs. chronic secondary pain syndromes.

Chronic primary pain syndromes: *pain in one or more anatomical regions characterized by significant emotional distress or functional disability*	Chronic secondary pain syndromes: *pain arising from another health or underlying medical condition*
Examples: - Fibromyalgia - Complex regional pain syndrome - Chronic primary headache - Chronic primary visceral pain - Nonspecific lower back pain	Subcategories: - Chronic cancer-related pain - Chronic postsurgical/post-traumatic pain - Chronic neuropathic pain - Chronic headache and orofacial pain - Chronic secondary visceral pain - Chronic secondary musculoskeletal pain

In contrast, chronic secondary pain syndromes arise from another health condition as the underlying cause. In these conditions, pain may have been a symptom of an underlying illness prior to becoming its own autonomous health condition. The diagnosis of chronic secondary pain syndrome may be prompted when the patient's pain requires its own care and treatment plan, or when the pain persists despite resolution of the initial underlying illness. It is important to exclude patients who have underlying conditions commonly associated with pain, but do not themselves meet criteria for a co-diagnosis of chronic pain.

Chronic secondary pain is further divided into six subcategories, all of which must still meet the minimum 3-month duration for chronic pain. These subcategories include chronic cancer-related pain, chronic postsurgical or post-traumatic pain, chronic neuropathic pain, chronic headache and orofacial pain, chronic secondary visceral pain, and chronic secondary musculoskeletal pain. Chronic cancer-related pain may be caused by cancerous growth or spread or by chemotherapy or radiation treatment. Meanwhile, pain related to surgical intervention for cancer falls under the chronic postsurgical or post-traumatic pain category. Notably, postsurgical pain often stems from a peripheral neuropathic etiology. Therefore, chronic neuropathic pain is a common co-diagnosis. Chronic daily headache is defined by the International Headache Society (IHS) as "15 or more headache episodes per month for at least three months [43]" Common secondary causes of chronic headache include central nervous system infections, tumors, hematomas, aneurysms, or vasculitis [44–48].

Medication overuse is also an important secondary cause of chronic headaches [49]. This subclass often overlaps with primary headache disorders such as migraines, tension headaches, and cluster headaches as precipitants to medication overuse. This is just one example of how important it is to screen patients for underlying primary disorders before initiating treatment based on the secondary cause. A similar pattern may be seen in chronic secondary visceral and secondary musculoskeletal pain. Patients whose chronic visceral or musculoskeletal pain is idiopathic or has an established functional mechanism should be treated for a primary chronic pain disorder. If it is determined that the patient's pain is truly secondary in nature, then chronic visceral and musculoskeletal pains may be further characterized by their etiologies, including, but not limited to, mechanical, vascular, or inflammatory mechanisms.

6. Somatosensory Assessments

Common chronic pain management seeks to initially rule out any treatable causes of the pain, and then to provide the patient with as high a quality of life as possible [50]. Somatosensory assessments of pain in a clinical setting often use cutaneous stimuli, such as touch and light pressure, or deep pressure stimuli, such as manually inflated cuffs or instruments for pressure. Most commonly, pain thresholds are evaluated by applying cutaneous and deep pressure stimuli to control sites and the sites of reported pain. Research has suggested the use of mechanical stimuli, such as touch or punctuate pressure, are predictive of pain intensity [51].

The current gold standard of chronic pain assessment is based on self-reports of sensory intensity. This can be used via categorical scales, numerical rating scales, visual analog scales, and descriptor scales, though numerical scales are the most used. This method relies on patient recall to define temporal features of pain, i.e., the variability of the pain: whether it is intermittent, constant, or changing in intensity. The recommended numerical rating scale asks patients to rank their pain on a 0–10 scale, with 0 as an indication of no pain and 10 equaling the worst possible pain [52].

Current guidelines for assessing somatosensory function in chronically ill patients have been outlined by the German Neuropathic Pain Network (DFNS) [53]. These include measures to evaluate for temporal and conditioned pain and are used to explore facilitators and inhibitors of pain. For young children or patients with limited verbal ability, it has been suggested that the use of a Faces Pain Scale may be a more accurate predictor, in which patients are shown pictures of facial expressions depicting pain and asked for the image they identify their pain with [54]. Quantitative sensory testing (QST) is another developing assessment that can be used to examine thermal (cold, warmth, etc.) and mechanical thresholds (touch and vibration) to characterize peripheral and central mechanisms of pain. This can used to predict propensity to develop chronic pain and sensitivity to treatment effects [55].

Pain biomarkers are a frequently considered method of evaluating chronic pain, as researchers seek specific neuronal activity that defines pain [56]. This accounts for two forms of pain biomarkers: pain selective and pain specific. Pain selective markers are graded neurons, visualized with higher activation during pain but also present in the absence of pain. Pain specific markers are based on an all-or-nothing response, firing only when the pain is present but never in the absence of pain. The challenge in this approach is the difficulty in defining pain specific markers to an exclusive mechanism of pain, as pain often shows activity within many neurons, and the pain biomarkers of a healthy brain may differ from those in a chronically ill patient [57]. Further evaluation of these biomarkers can help facilitate more personalized treatments for chronic pain.

7. Imaging and Clinical Prediction Models

Neuroimaging, such as MRIs, may also be used to assess chronic pain. The functional MRI (fMRI) measures changes in blood oxygenation levels and is an indirect indicator of brain activity. Resting state fMRIs are conducted to view the brain activity of a patient in chronic pain without additional external stimuli, to provide a baseline of the brain's functional connectivity [58]. This may be compared to the brain's activity when the chronic pain is exacerbated, specifically seeking alterations in brain networking of resting low oscillatory activity. Other methods of assessing cerebral brain flow for chronic pain include PET and arterial spin labelling[53]. Further methods to explore changes in brain networking include diffusion tensor imaging, which evaluates for variations in the structural connectivity of brain regions. Changes in brain structures are another commonly used means to assess chronic pain. Some investigators suggest reductions in gray matter volume or other changes in brain structure may be associated with pain [52].

Multivariate pattern analysis (MVPA) may additionally be used to compare healthy controls to individuals in pain. This requires patterns of brain activity in control versus chronic pain patients to specify brain structure or activity that may be contributing to pain. Over time, MVPA is anticipated to become a more widely acknowledged diagnostic tool to aid in defining prognoses and tailoring treatment to an individual's brain activity and structure [59]. Neuroimaging may be utilized in evaluating chronic pain as quantitative measurements which don't require external stimuli, as compared to measurements via stimuli-based abnormalities, such as the EEG. However, these methods are currently not as widely available for use by clinicians [60].

As the MRI assesses spatial resolution, it may be more accurate to combine neuroimaging with measurements of temporal resolutions, such as the EEG or MEG [59]. However, the expense and lack of specificity associated with neuroimaging limits the clinical use of this method, especially when compared to the practicality of self-reports. Further methods of quantifying chronic pain may include genotyping (identifying genetic markers of mechanisms that contribute to pain), pharmacological studies (clinical responses to drugs), and chemical neuroimaging (ligand-based imaging/magnetic resonance spectroscopy). Nonetheless, these methods remain of low clinical utility, as they are both nonspecific and expensive [52].

Several risk factors have been attributed to chronic pain, including socio-economic, psychological, clinical, and biological factors. Prior literature concluded that to prevent and reduce the impact of chronic pain, modifiable risk factors (e.g., nutrition, physical activity, and acute pain) need to be addressed [61]. Clinical prediction models for the future development of chronic pain have thus far been an ongoing challenge to the pain research community, especially due to the wide ranges of pain perception. One study examined chronic pain associated with nerve injuries after surgical and medical procedures; it found that the severity of chronic postoperative pain can be predicted by experimental pain assessment prior to surgery, specifically having the endogenous analgesia system tested with diffuse noxious inhibitory control (DNIC) [62]. There are more studies exploring the predictive value of presurgical psychosocial pain assessment for acute postoperative pain, yet fewer that study biomarkers predicting chronic pain.

8. Management of Chronic Pain

Conservative management of pain is generally the first intervention tried by patients when symptoms of pain first arise, and treatment strategies often include avoidance of triggers for pain, physical therapy, and often non-narcotic analgesics. Due to the multifactorial disease process and various parts of pathophysiology yet still unknown with chronic pain, multiple treatment modalities are needed to produce significant pain relief for patients [63,64]. A biopsychosocial approach to multidisciplinary pain management can coexist with use of analgesics, interventions, etc. [65]. Generally, opioids are less effective for chronic non-cancer pain compared to use on a short-term basis and at low doses used for acute postsurgical pain [66]. Besides pharmacological treatment for chronic pain, there have also been studies concluding there is an inverse dose–response association between physical activity and chronic pain [67].

Recent randomized controlled trials have also been more frequent in examining treatments tailored towards the biopsychosocial approach to managing chronic pain. For example [68], one clinical trial studying patients with chronic lower back pain found that sensorimotor retraining interventions resulted in improved pain intensity. Retraining focused on altering how patients thought about their pain, processed sensory information, and moved their back during activities. However, one weakness of this trial was that there was no double-blindingor the clinicians in either of the treatment arms, which would have reduced bias. Another meta-analysis [69] of individual cognitive functional therapy, compared to group-based exercise intervention, found no significant difference in pain intensity. Patients who underwent individualized cognitive functional therapy, however, reported greater long term improvements in disability associated with chronic pain.

Pharmacological treatment of chronic pain conditions primarily associated with nociception include acetaminophen, non-steroidal anti-inflammatory drugs (NSAIDs) and other neuroactive drugs for patients with neuropathy or central sensitization. Education, physical exercise, and cognitive behavioral therapy have been shown to be effective for almost any type of pain [70]. Neuromodulation techniques for pain management have also been on the rise [71–74]. Local anesthetics have also been used beyond intraoperative anesthesia and analgesia for treatment of both acute and chronic pain conditions [75,76]. There needs to be a strong therapeutic alliance between clinicians and patients, from diagnosing and classifying chronic pain to correctly imaging, assessing, and ultimately treating the disease.

Antidepressants have also been employed as an off-label treatment for chronic pain conditions such as fibromyalgia, neuropathic pain, and musculoskeletal pain. One meta-analysis [77] examining several antidepressants for chronic pain outcomes found duloxetine as the only option with effectiveness as a pain reliever. Medical cannabis is another treatment that has gained more popularity to treat chronic pain more refractory to other pharmacological and interventional methods. Thirty-two trials [78] consisting of over five thousand enrolled patients with chronic and cancer-related pain were reviewed and concluded that medical cannabis has utility for pain relief and improved sleep quality. Currently, there is a lack of assessment on the long term effects of medical cannabis, and no previous trial has followed patients more than five and a half months.

Interventional pain management and sometimes even surgical intervention may be indicated for chronic pain with a lumbar spine etiology. For example, therapeutic epidural injections—caudal, lumbar, interlaminar, and transforaminal—have been utilized to manage chronic lower back pain secondary to disc herniation. A systematic review [79] showed stronger evidence for short-term effects in alleviating pain and disability compared to long-term effects. There is a lack of trials with one year follow-up in patients who underwent epidural injection under fluoroscopy.

Radiofrequency ablation (RFA) is another interventional procedure using heat to treat chronic lower back pain associated with lumbar facet and sacroiliac joints. One review of eleven RCTs showed evidence for RFA as an effective short-term treatment but less so for the treatment of intervertebral (discogenic) pain [80]. There has been a recent interest and growing research into discogenic chronic lower back pain being treated with intraosseous basivertebral nerve (BVN) ablation. BVNs are thought to be responsible for transmitting pain signals from vertebral end plates often associated with discogenic disease [81]. One study [82] observing patients for two years following BVN ablation showed significant improvement of pain and function compared to the standard care arm of the trial. While this relatively new procedure is considered minimally invasive and safe, there should be a wave of upcoming research into any long term adverse effects such as potential vertebral compression fractures, especially in an elderly population who may already be predisposed to osteoporosis.

9. Conclusions

Pain medicine is a multidisciplinary and multimodal approach to help patients manage chronic pain. Over the recent years, the definition of chronic pain has evolved to become less "non-specific" and to help aid in the proper classification of the disease. While the term can often be too generalized when describing a wide array of conditions, the future of chronic pain diagnosis and treatment is becoming more personalized and precision based. More optimized and specific chronic pain diagnoses can help avoid pooling together heterogenous conditions. A further revision of ICD diagnoses for chronic pain is needed to better accomplish this goal.

Millions are affected by chronic pain physically, emotionally, and socially, with a tremendous impact on economic costs. A biopsychosocial assessment is most helpful in understanding all facets of chronic pain. In addition to recognizing the cognitive elements of pain, treatment for chronic pain will comprise pharmacological therapy, physical rehabilitation, and potentially interventional procedures for refractory pain.

Chronic pain also has a significant burden on older populations and is associated with lower socioeconomic status, lost productivity, and disability, along with its functional, emotional, and social impacts. In this review, a range of definitions of acute to chronic pain were outlined with the goal a more mechanistic approach to address the growing understanding of the anatomical and physiological processes involved. Pain subclassifications can assist in distinguishing primary and secondary pain syndromes, which is important in the screening phase prior to initiation of treatment. Proper classification of a patient's chronic pain can help treat the underlying cause of illness.

There is ongoing research in the field of somatosensory assessments for chronic pain ranging from self-reported measures of sensory intensity to the use of mechanical stimuli, even quantitative sensory testing to assess thermal and mechanical thresholds for pain. Clinical studies for chronic pain need to be more inclusive of feasible solutions. Policy makers and regulators need to be alerted to the economic and personal burden of this widely common disease to better diagnose and classify chronic pain conditions [83]. Additionally, there has been progress in learning more about pain selective and pain specific biomarkers, but there needs to be more research done to correlate them with exclusive mechanisms of chronic pain.

Delayed diagnosis can often lead to worse outcomes for patients with chronic pain, as is often seen with older adults. This increases the importance for correct diagnosis and classification of the disease process. Other imaging techniques like neuroimaging (fMRI) and multivariate pattern analysis (MVPA) help investigate the connections between chronic pain and structural and physiological changes in the brain. There is a need for more interest in developing more reliable clinical prediction models for chronic pain. More studies are also needed to examine biomarkers, which can predispose patients to chronic pain, and better understand related comorbid conditions.

The biopsychosocial model also helps facilitate current treatment modalities for chronic pain, which includes pharmacological treatment, physical therapy, neuromodulation, and neuraxial techniques. With the recent advent of opportunities for artificial intelligence in medicine [84–86], computer-aided diagnosis of extremely common chronic pain conditions like lower back pain may help improve diagnosis and treatment rates [87]. Earlier and more accurate diagnosis and classification can pave the road to improved outcomes and treatment for the many suffering from chronic pain. A paradigm shift like this will hopefully help spur efforts for more research into biological and clinical advances for patients suffering from chronic pain.

Funding: This research received no external funding.

Institutional Review Board Statement: Not applicable.

Informed Consent Statement: Not applicable.

Data Availability Statement: Not applicable.

Conflicts of Interest: The authors declare no conflict of interest.

References

1. Goldberg, D.S.; McGee, S.J. Pain as a global public health priority. *BMC Public Health* **2011**, *11*, 770. [CrossRef] [PubMed]

2. Rice, A.S.; Smith, B.H.; Blyth, F.M. Pain and the global burden of disease. *Pain* **2016**, *157*, 791–796. [CrossRef] [PubMed]
3. GBD 2021 Low Back Pain Collaborators. Global, regional, and national burden of low back pain, 1990–2020, its attributable risk factors, and projections to 2050: A systematic analysis of the Global Burden of Disease Study 2021. *Lancet Rheumatol.* **2023**, *5*, e316–e329. [CrossRef] [PubMed]
4. Chou, R. Low back pain (chronic). *BMJ Clin. Evid.* **2010**, *2010*, 1116. [PubMed]
5. Crofford, L.J. Chronic Pain: Where the Body Meets the Brain. *Trans. Am. Clin. Climatol. Assoc.* **2015**, *126*, 167–183. [PubMed]
6. Schwan, J.; Sclafani, J.; Tawfik, V.L. Chronic Pain Management in the Elderly. *Anesthesiol. Clin.* **2019**, *37*, 547–560. [CrossRef] [PubMed]
7. Brooks, A.K.; Udoji, M.A. Interventional Techniques for Management of Pain in Older Adults. *Clin. Geriatr. Med.* **2016**, *32*, 773–785. [CrossRef]
8. van Baar, M.E.; Dekker, J.; Oostendorp, R.A.; Bijl, D.; Voorn, T.B.; Lemmens, J.A.; Bijlsma, J.W. The effectiveness of exercise therapy in patients with osteoarthritis of the hip or knee: A randomized clinical trial. *J. Rheumatol.* **1998**, *25*, 2432–2439.
9. Costigan, M.; Scholz, J.; Woolf, C.J. Neuropathic pain: A maladaptive response of the nervous system to damage. *Annu. Rev. Neurosci.* **2009**, *32*, 1–32. [CrossRef]
10. Bonica, J.J. The management of pain of cancer. *J. Mich. State Med. Soc.* **1953**, *52*, 284–290.
11. Raja, S.N.; Carr, D.B.; Cohen, M.; Finnerup, N.B.; Flor, H.; Gibson, S.; Keefe, F.J.; Mogil, J.S.; Ringkamp, M.; Sluka, K.A.; et al. The revised International Association for the Study of Pain definition of pain: Concepts, challenges, and compromises. *Pain* **2020**, *161*, 1976–1982. [CrossRef] [PubMed]
12. Rief, W.; Kaasa, S.; Jensen, R.; Perrot, S.; Vlaeyen, J.W.; Treede, R.-D.; Vissers, K.C. The need to revise pain diagnoses in ICD-11. *Pain* **2010**, *149*, 169–170. [CrossRef] [PubMed]
13. Schug, S.A.; Lavand'Homme, P.; Barke, A.; Korwisi, B.; Rief, W.; Treede, R.-D.; IASP Taskforce for the Classification of Chronic Pain. The IASP classification of chronic pain for ICD-11: Chronic postsurgical or posttraumatic pain. *Pain* **2019**, *160*, 45–52. [CrossRef] [PubMed]
14. Zusman, M. Forebrain-mediated sensitization of central pain pathways: 'non-specific' pain and a new image for MT. *Man. Ther.* **2002**, *7*, 80–88. [CrossRef]
15. Goldenberg, D.L. The interface of pain and mood disturbances in the rheumatic diseases. *Semin. Arthritis Rheum.* **2010**, *40*, 15–31. [CrossRef] [PubMed]
16. Gatchel, R.J.; Peng, Y.B.; Peters, M.L.; Fuchs, P.N.; Turk, D.C. The biopsychosocial approach to chronic pain: Scientific advances and future directions. *Psychol. Bull.* **2007**, *133*, 581–624. [CrossRef] [PubMed]
17. Lumley, M.A.; Cohen, J.L.; Borszcz, G.S.; Cano, A.; Radcliffe, A.M.; Porter, L.S.; Schubiner, H.; Keefe, F.J. Pain and emotion: A biopsychosocial review of recent research. *J. Clin. Psychol.* **2011**, *67*, 942–968. [CrossRef] [PubMed]
18. Cohen, S.P.; Vase, L.; Hooten, W.M. Chronic pain: An update on burden, best practices, and new advances. *Lancet* **2021**, *397*, 2082–2097. [CrossRef]
19. Dahlhamer, J.; Lucas, J.; Zelaya, C.; Nahin, R.; Mackey, S.; DeBar, L.; Kerns, R.; Von Korff, M.; Porter, L.; Helmick, C. Prevalence of Chronic Pain and High-Impact Chronic Pain Among Adults—United States, 2016. *MMWR. Morb. Mortal. Wkly. Rep.* **2018**, *67*, 1001–1006. [CrossRef]
20. Nahin, R.L.; Feinberg, T.; Kapos, F.P.; Terman, G.W. Estimated Rates of Incident and Persistent Chronic Pain among US Adults, 2019–2020. *JAMA Netw. Open* **2023**, *6*, e2313563. [CrossRef]
21. Hoy, D.; Bain, C.; Williams, G.; March, L.; Brooks, P.; Blyth, F.; Woolf, A.; Vos, T.; Buchbinder, R. A systematic review of the global prevalence of low back pain. *Arthritis Rheum.* **2012**, *64*, 2028–2037. [CrossRef] [PubMed]
22. Kamper, S.J.; Henschke, N.; Hestbaek, L.; Dunn, K.M.; Williams, C.M. Musculoskeletal pain in children and adolescents. *Braz. J. Phys. Ther.* **2016**, *20*, 275–284. [CrossRef] [PubMed]
23. Hartvigsen, J.; Christensen, K.; Frederiksen, H. Back pain remains a common symptom in old age. a population-based study of 4486 Danish twins aged 70–102. *Eur. Spine J.* **2003**, *12*, 528–534. [CrossRef] [PubMed]
24. Larsson, C.; Hansson, E.; Sundquist, K.; Jakobsson, U. Chronic pain in older adults: Prevalence, incidence, and risk factors. *Scand. J. Rheumatol.* **2017**, *46*, 317–325. [CrossRef] [PubMed]
25. Tinnirello, A.; Mazzoleni, S.; Santi, C. Chronic Pain in the Elderly: Mechanisms and Distinctive Features. *Biomolecules* **2021**, *11*, 1256. [CrossRef] [PubMed]
26. Todd, J.; Austin, H.; Clarke, P.; Notebaert, L. Chronic Pain, Insomnia and their Mutual Maintenance: A Call for Cognitive Bias Research. *J. Pain* **2022**, *23*, 1530–1542. [CrossRef] [PubMed]
27. Pizzo, P.; Clark, N.M.; Carter-Pokras, O.; Christopher, M.; Farrar, J.T.; Follett, K.A.; Heitkemper, M.M.; Inturrisi, C.E.; Keefe, F.J.; Kerns, R.; et al. Relieving Pain in America: A Blueprint for Transforming Prevention, Care, Education, and Research. In *The National Academies Collection: Reports Funded by National Institutes of Health*; National Academies Press (US): Washington, DC, USA, 2011.
28. Yong, R.J.; Mullins, P.M.; Bhattacharyya, N. Prevalence of chronic pain among adults in the United States. *Pain* **2022**, *163*, e328–e332. [CrossRef] [PubMed]
29. Treede, R.-D.; Rief, W.; Barke, A.; Aziz, Q.; Bennett, M.I.; Benoliel, R.; Cohen, M.; Evers, S.; Finnerup, N.B.; First, M.B.; et al. Chronic pain as a symptom or a disease: The IASP Classification of Chronic Pain for the International Classification of Diseases (ICD-11). *Pain* **2019**, *160*, 19–27. [CrossRef]

30. Varenna, M.; Crotti, C.; Ughi, N.; Zucchi, F.; Caporali, R. Determinants of Diagnostic Delay in Complex Regional Pain Syndrome Type 1: An Observational Study of 180 Consecutive New Cases. *J. Clin. Rheumatol.* **2021**, *27*, e491–e495. [CrossRef]
31. Seo, M.R.; Baek, H.L.; Yoon, H.H.; Ryu, H.J.; Choi, H.-J.; Baek, H.J.; Ko, K.-P. Delayed diagnosis is linked to worse outcomes and unfavourable treatment responses in patients with axial spondyloarthritis. *Clin. Rheumatol.* **2015**, *34*, 1397–1405. [CrossRef]
32. Gendelman, O.; Amital, H.; Bar-On, Y.; Shor, D.B.-A.; Amital, D.; Tiosano, S.; Shalev, V.; Chodick, G.; Weitzman, D. Time to diagnosis of fibromyalgia and factors associated with delayed diagnosis in primary care. *Best Pract. Res. Clin. Rheumatol.* **2018**, *32*, 489–499. [CrossRef] [PubMed]
33. Vardeh, D.; Mannion, R.J.; Woolf, C.J. Toward a Mechanism-Based Approach to Pain Diagnosis. *J. Pain* **2016**, *17 (Supp. S9)*, T50–T69. [CrossRef]
34. Gallagher, R.M. Management of neuropathic pain: Translating mechanistic advances and evidence-based research into clinical practice. *Clin. J. Pain* **2006**, *22 (Supp. S1)*, S2–S8. [CrossRef]
35. Woolf, C.J.; Bennett, G.J.; Doherty, M.; Dubner, R.; Kidd, B.; Koltzenburg, M.; Lipton, R.; Loeser, J.D.; Payne, R.; Torebjork, E. Towards a mechanism-based classification of pain? *Pain* **1998**, *77*, 227–229. [CrossRef] [PubMed]
36. Woolf, C.J.; Mannion, R.J. Neuropathic pain: Aetiology, symptoms, mechanisms, and management. *Lancet* **1999**, *353*, 1959–1964. [CrossRef] [PubMed]
37. Kuner, R. Central mechanisms of pathological pain. *Nat. Med.* **2010**, *16*, 1258–1266. [CrossRef]
38. Goode, A.P.; Carey, T.S.; Jordan, J.M. Low back pain and lumbar spine osteoarthritis. How are they related? *Curr. Rheumatol. Rep.* **2013**, *15*, 305. [CrossRef] [PubMed]
39. Mayer, T.G.; Neblett, R.; Cohen, H.; Howard, K.J.; Choi, Y.H.; Williams, M.J.; Perez, Y.; Gatchel, R.J. The development and psychometric validation of the central sensitization inventory. *Pain Pract.* **2012**, *12*, 276–285. [CrossRef]
40. Peirs, C.; Williams, S.-P.G.; Zhao, X.; Walsh, C.E.; Gedeon, J.Y.; Cagle, N.E.; Goldring, A.C.; Hioki, H.; Liu, Z.; Marell, P.S.; et al. Dorsal Horn Circuits for Persistent Mechanical Pain. *Neuron* **2015**, *87*, 797–812. [CrossRef]
41. Finnerup, N.; Scholz, J.; Attal, N.; Baron, R.; Haanpää, M.; Hansson, P.; Raja, S.; Rice, A.; Rief, W.; Rowbotham, M.; et al. Neuropathic pain needs systematic classification. *Eur. J. Pain* **2013**, *17*, 953–956. [CrossRef]
42. Nicholas, M.; Vlaeyen, J.W.; Rief, W.; Barke, A.; Aziz, Q.; Benoliel, R.; Cohen, M.; Evers, S.; Giamberardino, M.A.; Goebel, A.; et al. The IASP classification of chronic pain for ICD-11: Chronic primary pain. *Pain* **2019**, *160*, 28–37. [CrossRef] [PubMed]
43. Murphy, C.; Hameed, S. Chronic Headaches. In *StatPearls*; StatPearls Publishing: St. Petersburg, FL, USA, 2023.
44. Aziz, Q.; Giamberardino, M.A.; Barke, A.; Korwisi, B.; Baranowski, A.P.; Wesselmann, U.; Rief, W.; Treede, R.-D.; IASP Taskforce for the Classification of Chronic Pain. The IASP classification of chronic pain for ICD-11: Chronic secondary visceral pain. *Pain* **2019**, *160*, 69–76. [CrossRef] [PubMed]
45. Bennett, M.; Kaasa, S.; Barke, A.; Korwisi, B.; Rief, W.; Treede, R.-D.; IASP Taskforce for the Classification of Chronic Pain. The IASP classification of chronic pain for ICD-11: Chronic cancer-related pain. *Pain* **2019**, *160*, 38–44. [CrossRef] [PubMed]
46. Benoliel, R.; Svensson, P.; Evers, S.; Wang, S.-J.; Barke, A.; Korwisi, B.; Rief, W.; Treede, R.-D.; IASP Taskforce for the Classification of Chronic Pain. The IASP-classification of chronic pain for ICD-11: Chronic secondary headache or orofacial pain. *Pain* **2019**, *160*, 60–68. [CrossRef] [PubMed]
47. Perrot, S.; Cohen, M.; Barke, A.; Korwisi, B.; Rief, W.; Treede, R.D.; IASP Taskforce for the Classification of Chronic Pain. The IASP classification of chronic pain for ICD-11: Chronic secondary musculoskeletal pain. *Pain* **2019**, *160*, 77–82. [CrossRef]
48. Scholz, J.; Finnerup, N.B.; Attal, N.; Aziz, Q.; Baron, R.; Bennett, M.I.; Benoliel, R.; Cohen, M.; Cruccu, G.; Davis, K.D.; et al. The IASP classification of chronic pain for ICD-11: Chronic neuropathic pain. *Pain* **2019**, *160*, 53–59. [CrossRef]
49. Wakerley, B.R. Medication-overuse headache. *Pract. Neurol.* **2019**, *19*, 399–403. [CrossRef]
50. Mills, S.; Torrance, N.; Smith, B.H. Identification and Management of Chronic Pain in Primary Care: A Review. *Curr. Psychiatry Rep.* **2016**, *18*, 22. [CrossRef]
51. Kersch, A.; Perera, P.; Mercado, M.; Gorrie, A.; Sainsbury, D.; McGrath, T.; Aouad, P.; Sarraf, S.; Jaaniste, T.; Champion, D. Somatosensory Testing in Pediatric Patients with Chronic Pain: An Exploration of Clinical Utility. *Children* **2020**, *7*, 275. [CrossRef]
52. Fillingim, R.B.; Loeser, J.D.; Baron, R.; Edwards, R.R. Assessment of Chronic Pain: Domains, Methods, and Mechanisms. *J. Pain* **2016**, *17 (Supp. S9)*, T10–T20. [CrossRef]
53. Maier, C.; Baron, R.; Tölle, T.R.; Binder, A.; Birbaumer, N.; Birklein, F.; Gierthmühlen, J.; Flor, H.; Geber, C.; Huge, V.; et al. Quantitative sensory testing in the German Research Network on Neuropathic Pain (DFNS): Somatosensory abnormalities in 1236 patients with different neuropathic pain syndromes. *Pain* **2010**, *150*, 439–450. [CrossRef] [PubMed]
54. Hunter, M.; McDowell, L.; Hennessy, R.; Cassey, J. An evaluation of the Faces Pain Scale with young children. *J. Pain Symptom Manag.* **2000**, *20*, 122–129. [CrossRef]
55. Treede, R.-D. The role of quantitative sensory testing in the prediction of chronic pain. *Pain* **2019**, *160*, S66–S69. [CrossRef] [PubMed]
56. Davis, K.D.; Aghaeepour, N.; Ahn, A.H.; Angst, M.S.; Borsook, D.; Brenton, A.; Burczynski, M.E.; Crean, C.; Edwards, R.; Gaudilliere, B.; et al. Discovery and validation of biomarkers to aid the development of safe and effective pain therapeutics: Challenges and opportunities. *Nat. Rev. Neurol.* **2020**, *16*, 381–400. [CrossRef] [PubMed]
57. Mouraux, A.; Iannetti, G.D. The search for pain biomarkers in the human brain. *Brain* **2018**, *141*, 3290–3307. [CrossRef] [PubMed]

58. Yin, Y.; He, S.; Xu, J.; You, W.; Li, Q.; Long, J.; Luo, L.; Kemp, G.J.; Sweeney, J.A.; Li, F.; et al. The neuro-pathophysiology of temporomandibular disorders-related pain: A systematic review of structural and functional MRI studies. *J. Headache Pain* **2020**, *21*, 78. [CrossRef] [PubMed]
59. Martucci, K.T.; Ng, P.; Mackey, S. Neuroimaging chronic pain: What have we learned and where are we going? *Futur. Neurol.* **2014**, *9*, 615–626. [CrossRef]
60. Davis, K.D.; Flor, H.; Greely, H.T.; Iannetti, G.D.; Mackey, S.; Ploner, M.; Pustilnik, A.; Tracey, I.; Treede, R.-D.; Wager, T.D. Brain imaging tests for chronic pain: Medical, legal and ethical issues and recommendations. *Nat. Rev. Neurol.* **2017**, *13*, 624–638. [CrossRef]
61. Mills, S.E.; Nicolson, K.P.; Smith, B.H. Chronic pain: A review of its epidemiology and associated factors in population-based studies. *Br. J. Anaesth.* **2019**, *123*, e273–e283. [CrossRef]
62. Yarnitsky, D.; Crispel, Y.; Eisenberg, E.; Granovsky, Y.; Ben-Nun, A.; Sprecher, E.; Best, L.-A.; Granot, M. Prediction of chronic post-operative pain: Pre-operative DNIC testing identifies patients at risk. *Pain* **2008**, *138*, 22–28. [CrossRef]
63. Chou, R.; Huffman, L.H.; American Pain Society; American College of Physicians. Nonpharmacologic therapies for acute and chronic low back pain: A review of the evidence for an American Pain Society/American College of Physicians clinical practice guideline. *Ann. Intern. Med.* **2007**, *147*, 492–504, Erratum in *Ann. Intern. Med.* **2008**, *148*, 247–248. [CrossRef] [PubMed]
64. Chou, R.; Turner, J.A.; Devine, E.B.; Hansen, R.N.; Sullivan, S.D.; Blazina, I.; Dana, T.; Bougatsos, C.; Deyo, R.A. The effectiveness and risks of long-term opioid therapy for chronic pain: A systematic review for a National Institutes of Health Pathways to Prevention Workshop. *Ann. Intern. Med.* **2015**, *162*, 276–286. [CrossRef] [PubMed]
65. Hylands-White, N.; Duarte, R.V.; Raphael, J.H. An overview of treatment approaches for chronic pain management. *Rheumatol. Int.* **2017**, *37*, 29–42. [CrossRef]
66. Littlejohn, C.; Baldacchino, A.; Bannister, J. Chronic non-cancer pain and opioid dependence. *J. R. Soc. Med.* **2004**, *97*, 62–65. [CrossRef] [PubMed]
67. Fjeld, M.K.; Årnes, A.P.; Engdahl, B.; Morseth, B.; Hopstock, L.A.; Horsch, A.; Stubhaug, A.; Strand, B.H.; Nielsen, C.S.; Steingrímsdóttir, Ó.A. Consistent pattern between physical activity measures and chronic pain levels: The Tromsø Study 2015 to 2016. *Pain* **2023**, *164*, 838–847. [CrossRef] [PubMed]
68. Bagg, M.K.; Wand, B.M.; Cashin, A.G.; Lee, H.; Hübscher, M.; Stanton, T.R.; O'connell, N.E.; O'hagan, E.T.; Rizzo, R.R.N.; Wewege, M.A.; et al. Effect of Graded Sensorimotor Retraining on Pain Intensity in Patients with Chronic Low Back Pain. *JAMA* **2022**, *328*, 430–439. [CrossRef]
69. O'Keeffe, M.; O'Sullivan, P.; Purtill, H.; Bargary, N.; O'Sullivan, K. Cognitive functional therapy compared with a group-based exercise and education intervention for chronic low back pain: A multicentre randomised controlled trial (RCT). *Br. J. Sports Med.* **2020**, *54*, 782–789. [CrossRef]
70. Clauw, D.J.; Essex, M.N.; Pitman, V.; Jones, K.D. Reframing chronic pain as a disease, not a symptom: Rationale and implications for pain management. *Postgrad. Med.* **2019**, *131*, 185–198. [CrossRef]
71. Knotkova, H.; Hamani, C.; Sivanesan, E.; Le Beuffe, M.F.E.; Moon, J.Y.; Cohen, S.P.; Huntoon, M.A. Neuromodulation for chronic pain. *Lancet* **2021**, *397*, 2111–2124. [CrossRef]
72. Huygen, F.J.; Kallewaard, J.W.; Nijhuis, H.; Liem, L.; Vesper, J.; Fahey, M.E.; Blomme, B.; Morgalla, M.H.; Deer, T.R.; Capobianco, R.A. Effectiveness and Safety of Dorsal Root Ganglion Stimulation for the Treatment of Chronic Pain: A Pooled Analysis. *Neuromodul. Technol. Neural Interface* **2020**, *23*, 213–221. [CrossRef]
73. Harden, R.N.; McCabe, C.S.; Goebel, A.; Massey, M.; Suvar, T.; Grieve, S.; Bruehl, S. Complex Regional Pain Syndrome: Practical Diagnostic and Treatment Guidelines, 5th Edition. *Pain Med.* **2022**, *23 (Supp. S1)*, S1–S53. [CrossRef]
74. Deer, T.R.; Levy, R.M.; Kramer, J.; Poree, L.; Amirdelfan, K.; Grigsby, E.; Staats, P.; Burton, A.W.; Burgher, A.H.; Obray, J.; et al. Dorsal root ganglion stimulation yielded higher treatment success rate for complex regional pain syndrome and causalgia at 3 and 12 months: A randomized comparative trial. *Pain* **2017**, *158*, 669–681. [CrossRef] [PubMed]
75. Shah, J.; Votta-Velis, E.G.; Borgeat, A. New local anesthetics. *Best Pract. Res. Clin. Anaesthesiol.* **2018**, *32*, 179–185. [CrossRef] [PubMed]
76. Kot, P.; Rodriguez, P.; Granell, M.; Cano, B.; Rovira, L.; Morales, J.; Broseta, A.; De Andrés, J. The erector spinae plane block: A narrative review. *Korean J. Anesthesiol.* **2019**, *72*, 209–220. [CrossRef] [PubMed]
77. Birkinshaw, H.; Friedrich, C.M.; Cole, P.; Eccleston, C.; Serfaty, M.; Stewart, G.; White, S.; Moore, R.A.; Phillippo, D.; Pincus, T. Antidepressants for pain management in adults with chronic pain: A network meta-analysis. *Cochrane Database Syst. Rev.* **2023**, *2023*, CD014682. [CrossRef]
78. Wang, L.; Hong, P.J.; May, C.; Rehman, Y.; Oparin, Y.; Hong, C.J.; Hong, B.Y.; AminiLari, M.; Gallo, L.; Kaushal, A.; et al. Medical cannabis or cannabinoids for chronic non-cancer and cancer related pain: A systematic review and meta-analysis of randomised clinical trials. *BMJ* **2021**, *374*, n1034. [CrossRef]
79. Manchikanti, L.; Benyamin, R.M.; Falco, F.J.E.; Kaye, A.D.; Hirsch, J.A. Do Epidural Injections Provide Short- and Long-term Relief for Lumbar Disc Herniation? A Systematic Review. *Clin. Orthop. Relat. Res.* **2015**, *473*, 1940–1956. [CrossRef]
80. Leggett, L.E.; Soril, L.J.; Lorenzetti, D.L.; Noseworthy, T.; Steadman, R.; Tiwana, S.; Clement, F. Radiofrequency Ablation for Chronic Low Back Pain: A Systematic Review of Randomized Controlled Trials. *Pain Res. Manag.* **2014**, *19*, e146–e153. [CrossRef]
81. Huang, J.; Delijani, K.; Jones, J.; Di Capua, J.; El Khudari, H.; Gunn, A.J.; Hirsch, J.A. Basivertebral Nerve Ablation. *Semin. Interv. Radiol.* **2022**, *39*, 162–166, Erratum in *Semin. Interv. Radiol.* **2022**, *39*, e1. [CrossRef]

82. Khalil, J.G.; Smuck, M.; Koreckij, T.; Keel, J.; Beall, D.; Goodman, B.; Kalapos, P.; Nguyen, D.; Garfin, S. A prospective, randomized, multicenter study of intraosseous basivertebral nerve ablation for the treatment of chronic low back pain. *Spine J.* **2019**, *19*, 1620–1632. [CrossRef]
83. The Lancet. Rethinking chronic pain. *Lancet* **2021**, *397*, 2023. [CrossRef] [PubMed]
84. Kim, E.E. Artificial Intelligence and Computer-aided Diagnosis in Medicine. *Curr. Med. Imaging Rev.* **2020**, *16*, 1. [CrossRef] [PubMed]
85. Galbusera, F.; Casaroli, G.; Bassani, T. Artificial intelligence and machine learning in spine research. *JOR Spine* **2019**, *2*, e1044. [CrossRef] [PubMed]
86. Hosny, A.; Parmar, C.; Quackenbush, J.; Schwartz, L.H.; Aerts, H.J.W.L. Artificial intelligence in radiology. *Nat. Rev. Cancer* **2018**, *18*, 500–510. [CrossRef]
87. D'antoni, F.; Russo, F.; Ambrosio, L.; Bacco, L.; Vollero, L.; Vadalà, G.; Merone, M.; Papalia, R.; Denaro, V. Artificial Intelligence and Computer Aided Diagnosis in Chronic Low Back Pain: A Systematic Review. *Int. J. Environ. Res. Public Health* **2022**, *19*, 5971. [CrossRef]

diagnostics

MDPI

Systematic Review

Effects of High-Intensity Interval Training (HIIT) on Patients with Musculoskeletal Disorders: A Systematic Review and Meta-Analysis with a Meta-Regression and Mapping Report

Ferran Cuenca-Martínez [1,†], Núria Sempere-Rubio [2,†], Clovis Varangot-Reille [1], Josué Fernández-Carnero [3,4,*], Luis Suso-Martí [1,*], Patricio Alba-Quesada [1] and Roy La Touche [4,5,6]

1 Exercise Intervention for Health Research Group (EXINH-RG), Department of Physiotherapy, University of Valencia, 46022 Valencia, Spain
2 UBIC, Department of Physiotherapy, Faculty of Physiotherapy, Universitat de València, 46010 Valencia, Spain
3 Department of Physical Therapy, Occupational Therapy, Rehabilitation and Physical Medicine, Rey Juan Carlos University, 28933 Madrid, Spain
4 Motion in Brains Research Group, Institute of Neuroscience and Sciences of the Movement (INCIMOV), Centro Superior de Estudios Universitarios La Salle, Universidad Autónoma de Madrid, 28049 Madrid, Spain
5 Departamento de Fisioterapia, Centro Superior de Estudios Universitarios La Salle, Universidad Autónoma de Madrid, 28049 Madrid, Spain
6 Instituto de Neurociencia y Dolor Craneofacial (INDCRAN), 28003 Madrid, Spain
* Correspondence: josue.fernandez@urjc.es (J.F.-C.); luis.suso@uv.es (L.S.-M.); Tel.: +34-914-88-88-00 (J.F.-C.); +34-963-98-38-55 (L.S.-M.)
† These authors contributed equally to this work.

Abstract: The aim was to assess the impact of high-intensity interval training (HIIT) on patients with musculoskeletal disorders. We conducted a search of Medline, Embase, PEDro, and Google Scholar. We conducted a meta-analysis to determine the effectiveness of HIIT on pain intensity, maximal oxygen consumption (VO_2 max), disability, and quality of life (QoL). We employed the GRADE and PEDro scales to rate the quality, certainty, and applicability of the evidence. Results showed significant differences in pain intensity, with a moderate clinical-effect (SMD = −0.73; 95% CI: −1.40–−0.06), and in VO_2 max, with a moderate clinical-effect (SMD = 0.69; 95% CI: 0.42–0.97). However, the meta-analysis showed no statistically significant results for disability (SMD = −0.34; 95% CI: −0.92–0.24) and QoL (SMD = 0.40; 95% CI: −0.80–1.60). We compared HIIT against other exercise models for reducing pain intensity and increasing VO_2 max. The meta-analysis showed no significant differences in favour of HIIT. Meta-regression analysis revealed that pain intensity scores were negatively associated with VO_2 max (R^2 = 82.99%, p = 0.003). There is low-moderate evidence that the HIIT intervention for patients with musculoskeletal disorders can reduce pain intensity and increase VO_2 max but has no effect on disability and QoL. Results also showed that HIIT was not superior to other exercise models in reducing pain intensity and increasing VO_2 max.

Keywords: high-intensity interval training; musculoskeletal pain; pain intensity; VO_2 max; disability; quality of life

1. Introduction

Musculoskeletal pain is an important public health issue because of its impact on quality of life (QoL) and the disability it can represent [1]. More than 20% of the world's population is affected by painful conditions, contributing to the high consumption of healthcare resources [2]. Pain management can be approached from several perspectives, both pharmacological and non-pharmacological, the latter of which includes physical agents, manual therapy, psychosocial interventions, patient education, and exercise training [3,4].

Exercise therapy has been reported to be highly effective in managing patients with musculoskeletal pain [5] and has been shown to produce hypoalgesia by releasing beta-endorphins or endocannabinoids [6–8]. Exercise therapy also interacts with the autonomic, cognitive, and affective aspects of pain [9,10]. For example, a recent meta-analysis found that aerobic exercise led to reduced pain intensity, duration, and frequency as well as improved QoL for patients with migraines [11].

The effects of high-intensity interval training (HIIT) on pain tolerance and threshold have sparked interest among the scientific community concerned with pain [12,13]. As described by Andreato, HIIT is a form of training that alternates high-intensity exercises at 90% or more of the maximal oxygen consumption (VO_2 max) (or ≥80% VO_2 max for the clinical population) with recovery periods, repeating the exercise several times [14]. A number of articles have recently shown that HIIT could improve pain-related clinical variables in patients with musculoskeletal disorders [15–17]. To date, systematic reviews on HIIT have mainly focused on patients with cardiovascular diseases, cancer, or obesity, where HIIT has shown great effectiveness in modifying cardiorespiratory variables [18–20]. Picavet et al. found that disability and quality of life are commonly affected in patients with musculoskeletal disorders [1]. This work prompted us to include these two variables in our study, with the objective of evaluating the role of this therapeutic exercise model on this clinical population of patients with musculoskeletal disorders. In addition to this, we wanted to include the pain intensity variable because almost 1/5 of the world's population lives with clinical conditions that involve pain [2]. Finally, we also wanted to include the variable VO_2 max because it is an objective variable and, in addition, it is the gold standard for assessing cardiorespiratory fitness, which seems to be affected in patients with musculoskeletal disorders with associated pain [21]. As far as we know, no published review has assessed the effects of HIIT on clinical and cardiorespiratory variables in patients with musculoskeletal disorders and pain.

Therefore, the main aim of the present study was to develop a systematic review and meta-analysis to assess the effectiveness of HIIT on pain intensity, maximal oxygen consumption, disability, and health-related QoL for patients with musculoskeletal disorders.

2. Materials and Methods

This systematic review and the meta-analysis were performed according to the Preferred Reporting Items for Systematic Reviews and Meta-analysis (PRISMA) guidelines described by Moher [22]. The protocol of this systematic review and meta-analysis was registered in an international registry prior to starting the review (Prospero: CRD42020216298 (5 November 2020)).

2.1. Inclusion Criteria

The selection criteria used in this systematic review and meta-analysis were based on methodological and clinical factors, such as the Population, Intervention, Control, Outcomes, and Study Design (PICOS) described by Stone [23].

2.1.1. Population

The participants selected for the studies were patients older than 18 years with any kind of musculoskeletal disorder. The participants' gender was irrelevant.

2.1.2. Intervention and Control

The intervention was the HIIT exercise modality, which could be given as an independent treatment, added to an existing intervention, or embedded in an existing intervention (e.g., usual care and treatment). For the control group, the comparators were minimal intervention, no intervention, and usual care (e.g., maintenance of the habitual daily physical activity profile, standard physical activity recommendations, physical exercise habits, and exercise intervention [excluding HIIT modality]) in combination or not with placebo interventions. In addition, we performed a sub-analysis to evaluate the effectiveness of HIIT compared with other therapeutic exercise models (e.g., moderate-intensity exercise, high-intensity continuous training, and home exercises) in those articles that, in addition to a control or comparator with no intervention or minimal intervention, presented an additional group that performed an exercise model.

2.1.3. Outcomes

The measures used to assess the results and effects were pain intensity, $VO_{2\,max}$, disability, and health-related QoL.

2.1.4. Study Design

We selected randomised controlled trials (RCTs), randomised parallel-design controlled trials, randomised cross-over trials, and prospective controlled clinical trials.

2.2. Search Strategy

The search for studies was performed using Medline (PubMed) (1950–2020), Embase (1950–2020), PEDro (1950–2020), and Google Scholar. The first search was run on the 8 November 2020 (however, the search was updated on 31 January 2022). We used a validated search filter for retrieving studies on measurement properties in PubMed; the same filter was adapted for all other databases [24]. In addition, the search was adapted and performed in Google Scholar due to its capacity to search for relevant articles and grey literature [25,26]. No restrictions were applied to any specific language as recommended by the international criteria [27]. The search strategy combined medical subject headings (MeSH) and non-MeSH terms, adding a Boolean operator (OR and/or AND) to combine them. The terms were as follows: "Hig- Intensity Interval Training", "High-Intensity Interval Trainings", "Interval Training, High-Intensity", "Interval Trainings, High Intensity", "Training, High-Intensity Interval", "Trainings, High-Intensity Interval", "High-Intensity Intermittent Exercise", "Exercise, High-Intensity Intermittent", "Exercises, High-Intensity Intermittent", "High-Intensity Intermittent Exercises", "Sprint Interval Training", "Sprint Interval Trainings", "Pain", "Chronic Pain", "Musculoskeletal Pain", "Pain intensity", "Disability", "Quality of Life", "VO_2 max", "Maximal Oxygen Consumption", and "Maximal Oxygen Uptake".

Two independent reviewers (F.C.-M. and J.F.-C.) conducted the search using the same methodology, and the differences were resolved by consensus. Additionally, meticulous manual searches were performed, including journals that have published articles related to the topic of this review as well as reference lists of the included studies. The reference sections of the original studies were screened manually. To remove duplicates, we employed the citation management software Mendeley (Mendeley desktop v1.17.4, Elsevier, New York, NY, USA) and hand-checked the citations [28].

2.3. Selection Criteria and Data Extraction

First, two independent reviewers (F.C.M. and L.S.M.), who assessed the relevance of the RCTs regarding the study questions and aims, performed a data analysis, which was performed based on information from the title, abstract, and keywords of each study. If there was no consensus or the abstracts did not contain sufficient information, the full text was reviewed. In the second phase of the analysis, the full text was used to assess whether the studies met all the inclusion criteria. Differences between the two independent reviewers were resolved by a consensus process moderated by a third reviewer [29]. Data described in the results were extracted by means of a structured protocol that ensured that the most relevant information was obtained from each study [30].

2.4. Methodological Quality Assessment

We used the Cochrane Handbook for Systematic Reviews of Interventions version 5.1.0 to assess the risk of bias in the included studies [30]. The assessment tool covers a total of 7 domains: (1) random sequence generation (selection bias), (2) allocation concealment (selection bias), (3) blinding of participants and personnel (performance bias), (4) blinding of outcome assessments (detection bias), (5) incomplete outcome data (attrition bias),

(6) selective reporting (reporting bias), and (7) other biases. Bias was assessed as low risk, high risk, or unclear risk.

The studies' methodological quality was assessed using the PEDro scale [31], which assesses the internal and external validity of a study and consists of 11 criteria: (1) specified study eligibility criteria, (2) random allocation of patients, (3) concealed allocation, (4) measure of similarity between groups at baseline, (5) patient blinding, (6) therapist blinding, (7) assessor blinding, (8) fewer than 15% dropouts, (9) intention-to-treat analysis, 10) intergroup statistical comparisons, and 11) point measures and variability data. The methodological criteria were scored as follows: yes (1 point), no (0 points), or do not know (0 points). The PEDro score for each selected study provided an indicator of the methodological quality (9–10 = excellent; 6–8 = good; 4–5 = fair; 3–0 = poor) [32]. We used the data obtained from the PEDro scale to map the results of the quantitative analyses.

Two independent reviewers (F.C.-M. and L.S.-M.) examined the quality of all the selected studies using the same methodology. Disagreements between the reviewers were resolved by consensus with a third reviewer. The concordance between the results (inter-rater reliability) was measured using Cohen's kappa coefficient (κ) as follows: (1) $\kappa > 0.7$ indicated a high level of agreement between assessors; (2) $\kappa = 0.5$–0.7 indicated a moderate level of agreement; and (3) $\kappa < 0.5$ indicated a low level of agreement) [33].

2.5. Evidence Map

We created a visual map of the scientific evidence for each article to visually display the information as a bubble plot. The review information is based on 3 dimensions:

1. Type of outcome measure (bubble colour): The bubble colour represents the variables (pain intensity, blue; $VO_{2\,max}$, violet; disability, green; QoL, black).
2. Variable (x-axis): We employed the calculation of effect sizes.
3. Effect (y-axis): Each of the reviews was classified according to its methodological quality using the PEDro scale.
4. Statistically significant differences: Articles with statistically significant differences were marked with white dots.

2.6. Certainty of Evidence

The certainty of evidence analysis was based on classifying the results into levels of evidence according to the Grading of Recommendations, Assessment, Development, and Evaluation (GRADE) framework, which is based on five domains: study design, imprecision, indirectness, inconsistency, and publication bias [34]. The assessment of the five domains was conducted according to GRADE criteria [35,36]. Evidence was categorised into the following four levels accordingly: (a) High quality. Further research is very unlikely to change our confidence in the effect estimate. All five domains are also met; (b) Moderate quality. Further research is likely to have an important impact on our confidence in the effect estimate and might change the effect estimate. One of the five domains is not met; (c) Low quality. Further research is very likely to have a significant impact on our confidence in the effect estimate and is likely to change the estimate. Two of the five domains are not met; and, finally, (d) Very low quality. Any effect estimates are highly uncertain. Three of the five domains are not met [35,36].

For the study design domain, the recommendations were downgraded one level in the event there was an uncertain or high risk of bias and serious limitations in the effect estimate (more than 25% of the participants were from studies with fair or poor methodological quality, as measured by the PEDro scale). In terms of inconsistency, the recommendations were downgraded one level when the point estimates varied widely among studies, the confidence intervals showed minimal overlap, or when the I^2 was substantial or large (greater than 50%). At indirectness domain recommendations were downgraded when severe differences in interventions, study populations or outcomes were found (the recommendations were downgraded in the absence of direct comparisons between the interventions of interest or when there are no key outcomes, and the recommendation is based only on intermediate outcomes or if more than 50% of the participants were outside the target group). For the imprecision domain, the recommendations were downgraded by one level if there were fewer than 300 participants for the continuous data [37].

2.7. Data Synthesis and Analysis

The statistical analysis was conducted using MetaXL software (version 5.3 (EpiGear International, Sunrise Beach, Queensland, Australia) [38]. To compare the outcomes reported by the studies, we calculated the standardised mean difference (SMD) over time and the corresponding 95% confidence interval (CI) for the continuous variables. The statistical significance of the pooled SMD was examined as Hedges' g to account for a possible overestimation of the true population effect size in the small studies [39].

We used the same inclusion criteria for the systematic review and the meta-analysis and included three additional criteria: (1) In the results, there was detailed information regarding the comparative statistical data of the exposure factors, therapeutic interventions, and treatment responses; (2) the intervention was compared with a similar control group; and (3) data on the analysed variables were represented in at least three studies.

The estimated SMDs were interpreted as described by Hopkins et al. [40], that is, we considered that an SMD of 4.0 represented an extremely large clinical effect, 2.0–4.0 represented a very large effect, 1.2–2.0 represented a large effect, 0.6–1.2 represented a moderate effect, 0.2–0.6 represented a small effect, and 0.0–0.2 represented a trivial effect. We estimated the degree of heterogeneity among the studies using Cochran's Q statistic test (a p-value < 0.05 was considered significant) and the inconsistency index (I^2) [40]. We considered that an $I^2 > 25\%$ represented small heterogeneity, $I^2 > 50\%$ represented medium heterogeneity, and $I^2 > 75\%$ represented large heterogeneity [41]. The I^2 index is a complement to the Q test, although it has the same problems of power with a small number of studies [41]. When the Q-test was significant ($p < 0.1$) and/or the result of I^2 was >75%, there was heterogeneity among the studies, and the random-effects model was conducted in the meta-analysis. To detect publication bias and to test the influence of each individual study, we performed a visual evaluation of the Doi plot [42], seeking asymmetry. We also performed a quantitative measure of the Luis Furuya-Kanamori (LFK) index, which has been shown to be more sensitive than the Egger test in detecting publication bias in a meta-analysis of a low number of studies [43]. An LFK index within ± 1 represents no asymmetry, exceeding ± 1 but within ± 2 represents minor asymmetry, and exceeding ± 2 involves major asymmetry. To test each study's influence, we visually examined the forest plot and performed an exclusion sensitivity analysis. Lastly, we applied a meta-regression analysis to analyse the relationship between pain intensity and VO_2 max variables using a random effects model employing the effect size statistic (Hedges' g) of the pain intensity scores to correlate with the VO_2 max scores [44].

3. Results

The study search strategy was presented in the form of a flow diagram (Figure 1).

3.1. Characteristics of the Included Studies

The patients were diagnosed with a persistent musculoskeletal pain condition [2 knee osteoarthritis studies [45,46], two axial spondylarthritis studies [16,47], three studies on chronic nonspecific low back pain [17,48,49], one study on episodic migraineurs [50], one study on fibromyalgia [15], one study on subacromial pain syndrome [51], one study on rheumatoid arthritis and adult-juvenile idiopathic arthritis [52], and one study on general persistent pain condition with previous trauma [53], and all of them evaluated pain intensity, VO_2 max, disability, and health-related QoL. Table 1 lists the descriptive characteristics of the included studies.

3.2. Interventions

In all groups, HIIT was compared to other types of training or interventions (including controls and no interventions), with the exception of Bressel et al. [45], which studied a single HIIT and balance training group, and Sveaas et al. (2014 & 2019) [16,47], which included an HIIT and moderate-intensity continuous training (MICT) group and another no exercise group. Of the studies referred to above, three had two groups: one HIIT group and one MICT group [15,17,46]. Atan and Karavelioğlu [15] included a third standard care group. Two other studies had only one HIIT and one standard care group [48,51]. Two studies had an HIIT group and another group that maintained the activities of daily living [52] and their usual physical activity [54]. Flehr et al. [53] had one HIIT group and one yoga group, while Verbrugghe et al. [49] studied four groups with different types of HIIT. The total duration of the intervention ranged from 6 to 12 weeks, with most studies having a frequency of two to three times per week, except for Keogh et al. [46] and Atan and Karavelioğlu [15], which had frequencies of four and five times per week, respectively. Table 2 presents extensive details on the intervention characteristics of the included studies.

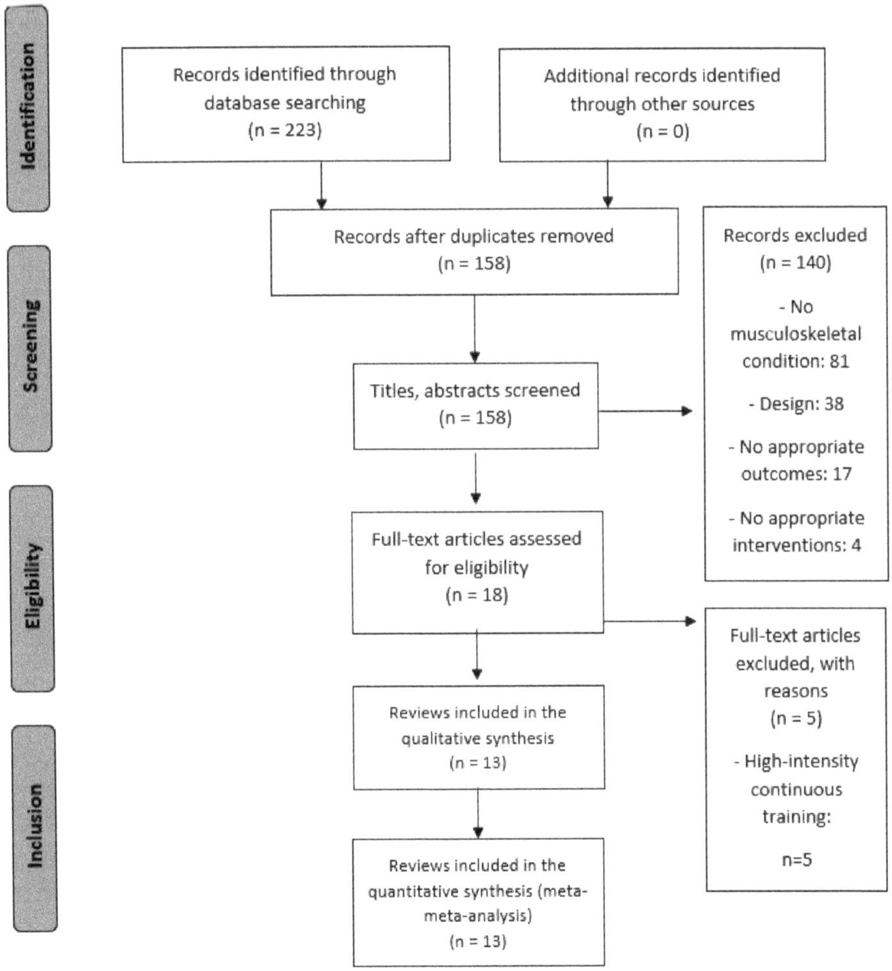

Figure 1. PRISMA Flowchart for selecting studies.

Table 1. Characteristics of the included studies.

Author, Year Country	Population Disease (*n*) Age (Years) Sex (%) Diagnostic Criteria Disease Duration (Years)	Study Design—Duration Intervention(s) and Control Group (*n*)	Outcome Measured (Instrument)	Results
Atan et al., 2020 [15] Turkey	Fibromyalgia (n = 55) *Age*, 48.7 ± 9.1 y 100% F American College of Rheumatology 2016 diagnostic criteria *Duration*, 2.5 ± 1.6 y	Pilot ROT—6 weeks *Intervention* - HIIT (n = 19) - MICT (n = 19) *Control* Usual care (n = 17)	- Pain Intensity (VAS) - HRQoL (SF-36 PF, PRL, Pain, GH, V, SF, ER, MH, EWB, E/F, HC) - $VO_{2\,max}$ (mL/kg/min)	HIIT showed significant differences compared with a control group on pain intensity, $VO_{2\,max}$, and SF-36 PF, PRL, ER, E/F, EWB, GH, and HC ($p < 0.05$) but no significant difference compared with MCT.
Berg et al., 2020 [50] Norway	Chronic SAPS (n = 21) *Age*, 48.1 ± 12.5 y 48% F/52% M Clinical criteria *Duration*, 3.5 ± 4.8 y	RCT—8 weeks *Intervention* HIIT + Home-exercise (n = 13) *Control* Home-exercise (n = 8)	- Pain intensity (NPA) - Disability (SPADI)	HIIT showed significant intragroup ($p < 0.05$) and intergroup differences ($p < 0.05$) compared with a control group in terms of disability but no significant difference in pain intensity.
Bressel et al., 2014 [44] United States	Knee OA (n = 18) *Age*, 64.5 ± 10.2 y 89% F/11% M Clinical and radiological criteria *Duration*, 6.8 ± 7.4 y	Pre-post study—6 weeks *Intervention* - HIIT + Balance training (n = 18) *Control* No intervention (n = 18)	Pain Intensity (VAS)	HIIT showed a significant improvement in pain intensity ($p < 0.05$).
Flehr et al., 2019 [52] Australia	Persistent pain condition (n = 32) *Age*, 30.2 ± 8 y 100% F N/R *Duration*, More than 12 months	RCT—8 weeks *Intervention* HIIT (n = 15) *Control* Bikram Yoga (n = 17)	- Pain Intensity (BPI) - HRQoL (SF-36 PF, PRL, Pain, GH, V, SF, ER, MH)	No significant difference between HIIT and Bikram Yoga in pain intensity. There was a significant intergroup difference on quality of life (SF-36 PF: $p = 0.019$; SF-36 MH: $p = 0.005$), with yoga showing higher improvement (SF-36 PF: M = 80.91; SF-36 MH: M= 63.94).
Hanssen et al., 2018 [49] Switzerland	Episodic migraine without aura (n= 36) *Age*, 36.8 ± 10.3 y 81% F/19% M International classification of headache disorders, 3rd ed. *Duration*, N/R	RCT—12 weeks *Intervention* - HIIT (n = 13) - MICT (n = 11) *Control Group* No intervention (n = 12)	$VO_{2\,max}$ (mL/kg/min)	No group × time interaction between the three groups ($p = 0.14$).

Table 1. *Cont.*

Author, Year Country	Population Disease (*n*) Age (Years) Sex (%) Diagnostic Criteria Disease Duration (Years)	Study Design—Duration Intervention(s) and Control Group (*n*)	Outcome Measured (Instrument)	Results
Keogh et al., 2018 [45] Australia	Knee OA ($n = 17$) *Age*, 62.4 ± 8.3 y 76% F/24% M Diagnosis by an orthopaedic surgeon *Duration*, 4.7 ± 4.6 y	Pilot RCT—8 weeks *Intervention* HIIT ($n = 9$) *Control* MICT ($n = 8$)	- Disability (WOMAC, Lequesne Index)	Both interventions demonstrated significant benefits on the WOMAC (HIIT: $p = 0.05$; MICT: $p = 0.006$) but without intergroup differences. No patient had significant improvement in the Lequesne index.
Sandstad et al., 2015 [51] Norway	RA and JIA ($n = 27$) *Age*, 33.0 ± 8.1 y 100% F Diagnosis by a rheumatologist *Duration*, N/R	Cross-over trial—10 weeks *Intervention* HIIT ($n = 12$) *Control* No intervention ($n = 15$)	- Pain Intensity (VAS) - Disability (MHAQ) - $VO_{2\ max}$ (mL/kg/min)	HIIT had a significant improvement in $VO_{2\ max}$ ($p < 0.001$) but no difference in pain intensity and disability.
Sveaas et al., 2014 [49] Norway	axSpA ($n = 24$) *Age*, 48.5 ± 12.0 y 50% F/50% M Spondyloarthritis International Society criteria *Duration*, 24.9 ± 15.8 y	Pilot RCT—12 weeks *Intervention* HIIT ($n = 10$) *Control* Usual care ($n = 14$)	$VO_{2\ max}$ (mL/kg/min)	HIIT had a significantly higher $VO_{2\ max}$ at 12 weeks than the control group ($p < 0.001$)
Sveaas et al., 2019 [16] Norway	axSpA ($n = 97$) *Age*, 46.2 ± N/R y 53% F/47% M Spondyloarthritis International Society criteria Duration, N/R	RCT—12 weeks *Intervention* HIIT ($n = 48$) *Control* No intervention ($n = 49$)	- Pain intensity (BASDAI neck/back/hip and peripheral pain) - $VO_{2\ max}$ (mL/kg/min)	HIIT significantly improves the neck/back/hips, and peripheral pain intensity, and the $VO_{2\ max}$ more than the control group ($p < 0.001$; $p = 0.016$; $p < 0.001$).
Thomsen et al., 2019 [53] Norway	PsA ($n = 67$) *Age*, 48.0 ± 11.5 y 64% F/36% M Classification of psoriatic arthritis Study group criteria *Duration*, N/R	RCT—11 weeks *Intervention* HIIT ($n = 32$) *Control* No intervention ($n = 35$)	- Pain Intensity (VAS)	HIIT showed no clear effect on pain intensity at the end of the intervention and at 9 months of follow-up.

Table 1. *Cont.*

Author, Year Country	Population Disease (*n*) Age (Years) Sex (%) Diagnostic Criteria Disease Duration (Years)	Study Design—Duration Intervention(s) and Control Group (*n*)	Outcome Measured (Instrument)	Results
Verbrugghe et al., 2018 [47] Belgium	Nonspecific Chronic LBP ($n = 20$) *Age*, N/R 55% F/45% M Clinical criteria *Duration*, N/R	CCT—6 weeks *Intervention* HIIT ($n = 10$) *Control* Usual care ($n = 10$)	- Pain Intensity (NPRS) - Disability (RMDQ) - HRQoL (SF-36 PF, PRL, ER, E/F, EWB, SF, Pain, GH) - $VO_{2\,max}$ (mL/kg/min)	Both groups had a reduction in disability ($p < 0.05$) with no intergroup difference. HIIT improved significantly HRQoL (SF-36 PRL, ER, SF, and Pain) ($p < 0.05$) but with no intergroup differences.
Verbrugghe et al., 2019 [17] Belgium	Nonspecific Chronic LBP ($n = 36$) *Age*, 44.2 ± 9.8 y 68% F/32% M Clinical criteria *Duration*, 11.1 ± 7.7 y	RCT—12 weeks *Intervention* HIIT ($n = 18$) *Control* MIT ($n = 18$)	- Pain Intensity (NPRS) - Disability (MODI) - $VO_{2\,max}$ (mL/kg/min)	HIIT significantly improved disability and $VO_{2\,max}$ more than MIT ($p < 0.05$). HIIT significantly reduced pain intensity ($p < 0.05$) but with no significant differences with MIT.
Verbrugghe et al., 2020 [48] Belgium	Nonspecific chronic LBP ($n = 80$) *Age*, 44.1 ± 9.7 y 58% F/42% M Clinical criteria *Duration*, 13.4 ± 9.1 y	RCT—12 weeks *Intervention* - HITCOM ($n = 19$) - HITSTRE ($n = 21$) - HITSTAB ($n = 20$) - HITMOB ($n = 20$)	- Pain Intensity (NPRS) - Disability (MODI) - $VO_{2\,max}$ (mL/kg/min)	All four HIIT groups significantly reduced pain intensity and disability and increased $VO_{2\,max}$ ($p < 0.05$), with no intergroup differences.

axSpA, axial spondyloarthritis; BPI, Brief Pain Inventory; CCT, Controlled clinical trial; E/F, energy/fatigue; ER, emotional role limitation; EWB, emotional well-being; GH, general health; HC, health change; HIIT, high-intensity interval training; HITCOM, high-intensity general resistance training, and high-intensity core strength training; HITMOB, trunk mobility exercises; HITSTAB, high-intensity core strength training; HITSTRE, high-intensity general resistance training; HRQoL, health-related quality of life; JIA, juvenile idiopathic arthritis; LBP, low back pain; MCT, moderate continuous training; MH, mental health; MHAQ, Modified Health Assessment Questionnaire; MICT, moderate-intensity continuous training; MIT, moderate-intensity training; MODI, Modified Oswestry Index; MPQ, McGill Pain Questionnaire; N/R, not reported; NPRS, Numeric Pain Rating Scale; OA, osteoarthritis; ODI, Oswestry Disability Index; PF, physical functioning; PRL, physical role limitation; PsA, psoriatic arthritis; RA, rheumatoid arthritis; RCT, randomised control trial; RMDQ, Roland-Morris Disability Questionnaire; SF-36, Short Form-36 Health Survey; SAPS, subacromial pain syndrome; SF, social functioning; SPADI, Shoulder Pain and Disability Index; V, vitality; VAS, visual analogue scale; WOMAC, Western Ontario and McMaster Universities Osteoarthritis Index.

Table 2. Prescription parameters extracted from each included study.

Trial	Group	Exercise Protocol (Distribution and Exercise Type)	Intensity (Pain Control during Training)	Frequency and Duration	Exercise Testing
Atan et al., 2020 [15]	HIIT (AerT) + StrT + Stretching	*Total exercise duration:* 35 min *Warmup and cooldown:* 5 min stationary cycling. *HIIT protocol:* 4 × 4 min of high-intensity stationary cycling interval alternating with 3 min cycling recovery periods. *Work/rest ratio:* [1:0.75] Followed by 10 min full body (shoulder, arm, leg, and hip) StrT, using 1–3-kg weights (1 × 8–10 rep) and 5 min stretching (4–5 × 20–30 s for each muscle group).	*Measurement:* HR_{max} (Monitorisation: N/R) *Warmup and cooldown:* 50% HR_{max} *HIIT:* *Interval:* 80–95% HR_{max} *Active Rest:* 70% HR_{max} *StrT:* N/R *Pain:* N/R	5×/week 6 weeks	Maximal cardiopulmonary test on a cycloergometer at baseline and follow-up. HR_{max}, VO_2 max, BP, workload, MET and duration-of-test were recorded.
	MICT (AerT) + StrT + Stretching	*Total exercise duration:* 55 min. *Warmup and cooldown:* 5 min stationary cycling. *MICT protocol:* 45 min continuous stationary cycling Followed by 10 min full body (shoulder, arm, leg, and hip) StrT, using 1–3-kg weights (1 × 8–10 rep) and 5 min stretching (4–5 × 20–30 s for each muscle group).	*Measurement:* HR_{max} (Monitorisation: N/R) *Warmup and cooldown:* 50% HR_{max} *MICT:* 65–70% HR_{max} *StrT:* N/R *Pain:* N/R		
	Usual Care	Recommendations regarding exercise for fibromyalgia.	N/A		
Berg et al., 2020 [50]	HIIT (StrT) + Usual Care	*HIIT protocol:* 4 × 4 min shoulder abduction-adduction at 2 Hz intervals alternating with 3 min walking rest periods *Work/Rest Ratio:* [1:0.75] If the patient was able to continue the final interval for one additional minute, the workload was increased by 250 g in the following session. *Home-based exercises:* Scapular stabilising, rotator cuff, and pain-free ROM exercises.	*Measurement:* WR_{max} *Interval:* 80% WR_{max} *Rest:* N/R *Pain:* When pain exceeds 5/10, session was ended.	3×/week 8 weeks	Time to exhaustion test during shoulder abduction-adduction. WR_{max} was recorded.
	Usual Care	*Home-based exercises:* Scapular stabilising, rotator cuff, and pain-free ROM exercises.	N/R		
Bressel et al., 2014 [44]	BalanceT + HIIT (AerT)	*Balance training:* Perturbations with water jets. Followed by: *HIIT protocol:* (Progressive increase from 1st to 6th week) 3 to 6 × 0.5 to 2.5 min walking (1.3 to 2.1 m/s) on an underwater treadmill interval alternating with 1 to 2.5 min walking (1.3 to 1.8 m/s) rest periods. (depth: xiphoid process) *Work/rest ratio:* [1:2; 1:1.3; 1:1; 1:1; 1:1; 1:1]	*Measurement:* RPE (Borg Scale/20) *BalanceT:* Progressive increase (from 1st to 6th week) from 11 to 18/20. *HIIT:* *Interval:* Progressive increase (from 1st to 6th week) from 13 to 19/20. *Rest:* 10/20 *Pain:* N/R	3×/week 6 weeks	N/A

Table 2. *Cont.*

Trial	Group	Exercise Protocol (Distribution and Exercise Type)	Intensity (Pain Control during Training)	Frequency and Duration	Exercise Testing
Flehr et al., 2019 [52]	HIIT (StrT + AerT)	45 min functional training incorporating running, throwing, standing from a seated position, placing items overhead, and picking items up. *Warmup and demonstration:* 15 min. *Movement learning*: 15 min *HIIT protocol:* 15 min reproduction of the movement at high intensity. Four formats possible: As fast as possible, 8-exercises Tabata intervallic training followed by AerT, Maximum reps or load in a set time, or as many rounds as possible in 12 min followed by AerT	N/R *Interval:* N/R *Rest:* N/R *Pain:* N/R	3× /week 8 weeks	N/R
	Yoga	90 min Bikram Yoga class (Room at 40 °C and 40% humidity): Deep breathing, 45 to 50 min standing, stretching, and relaxation postures.	Light to moderate (according to ACSM) and sometimes vigorous. *Pain:* N/R		
Hanssen et al., 2018 [49]	HIIT (AerT)	*Warmup:* 400 m of light running on a treadmill and 2 skipping exercises *HIIT protocol:* 4 × 4 min high-intensity running on a treadmill, interval alternating with 3 min running recovery periods. *Work/rest ratio:* [1:0.75] *Cooldown:* 400 m of light running and stretching	*Measurement:* HR_{max} (HR checked using HR monitor) *Interval:* 90% to 95% HRmax (±5 bpm) *Rest:* 70% of HRmax *Pain:* N/R	2× /week 12 weeks	Maximal Cardiopulmonary test on a treadmill. Anaerobic lactate-threshold, HR_{max}, RPE, and VO_2 max were recorded.
	MICT (AerT)	*Warmup:* 400 m of light running on a treadmill and 2 skipping exercises *MICT protocol:* 45 min continuous running on a treadmill. *Cooldown:* 400 m of light running and stretching	*Measurement:* HR_{max} (HR checked using HR monitor) *MICT:* 70% HRmax (± 5 bpm) *Pain:* N/R		
	Maintain their habitual daily physical activity	N/A	N/A		
Keogh et al., 2018 [45]	HIIT (AerT)	*Warmup:* 7 min stationary cycling, with progressively increasing intensity *HIIT protocol:* 5 × 45 s high-cadence stationary cycling interval alternating with 90 s low-intensity recovery cycling. Work/Rest Ratio: [1:2] *Cooldown:* 6–7 min of light to moderate cycling.	*HIIT:* *Interval:* 110 rpm with a resistance similar or slightly higher than the rest. Intensity was defined as "an intensity at which you felt it was quite difficult to complete sentences during the exercise". *Rest:* ~70 rpm To avoid pain, progressive increase in initial sessions.	4× /week 8 weeks	N/R
	MICT (AerT)	*Warmup and cooldown:* Light intensity cycling for 3 min and 2 min, respectively. *MICT protocol:* 20 min continuous cycling.	*MICT:* 60–80 rpm. Intensity was defined as "An intensity at which you are able to speak in complete sentences during the exercise". To avoid pain, progressive increase in initial sessions		

Table 2. *Cont.*

Trial	Group	Exercise Protocol (Distribution and Exercise Type)	Intensity (Pain Control during Training)	Frequency and Duration	Exercise Testing
Sandstad et al., 2015 [51]	HIIT (AerT)	*Warmup:* 10 min stationary cycling at moderate intensity *HIIT protocol:* 4 × 4 min high-intensity stationary cycling interval alternating with 3 min cycling recovery periods. The speed and workload were adjusted continuously.	*Measurement:* HR_{max} (HR checked using HR monitor) *Warmup:* ~70% *Interval:* 85–95% of HRmax *Rest:* ~70% of HRmax *Pain:* N/R	2×/week 10 weeks	Maximal cardiopulmonary test on a bike. VO_2 max and HR_{max} (defined as the highest HR during the test plus 5 bpm).
	Maintain daily life activities	N/A	N/A		
Sveaas et al., 2014 and 2019 [16,49]	HIIT (AerT) + StrT + MICT (AerT)	Twice a week, supervised HIIT and StrT: - *HIIT protocol:* 4 × 4 min walking/running on a treadmill interval alternating with 3 min of active resting. - *StrT protocol*: 20 min with external load (2–3 × 8–10 rep): Bench press or chest press machine, weighted squat or leg press machine, rowing with weights, triceps and biceps machine, and abdominal bridge. Once a week, individual interval training or MICT: 40 min of either interval training or MICT.	*Measurement:* HR_{max} (HR checked using HR monitor) *HIIT-* *Interval:* 90–95% HR_{max} Rest: 70% HR_{max} *MICT intensity:* >70% HR_{max} *Pain*: Exercises were adapted if pain was ≥ 5/10	3×/week 12 weeks	Cardiopulmonary test on a walking treadmill (modified Balke protocol). VO_2 max and HR_{max} were recorded.
	Asked to not start exercise	N/A	N/A		
Thomsen et al., 2019 [53]	HIIT (AerT)	*Warmup:* 10 min. *HIIT protocol:* 4 × 4 min high-intensity stationary cycling interval alternating with a 3 min cycling recovery period. *Work/rest ratio:* [1:0.75] Supervised twice a week and individually once a week. Participants were instructed in using the HIIT concept by, for example, running, bicycling, or walking uphill.	*Measurement:* HR_{max} (HR checked using HR monitor) *Interval:* 85–95% HR_{max} *Rest:* 70% HR_{max} *Pain:* N/R	3×/week 11 weeks	Maximal cardiopulmonary test on a bike. VO_2 max and HR_{max} (defined as the highest HR during the test more 5 bpm).
	Maintain daily physical activity	N/A	N/A		

Table 2. *Cont.*

Trial	Group	Exercise Protocol (Distribution and Exercise Type)	Intensity (Pain Control during Training)	Frequency and Duration	Exercise Testing
Verbrugghe et al., 2018 [47]	HIIT (AerT) + High Intensity StrT	*HIIT protocol:* *-Warmup:* 5 min *-Followed by HIIT training:* 5 × 1 min high-intensity stationary cycling interval alternating with 1 min of rest. Weekly increase of interval duration by 10 s until week 6. *Work/rest ratio:* [1:1; 1.2:1; 1.3:1; 1.5:1; 1.7:1; 1.8:1] *High load whole body StrT training protocol:* 3 upper body (pulley biceps curl, pulley chest press, and pulley vertical traction behind the neck) and 3 lower body exercises (leg press, leg extension, and leg curl) with external load: 1 to 2 × 8–12 rep.	*Measurement:* VO_2 max and 1RM (Monitorisation: N/R) *Interval:* VO_2 max workload *Rest:* N/R *StrT:* 80% 1RM *Pain:* N/R	2×/week 6 weeks	Maximal cardiopulmonary testing (Graded exercise test) on a bike. VO_2 max, expiratory volume, respiratory exchange ratio, and HR were recorded A 1RM test was performed for every exercise.
	Usual Physiotherapy Care	*MICT protocol:* 50 min continuous cycling, cross-training, and/or treadmill walking. *Control motor exercise:* Addressing lumbopelvic motor control impairments. *Trunk StrT:* Unstable posture corrections, plank, and bridge variations	*Measurement:* HR_{max} (Monitorisation: N/R) *MICT:* 60–65% HR_{max} *Pain:* N/R		
Verbrugghe et al., 2019 [17]	HIIT (AerT) + High-intensity Global and Core StrT	*HIIT protocol:* *-Warmup:* 5 min cycling *-HIIT Training:* 5 × 1 min high-intensity cycling interval alternating with a 1 min cycling recovery period. Weekly increase of interval duration of 10 s until week 6. *Work/rest ratio:* [1:1; 1.2:1; 1.3:1; 1.5:1; 1.7:1; 1.8:1] *High-intensity StrT:* 3 upper body (vertical traction, chest press, arm curl) and 3 lower body exercises (leg curl, leg press, leg extension) executed with external load on machines: 1 × maximum 12 rep *Core muscle training:* 6 static core exercises [glute bridge, resistance band glute clam, lying diagonal back extension, adapted knee plank, adapted knee side plank, elastic band shoulder retraction with hip hinge): 1 × 10 rep of a 10 s static hold.	*Measurement:* % VO_2 max, %1RM and %MVC (Monitorisation: N/R) *HIIT:* *Interval:* 110 rpm at 100% VO_2 max workload *Rest:* 75 rpm at 50% VO_2 max workload *StrT:* 80% 1RM 5% workload increase when the participant was able to perform more than 10 reps on 2 consecutive sessions. *Core:* Between 17% and 100% MVC of m. transversus abdominis, m. multifidus, m. gluteus. Progressive increase of time and load (body weight bearing, elastic or weights). *Pain:* N/R	2×/week 12 weeks	Maximal cardiopulmonary test on a bicycle. VO_2 max, Maximal workload, LA, and HR were recorded. Workload was updated, with a complementary cardiopulmonary test, for the last 6 weeks. 1RM testing was performed for every exercise.
	MICT (AerT) + Moderate intensity Global and Core STrT	*MICT protocol:* Cycling on a cycle ergometer. *- Warmup:* 5 min. *- MICT:* Continuous 14 min cycling at moderate intensity. Duration increased by 100 s every 2 sessions up to 22 min 40 s. *Moderate intensity Global StrT:* Same exercises as above, but at moderate intensity: 1 × 15 rep. *Moderate intensity core training:* Same exercises as above but at moderate intensity: 1 × 10 repetitions of a 10 s static hold.	*Measurement:* % VO_2 max, %1RM and %MVC (Monitorisation: N/R) *MICT:* 90 rpm at 60% VO_2 max workload *StrT:* 60% of 1RM *Core training:* N/R *Pain:* N/R		

Table 2. *Cont.*

Trial	Group	Exercise Protocol (Distribution and Exercise Type)	Intensity (Pain Control during Training)	Frequency and Duration	Exercise Testing
Verbrugghe et al., 2020 [48]	HIIT (AerT) + Global StrT	*HIIT protocol:* - *Warmup:* 5 min cycling - *HIIT Training:* 5 × 1 min high-intensity cycling interval alternating with a 1 min cycling recovery period. Weekly increase of interval duration, of 10 s, until week 6. *Work/rest ratio:* [1:1; 1.2:1; 1.3:1; 1.5:1; 1.7:1; 1.8:1] *High-intensity StrT:* 3 upper body (vertical traction, chest press, arm curl) and 3 lower body exercises (leg curl, leg press, leg extension) executed with external load on machines: 2 × maximum 12 rep	*Measurement:* % VO_2 max and %1RM (Monitorisation: N/R) *HIIT:* *Interval:* 110 rpm at 100% VO_2 max workload *Rest:* 75 rpm at 50% VO_2 max workload *StrT:* 80% 1 RM Weight was increased when the participant was able to perform more than 10 reps on 2 consecutive sessions. *Pain:* N/R	2×/week 12 weeks	Maximal cardiopulmonary test on a bicycle. VO_2 max, expiratory volume, respiratory exchange ratio, and HR were recorded. Parameters were adapted at 6 weeks with another cardiopulmonary test. 1RM testing was performed for every exercise.
	HIIT (AerT) + Core StrT	*HIIT protocol:* Same HIIT protocol as above. *Core muscle training:* 6 static core exercises [glute bridge, resistance band glute clam, lying diagonal back extension, adapted knee plank, adapted knee side plank, elastic band shoulder retraction with hip hinge): 2 × 10 rep of a 10 s static hold.	*Measurement:* % VO_2 max and %MVC (Monitorisation: N/R) *HIIT:* *Interval:* 110 rpm at 100% VO_2 max workload *Rest:* 75 rpm at 50% VO_2 max workload *Core:* 40–60% of the MVC of m. transversus abdominis, m. multifidus, m. gluteus Progressive increase of time and load. *Pain:* N/R		
	HIIT (AerT)+ Global and Core StrT	*HIIT protocol:* Same HIIT protocol as above. *High intensity StrT:* Same exercise as above: 1 × maximum 12 rep *Core muscle training:* Same exercise as above: 1 × 10 rep of a 10 s static hold.	*Measurement:* % VO_2 max, %1RM and %MVC (Monitorisation: N/R) *HIIT:* *Interval:* 110 rpm at 100% VO_2 max workload *Rest:* 75 rpm at 50% VO_2 max workload *StrT:* 80% 1 RM Weight was increased when the participant was able to perform more than 10 reps on 2 consecutive sessions. *Core:* 40–60% of the MVC of m. transversus abdominis, m. multifidus, m. gluteus. Progressive increase in time and load *Pain:* N/R		

Table 2. *Cont.*

Trial	Group	Exercise Protocol (Distribution and Exercise Type)	Intensity (Pain Control during Training)	Frequency and Duration	Exercise Testing
	HIIT (AerT)+ Mobility	*HIIT protocol:* Same HIIT protocol as above. *Mobility Training*: 6 mobility exercises (hamstrings stretch, gluteus medius stretch, lower back rotation mobilisation, back extension stretch, hip flexor stretch, and mid-back extension mobilisation): Stretches were held on each side 2 × 30 s, and mobilisations were performed 2 × 10 rep.	*HIIT:* *Interval:* 110 rpm at 100% VO_2 max workload *Rest:* 75 rpm at 50% VO_2 max workload *Mobility:* N/R *Pain:* N/R		

1RM, one-repetition maximum; ACSM, American College of Sports Medicine; AerT, aerobic training; BalanceT, balance training; bpm, beats per min; HIIT, high-intensity interval training; HR, heart rate; HR_{max}, maximal heart rate; HRR, heart rate reserve; LA, lactate level; MICT, moderate-intensity continuous training; MVC, maximal voluntary contraction; N/A, not applicable; N/R, not reported; RPE, rating of perceived exertion; rpm, revolutions per minute; StrT, strength training; VO_2 max, maximal oxygen uptake; WR_{max}, highest work rate.

3.3. Methodological Quality Results

We evaluated the studies' quality with the Cochrane assessment tool. Most of the studies had a low risk of selective reporting bias. The domain with the highest percentage of studies with a high risk of bias was the blinding of participants and personnel (performance bias). Figure 2 shows the risk of bias summary and risk of bias graph. The inter-rater reliability of the methodological quality assessment was high (κ = 0.787). All of the studies had an excellent or good methodological quality, except the one by Bressel et al. [45] Due to the nature of the interventions, none of the studies performed blinding of the patients or evaluators. Table 3 lists the PEDro scores for each study. The inter-rater reliability of the methodological quality assessment between assessors was high (κ = 0.815).

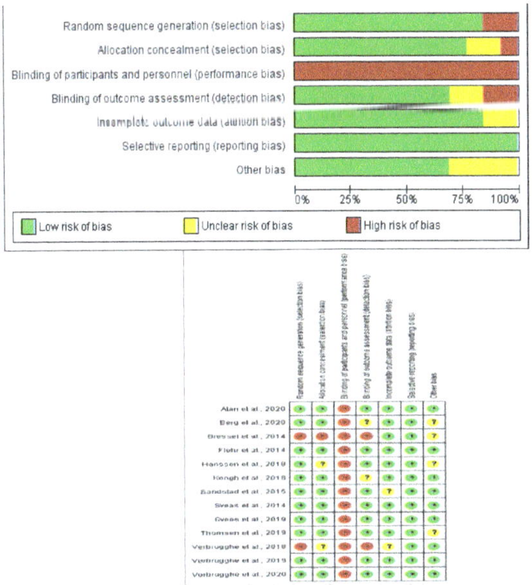

Figure 2. Risk of bias summary. Review authors' judgements about each risk of bias item for each included study (Risk of Bias scale) and risk of bias graph. Review authors' judgements about each risk of bias item presented as percentages across all included studies (Risk of Bias scale).

Table 3. Assessment of the studies' quality based on the PEDro Scale.

	Items											
	1	2	3	4	5	6	7	8	9	10	11	Total
Atan et al., 2020 [15]	1	1	1	1	0	0	1	1	1	1	1	8
Berg et al., 2020 [50]	1	1	1	0	0	0	0	1	1	1	1	6
Bressel et al., 2014 [44]	1	0	0	1	0	0	0	1	1	1	1	5
Flehr et al., 2019 [52]	1	1	1	1	0	0	1	1	1	1	1	8
Hanssen et al., 2018 [49]	1	1	1	1	0	0	1	1	1	1	1	8
Keogh et al., 2018 [45]	1	1	1	1	0	0	0	1	1	1	1	7
Sandstad et al., 2015 [51]	1	1	1	1	0	0	0	1	1	1	1	7
Sveas et al., 2014 [16]	1	1	1	1	0	0	1	1	1	1	1	8
Sveas et al., 2019 [49]	1	1	1	1	0	0	1	1	1	1	1	8
Thomsen et al., 2019 [53]	1	1	1	1	0	0	1	1	1	1	1	8
Verbrugghe et al., 2018 [47]	1	0	0	1	0	0	1	1	1	1	1	6
Verbrugghe et al., 2019 [17]	1	1	1	1	0	0	0	1	1	1	1	7
Verbrugghe et al., 2020 [48]	1	1	1	1	0	0	0	1	1	1	1	7

1, patient choice criteria are specified; 2, random assignment of patients to groups; 3, hidden assignment; 4, groups were similar at baseline; 5, all patients were blinded; 6, all therapists were blinded; 7, all evaluators were blinded; 8, measures of at least one of the key outcomes were obtained from more than 85% of baseline patients; 9, intention-to-treat analysis was performed; 10, results from statistical intergroup comparisons were reported for at least one key outcome; 11, the study provides point and variability measures for at least one key outcome.

3.4. Evidence Map

Figure 3 presents the results of the evidence map for the included studies.

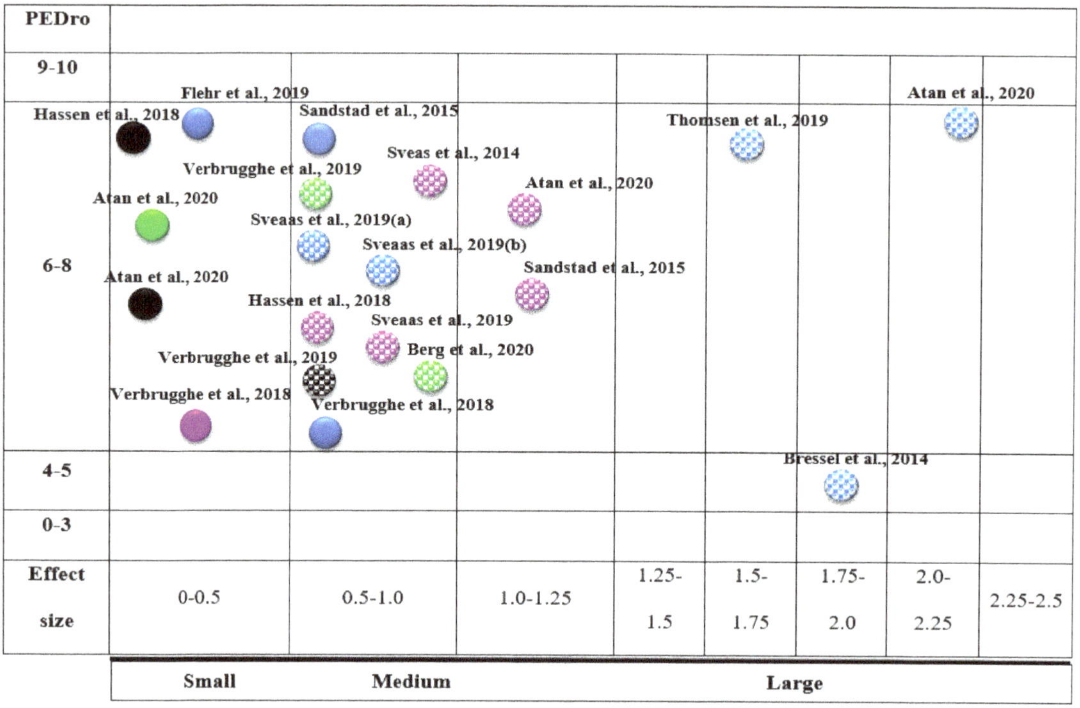

Figure 3. A mapping of included studies based on effect size. Blue, Pain intensity; Violet, $VO_{2\ max}$; Green, Disability; Black, Quality of Life. Bubbles marked with white dots indicate statistically significant differences ($p < 0.05$).

3.5. Meta-Analysis Results

3.5.1. Pain Intensity

The meta-analysis showed statistically significant differences for the HIIT intervention, with a moderate clinical effect in seven studies (SMD: −0.73; 95% CI −1.40–−0.06; $p < 0.05$) but with evidence of significant heterogeneity (Q = 32.57, $p < 0.001$, $I^2 = 82\%$). The shape of the funnel and DOI plot did not present asymmetry, and the LFK index showed minor asymmetry (LFK, −1.73) indicating a low risk of publication bias (Figures 4A and A1). The certainty of the evidence was low, showing that HIIT likely decreases pain intensity, having been downgraded due to imprecision (sample size < 300) and inconsistency ($I^2 = 82\%$) (Table 4).

Regarding the sub-analysis comparing HIIT against other therapeutic exercise models, the meta-analysis showed no significant differences for the HIIT intervention in 3 studies (SMD: −0.35; 95% CI −0.76–0.06, $p \geq 0.05$) with no evidence of significant heterogeneity (Q = 1.37, $p = 0.5$, $I^2 = 0\%$). The shape of the funnel and DOI plot did not present asymmetry, and the LFK index showed no asymmetry (LFK, 0.67) indicating a very low risk of publication bias (Figures 4B and A2).

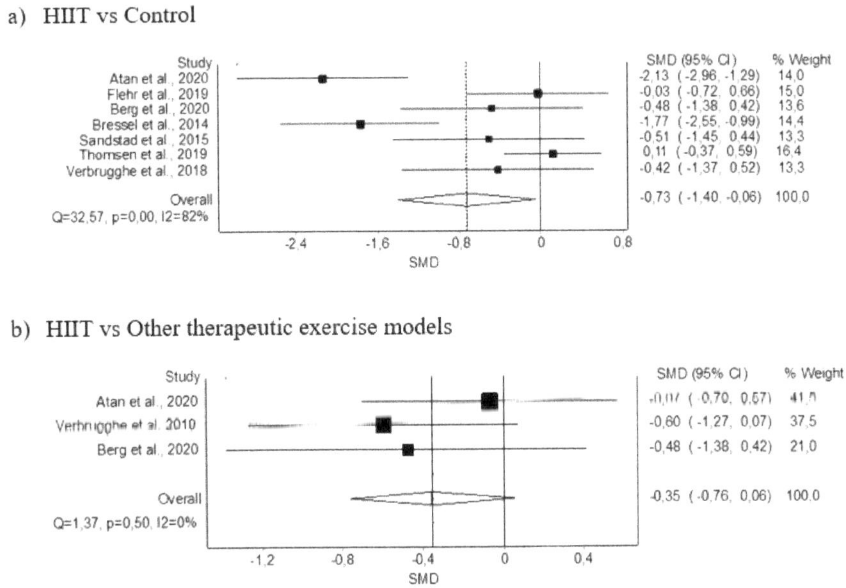

Figure 4. Synthesis forest plot of pain intensity variable. The forest plot summarises the results of the included studies (sample size, standardised mean differences [SMDs], and weight). The small boxes with the squares represent the point estimate of the effect size and sample size. The lines on either side of the box represent a 95% confidence interval (CI).

Table 4. Summary of findings and quality of evidence (GRADE).

Certainty Assessment						No. of Participants		Effect		Certainty	Importance
Outcome (No. of Studies)	**Study Design**	**Risk of Bias**	**Inconsistency**	**Indirectness**	**Imprecision**	**HIIT**	**Control**	**Relative (95% CI)**	**Absolute (95% CI)**		
Pain intensity (7)	RCT	Not serious	Serious	Not serious	Serious	119	120	-	−0.73 (1.40–−0.06)	Low (+) (+)	Critical
$VO_{2\,max}$ (6)	RCT	Not serious	Not serious	Not serious	Serious	112	118	-	0.69 (0.42–0.97)	Moderate (+) (+) (+)	Critical
Disability (4)	RCT	Not serious	Not serious	Not serious	Serious	35	33	-	−0.34 (−0.92–0.24)	Moderate (+) (+) (+)	Critical
Quality of life (4)	RCT	Not serious	Serious	Not serious	Serious	53	44	-	0.40 (−0.80–1.60)	Low (+) (+)	Critical

CI, confidence interval; RCT, randomised controlled trial.

3.5.2. $VO_{2\,max}$

The meta-analysis showed significant differences for the HIIT intervention, with a moderate clinical effect in six studies (SMD: 0.69; 95% CI 0.42–0.97, $p < 0.05$), with no evidence of significant heterogeneity ($Q = 4.06$, $p = 0.54$, $I^2 = 0\%$). The shape of the funnel and DOI plot did not present asymmetry, and the LFK index showed minor asymmetry (LFK, 1.33) indicating a low risk of publication bias (Figures 5A and A2). The certainty of the evidence was moderate, showing that HIIT probably increases VO_2 max, having been downgraded due to imprecision (sample size < 300) (Table 4).

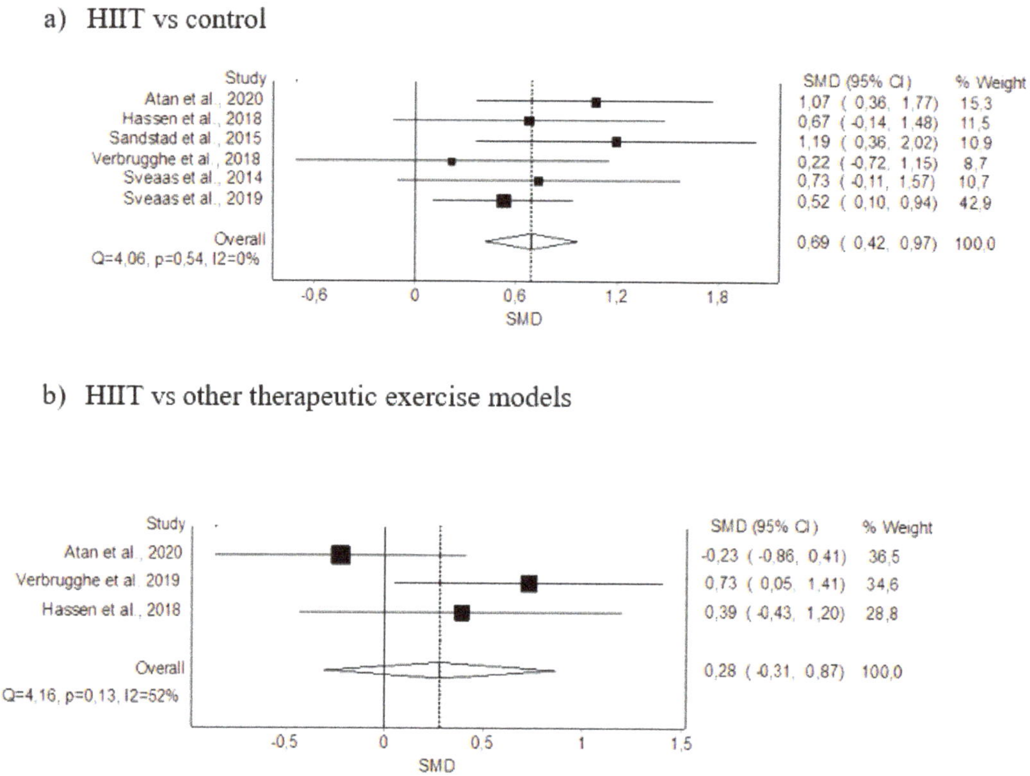

Figure 5. Synthesis forest plot of $VO_{2\ max}$ variable. The forest plot summarises the results of the included studies (sample size, standardised mean differences [SMDs], and weight). The small boxes with the squares represent the point estimate of the effect size and sample size. The lines on either side of the box represent a 95% confidence interval (CI).

Regarding the subanalysis comparing HIIT against other therapeutic exercise models, the meta-analysis showed no statistically significant differences for the HIIT intervention in three studies (SMD: 0.28; 95% CI −0.31–0.87, $p \geq 0.05$), with no evidence of significant heterogeneity (Q = 4.16, $p = 0.13$, $I^2 = 52\%$). The shape of the funnel and DOI plot did not present asymmetry, and the LFK index showed no asymmetry (LFK, −0.31) indicating a very low risk of publication bias (Figures 5B and A2).

3.5.3. Disability

The meta-analysis showed no statistically significant differences for the HIIT intervention in three studies (SMD: −0.34; 95% CI −0.92–0.24, $p \geq 0.05$), with no evidence of significant heterogeneity (Q = 4.55, $p = 0.21$, $I^2 = 34\%$). The shape of the funnel and DOI plot did not present asymmetry, and the LFK index showed minor asymmetry (LFK, −1.68) indicating a low risk of publication bias (Figures 6A and A3). The certainty of the evidence was moderate, showing that HIIT probably does not decrease disability, being downgraded due to imprecision (sample size <300) (Table 4).

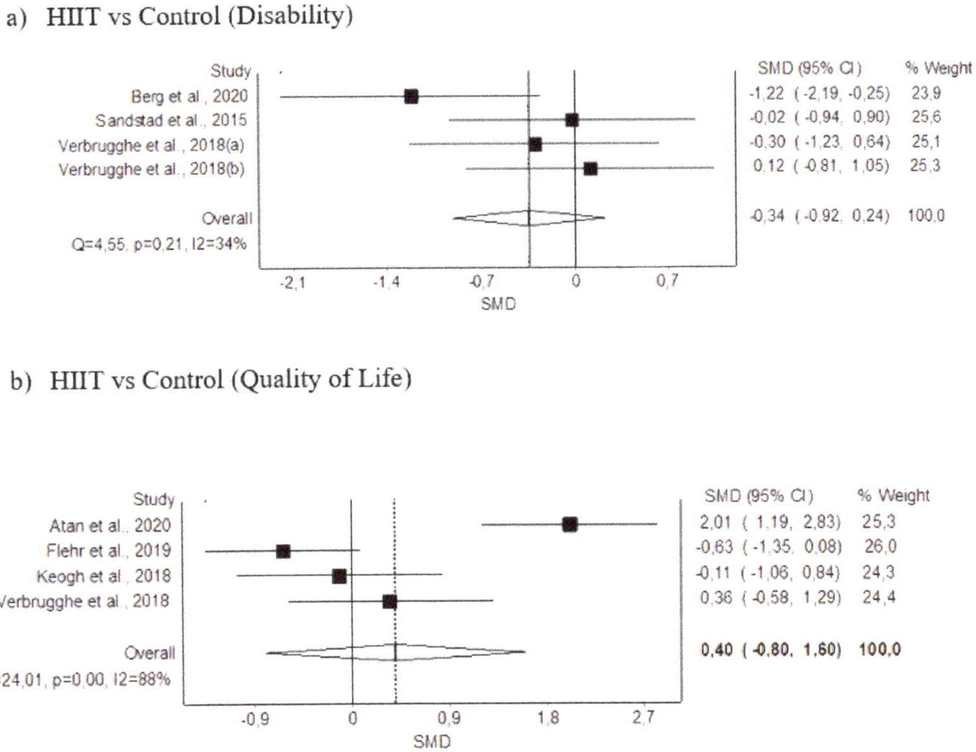

Figure 6. Synthesis forest plot of disability and quality-of-life variables. The forest plot summarises the results of the included studies (sample size, standardised mean differences [SMDs], and weight). The small boxes with the squares represent the point estimate of the effect size and sample size. The lines on either side of the box represent a 95% confidence interval (CI).

3.5.4. Quality of Life

The meta-analysis showed no significant differences for the HIIT intervention in 4 studies (SMD: 0.40; 95% CI −0.80–1.60, $p \geq 0.05$), with evidence of significant heterogeneity (Q = 24.01, $p < 0.001$, $I^2 = 88\%$). The shape of the funnel and DOI plot did not present asymmetry, and the LFK index showed minor asymmetry (LFK, 1.43), indicating a low risk of publication bias (Figures 6B and A3). The certainty of the evidence was low, showing that HIIT likely does not increase QoL, being downgraded due to imprecision (sample size < 300) and inconsistency ($I^2 = 88\%$) (Table 4).

3.6. Meta-Regression Analysis

In the meta-regression analysis, we explored the role of pain intensity scores in improving VO_2 max function. The results showed that pain intensity was significantly and negatively correlated with VO_2 max ($\beta = -0.91$; $Z = -3.02$; $p = 0.003$ and $R^2 = 82.99\%$) (Figure 7).

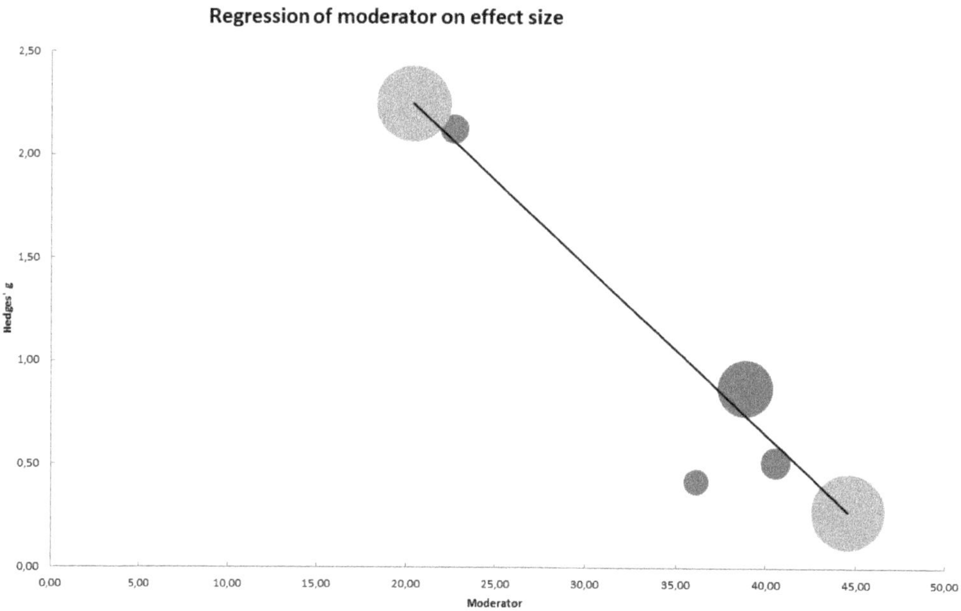

Figure 7. Meta-regression of pain intensity and $VO_{2\,max}$ scores. The meta-regression approach uses regression analysis to determine the influence of selected variables (the independent variables) on the effect size (the dependent variable). The large bubbles, together with the line, indicate the relationship of our model, and the small bubbles indicate their position, the relationship in the map of the effect size on the decrease in pain, on the score in the variable of maximal oxygen consumption.

4. Discussion

Our main goal was to analyse the effect of HIIT on the $VO_{2\,max}$, pain intensity, disability, and QoL of patients with musculoskeletal disorders. Our results suggest that HIIT has a significant moderate effect size on $VO_{2\,max}$ and pain intensity but does not seem to improve the disability and QoL of patients with musculoskeletal disorders. We also found that pain intensity was negatively associated with VO_2 max.

We found a moderate certainty of evidence of a moderate effect size of HIIT on $VO_{2\,max}$ when compared with no intervention. Several authors also found that HIIT was superior to usual care or no intervention in improving $VO_{2\,max}$ among patients with cardiovascular disorders or cancer [18,19,55]. We did not find that HIIT was superior to another exercise intervention on VO_2 max; however, the results across systematic reviews differ [19,56,57]. It has been previously reported that HIIT induces muscular adaptations, such as mitochondrial biogenesis and increased intramuscular capillarisation [58,59] vascular adaptations, such as increased blood cell volume [60], and cardiac adaptations, such as increased cardiac output and contractility [59,61]. All of these mechanisms have been shown to play a role in $VO_{2\,max}$ [62].

We found that the patients' pain intensity scores were negatively associated with $VO_{2\,max}$, which is an important predictor of all-cause mortality and cardiovascular disease [63,64]. It should be noted that patients with chronic pain and musculoskeletal disorders have shown an increased risk of cardiovascular and chronic disease and an increased risk of mortality due to cardiac disease [65,66]. An improvement in cardiorespiratory capacity has been shown to decrease the mortality risk by up to 16% [67,68]. HIIT appears to be an effective solution for improving patients' cardiorespiratory capacity.

We found a low certainty of evidence of a moderate effect size of HIIT on pain intensity compared with no intervention. Geneen et al. found that physical activity appears to induce exercise-induced hypoalgesia in patients with chronic pain; however, the results were inconsistent across the various exercise modalities [69]. When compared with another exercise intervention, HIIT did not show a greater effect. It has been shown that exercise-induced hypoalgesia acts through the activation of nociceptive inhibitory pathways that release endogenous opioids and endocannabinoids [70]; however, populations with chronic pain often have exercise-induced hypoalgesia dysfunction [70,71]. Nonetheless, we found that HIIT appeared to be an effective modality for decreasing pain intensity. Patients with musculoskeletal disorders often present central sensitisation, a facilitation of the nociceptive signal in the central nervous system [72]. Quantitative sensory testing is employed to evaluate central nervous system nociceptive modulation [72]. HIIT has shown an intensity-dependent [12,13] positive effect on pain tolerance [13] and pain thresholds [12,73]. In certain conditions, the presence of an inflammatory state can increase nociceptor activity and has been associated with pain intensity [71,74–76]. After performing HIIT, a number of authors have found a decrease in inflammatory markers [77–79], such as C-reactive protein, tumour necrosis factor-alpha and interleukin-6 (IL-6), and a release of anti-inflammatory cytokines, such as IL-10 [79]. In contrast, other authors have found that HIIT induced an acute increase in IL 6 levels [80,81]; however, Pedersen proposed that this acute liberation will then induce an anti-inflammatory response [82]. Shanaki et al. observed a decrease in pro-inflammatory M1-macrophage markers and an increase in anti-inflammatory M2-macrophage markers in mice after HIIT [83]. However, not all musculoskeletal conditions show reduced pain intensity in parallel with a decrease in pro-nociceptive or inflammatory serum markers [76,84], and not all musculoskeletal conditions progress with an increased inflammatory state [76].

We found a low level of evidence of no significant effect of HIIT on QoL compared with no intervention or usual care. Mugele et al. systematically reviewed the effect of HIIT on QoL, compared with usual care, and found unclear results [19]. QoL appears to be more closely related to interpretation and catastrophising than pain intensity [85], which might explain why we observed a decrease in pain intensity with no improvement in QoL. Monticone et al. found that a multidisciplinary treatment involving cognitive-behavioural therapy and exercise results in a significant improvement in QoL, while exercise alone resulted in little change [86]. We also found moderate certainty evidence of no significant effect of HIIT on disability compared with no intervention or usual care. Kamper et al. found that a treatment involving a physical and a psychological or social component had a greater effect on disability than physical therapy alone for patients with chronic low back pain. HIIT alone might be insufficient for improving disability or QoL in musculoskeletal disorders [87].

Time constraints and pain are two of the main barriers to physical activity for patients with musculoskeletal disorders [88–90]. Despite similar effects on $VO_{2\,max}$ and pain intensity with other exercise types, HIIT requires less training volume to achieve similar effects in the included studies that provide the control group's training duration [15,50]. Wewege et al. found that the most common adverse effects in patients with cardiovascular disease were musculoskeletal complaints; however, we observed that HIIT presented similar or almost no additional major or minor adverse events or pain flare-ups than no intervention or other exercise modalities [91]. Major cardiac adverse events during HIIT appear at a rate of 1 per 11,333 HIIT h in patients with cardiovascular disease [91] but with no significant difference in the overall adverse events rate between HIIT and MICT [91]. As recommended by Weston et al. if health professionals want to implement HIIT, they should evaluate patients on a case-by-case basis depending on their cardiac history [20]. Heisz et al. found that participants rated HIIT more enjoyable than MICT and that enjoyment increased with repeated HIIT when it remained constant with repeated MICT [92]. Health professionals should include HIIT in the management of musculoskeletal disorders, given that HIIT is a time-efficient, enjoyable, effective, and safe form of exercise. Finally, it is relevant to stress that it is important to prescribe exercise specifically for each patient and for each clinical condition, although in this work it has been grouped by variables, rather than by populations.

Limitations

We found low-to-moderate quality evidence for our results. Further studies are needed on the effects of HIIT on musculoskeletal disorders to confirm our results. The sample sizes of the included studies were often very small. Future studies should include larger sample sizes to improve the quality of the evidence. Due to the lack of sufficient data and the heterogeneity among the interventions (e.g., frequency, intervention duration), we could not establish the specific effect on each musculoskeletal disorder and the optimal HIIT parameters. Due to the small number of trials, we pooled the aerobic and anaerobic HIIT training studies; future systematic reviews should evaluate them separately. Only a few studies compared the effect of HIIT against high-intensity continuous training or other types of exercise; future studies should include this type of high-intensity training.

As recommended by the American Thoracic Society/American College of Chest Physicians Statement on Cardiopulmonary Exercise Testing, we included VO_2 peak and $VO_{2\,max}$ and used them interchangeably [93]. Quantitative sensory testing (e.g., pain pressure or thermal threshold, conditioned pain modulation, and temporal summation) is essential in pain research; future studies evaluating the effects of HIIT on musculoskeletal disorders should include these variables. In addition, no further meta-regression analysis could be performed due to the small number of articles sharing the outcomes of interest. Lastly, it is important to stress that there were 3 studies where HIIT was embedded in other exercise interventions such as balance exercise and continuous exercise. This is a clear limitation that should be considered when extrapolating the results [16,45,47].

5. Conclusions

There is low to moderate quality evidence that the HIIT intervention for patients with musculoskeletal disorders can improve pain intensity and $VO_{2\,max}$ but not disability and QoL. The results of the subanalyses showed that HIIT was not superior to other exercise models in improving pain intensity and $VO_{2\,max}$. Clinically, this tells us that we can implement high-intensity interval exercise models if our goal is to improve pain intensity or increase cardiorespiratory fitness through maximal oxygen consumption. However, it is important to keep in mind two aspects: changes in pain intensity may not be accompanied by improvements in the subjective perception of quality of life or disability, at least, based on the data we currently have, and second, that this exercise model was not superior to other exercise models with respect to eliciting these clinical changes. This should be considered clinically. Low sample sizes and lack of prescription parameters emphasise the need for further research on HIIT in musculoskeletal disorders for its implementation in a clinical context.

Author Contributions: Conceptualization, F.C.-M.; methodology, F.C.-M., N.S.-R., C.V.-R. and R.L.T.; software, F.C.-M. and R.L.T.; validation, N.S.-R., L.S.-M., P.A.-Q. and J.F.-C.; formal analysis, F.C.-M. and R.L.T.; investigation, all authors; resources, J.F.-C.; data curation, F.C.-M., C.V.-R. and R.L.T.; writing—original draft preparation, all authors; writing—review and editing, all authors; visualization, all authors; supervision, F.C.-M.; project administration, F.C.-M. and N.S.-R.; funding acquisition, not applicable. All authors have read and agreed to the published version of the manuscript.

Funding: This research received no external funding.

Institutional Review Board Statement: Not applicable.

Informed Consent Statement: Not applicable.

Data Availability Statement: Not applicable.

Acknowledgments: The authors would like to thank the CSEU La Salle for its services in editing this manuscript.

Conflicts of Interest: The authors declare no conflict of interest.

Appendix A

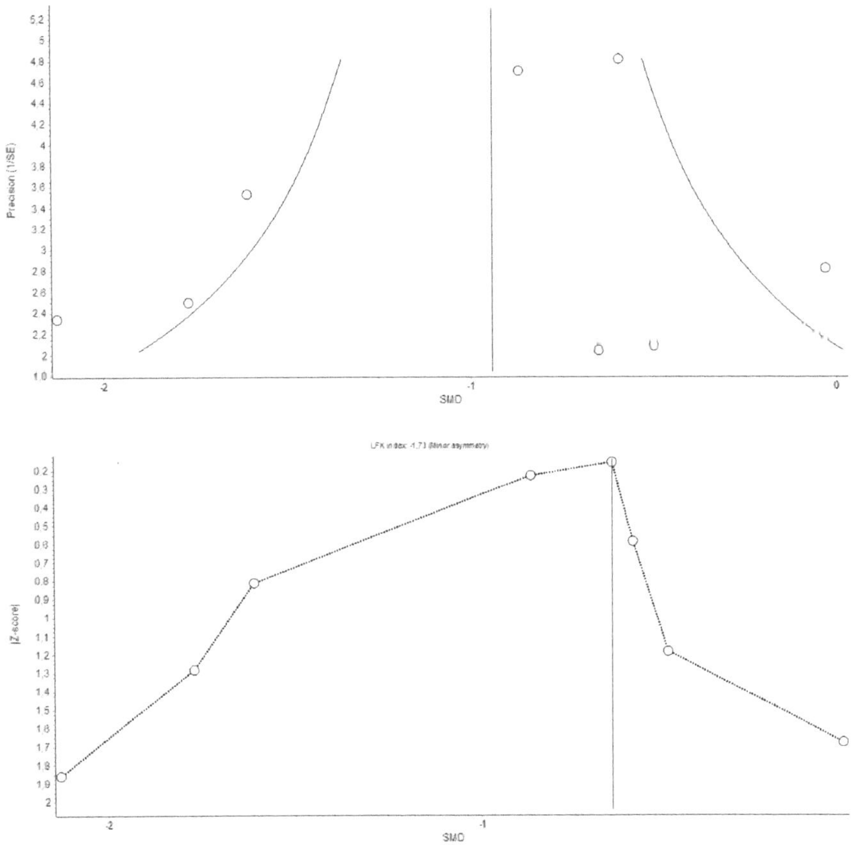

(**a**) HIIT vs. control

Figure A1. *Cont.*

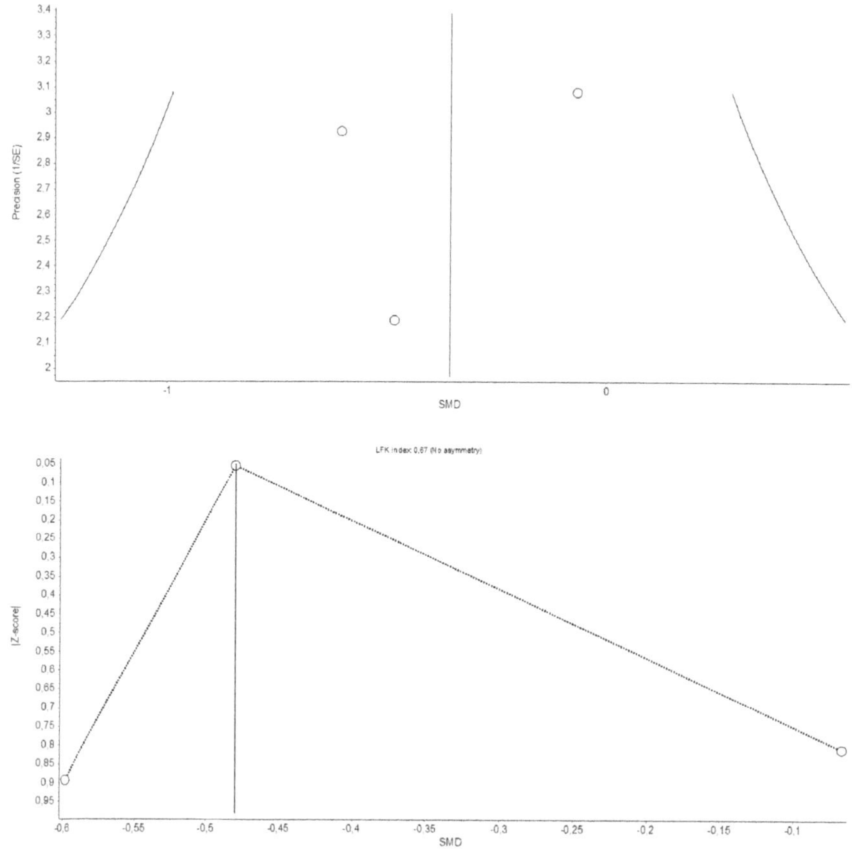

(**b**) HIIT vs. Other therapeutic exercise models

Figure A1. Synthesis funnel and Doi plot (LFK index) for pain intensity to assess the presence of publication bias.

Appendix B

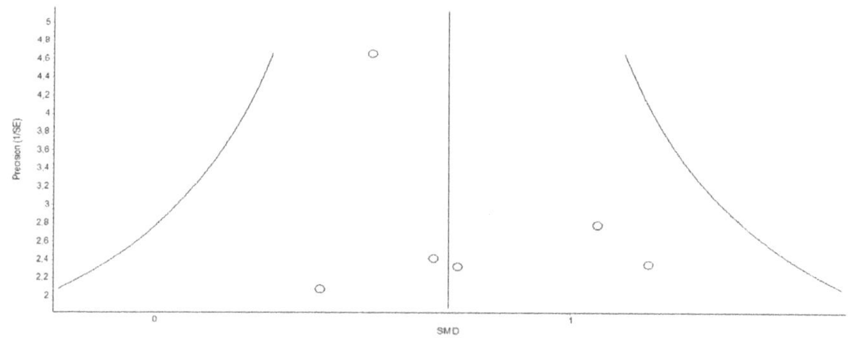

Figure A2. *Cont.*

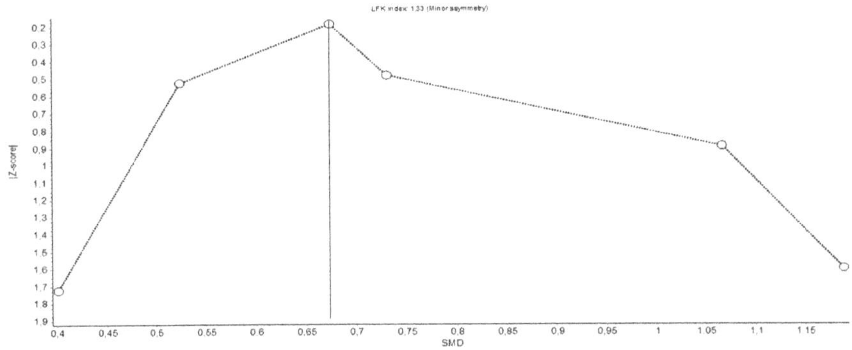

(a) HIIT vs. control

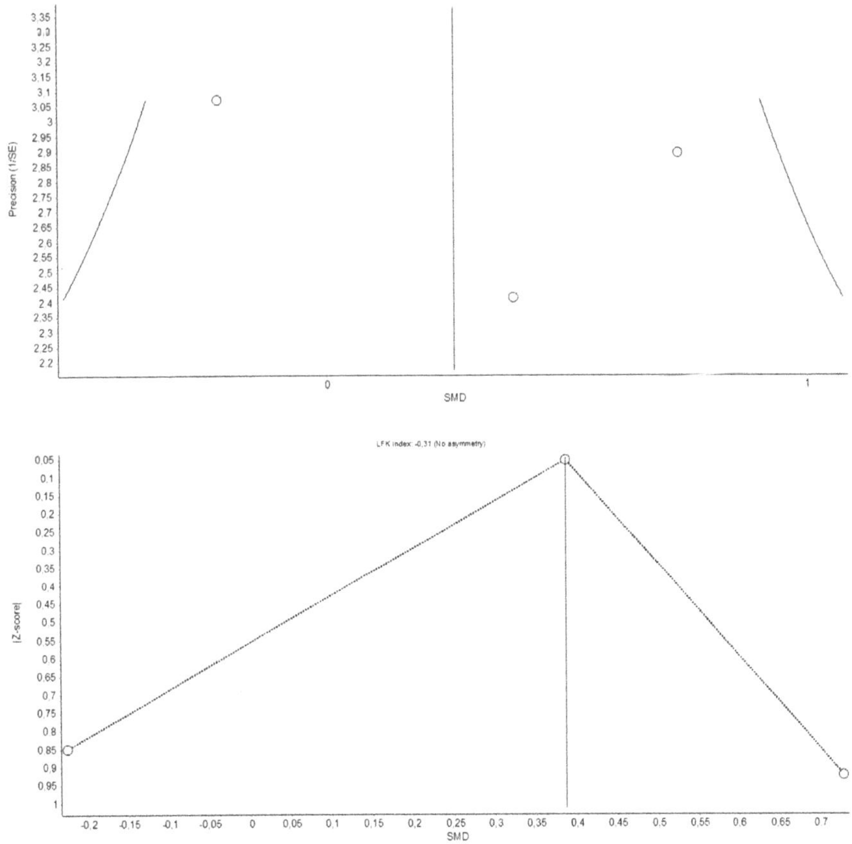

(b) HIIT vs. other therapeutic exercise models

Figure A2. Synthesis funnel and Doi plot (LFK index) for VO_2 max to assess the presence of publication bias.

Appendix C

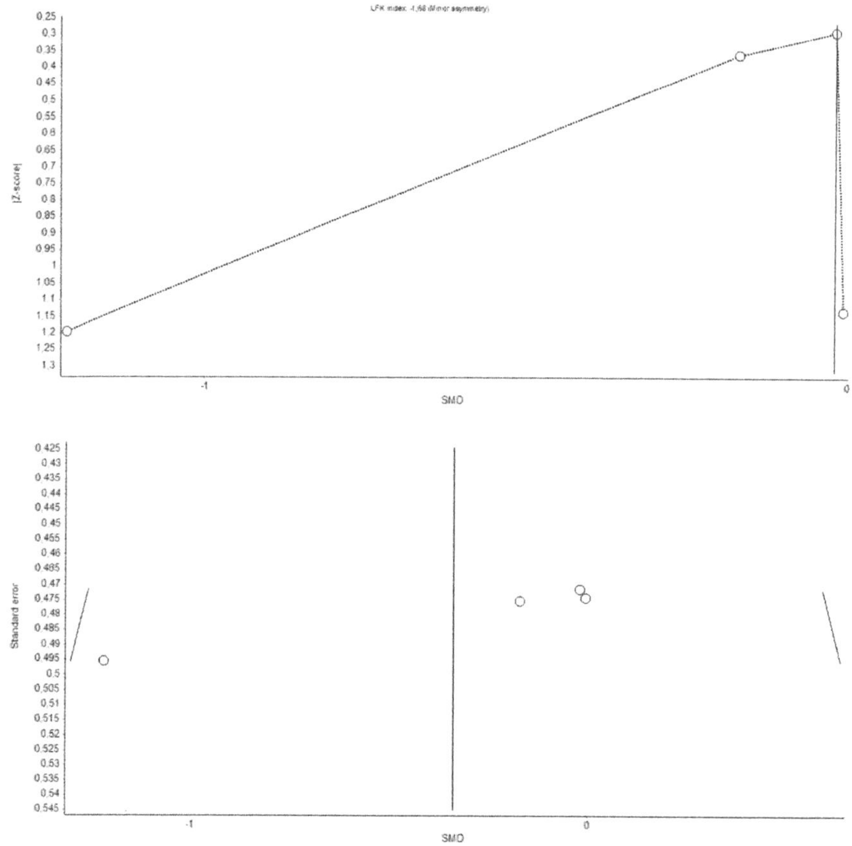

(**a**) HIIT vs. control (disability)

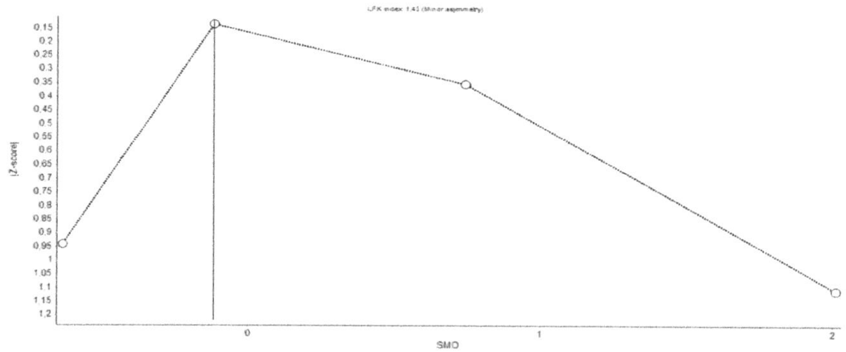

Figure A3. *Cont.*

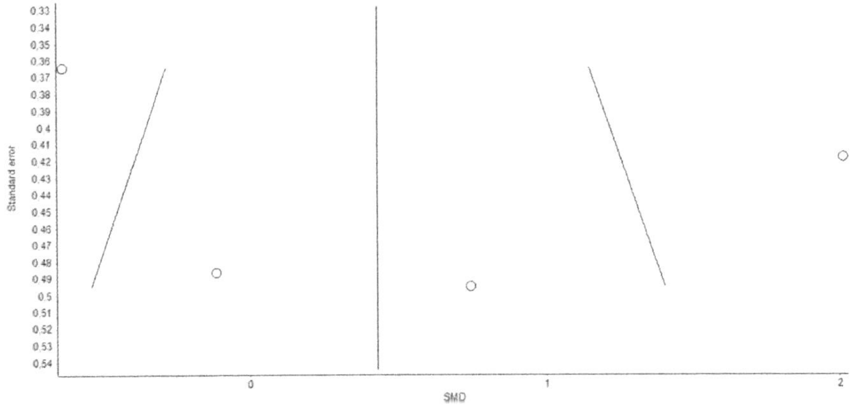

(**b**) HIIT vs. control (quality of life)

Figure A3. Synthesis Funnel and Doi plot (LFK index) for disability and quality-of-life variables to assess the presence of publication bias.

References

1. Picavet, H.S.J.; Schouten, J.S.A.G. Musculoskeletal pain in the Netherlands: Prevalences, consequences and risk groups, the DMC3-study. *Pain* **2003**, *102*, 167–178. [CrossRef]
2. Silva, A.G.; Alvarelhão, J.; Queirós, A.; Rocha, N.P. Pain intensity is associated with self-reported disability for several domains of life in a sample of patients with musculoskeletal pain aged 50 or more. *Disabil. Health J.* **2013**, *6*, 369–376. [CrossRef] [PubMed]
3. Nielson, W.R.; Weir, R. Biopsychosocial Approaches to the Treatment of Chronic Pain. *Clin. J. Pain* **2001**, *17*, S114–S127. [CrossRef] [PubMed]
4. Wright, A.; Sluka, K.A. Nonpharmacological Treatments for Musculoskeletal Pain. *Clin. J. Pain* **2001**, *17*, 33–46. [CrossRef]
5. Babatunde, O.O.; Jordan, J.L.; Van Der Windt, D.A.; Hill, J.C.; Foster, N.E.; Protheroe, J. Effective treatment options for musculoskeletal pain in primary care: A systematic overview of current evidence. *PLoS ONE* **2017**, 12. [CrossRef]
6. Dietrich, A. Endocannabinoids and exercise. *Br. J. Sports Med.* **2004**, *38*, 536–541. [CrossRef]
7. Goldfarb, A.H.; Jamurtas, A.Z. Beta-Endorphin Response to Exercise—An update. *Sports Med.* **1997**, *24*, 8–16. [CrossRef]
8. Naugle, K.M.; Fillingim, R.B.; Riley, J.L., III. A meta-analytic review of the hypoalgesic effects of exercise. *J. Pain* **2012**, *13*, 1139–1150. [CrossRef]
9. Booth, J.; Moseley, G.L.; Schiltenwolf, M.; Cashin, A.; Davies, M.; Hübscher, M. Exercise for chronic musculoskeletal pain: A biopsychosocial approach. *Musculoskelet. Care* **2017**, *15*, 413–421. [CrossRef]
10. Smith, B.E.; Hendrick, P.; Bateman, M.; Holden, S.; Littlewood, C.; Smith, T.O.; Logan, P. Musculoskeletal pain and exercise-challenging existing paradigms and introducing new. *Br. J. Sports Med.* **2019**, *53*, 907–912. [CrossRef]
11. La Touche, R.; Fernández Pérez, J.J.; Proy Acosta, A.; González Campodónico, L.; Martínez García, S.; Adraos Juárez, D.; Serrano García, B.; Angulo-Díaz-Parreño, S.; Cuenca-Martínez, F.; Suso-Martí, L.; et al. Is aerobic exercise helpful in patients with migraine? A systematic review and meta-analysis. *Scand. J. Med. Sci. Sports* **2020**, *30*, 965–982. [CrossRef] [PubMed]
12. Hakansson, S.; Jones, M.D.; Ristov, M.; Marcos, L.; Clark, T.; Ram, A.; Morey, R.; Franklin, A.; McCarthy, C.; Carli, L.D.; et al. Intensity-dependent effects of aerobic training on pressure pain threshold in overweight men: A randomized trial. *Eur. J. Pain* **2018**, *22*, 1813–1823. [CrossRef] [PubMed]
13. O'Leary, T.J.; Collett, J.; Howells, K.; Morris, M.G. High but not moderate-intensity endurance training increases pain tolerance: A randomised trial. *Eur. J. Appl. Physiol.* **2017**, *117*, 2201–2210. [CrossRef] [PubMed]
14. Andreato, L.V. High-Intensity Interval Training: Methodological Considerations for Interpreting Results and Conducting Research. *Trends Endocrinol. Metab.* **2020**, *31*, 812–817. [CrossRef] [PubMed]
15. Atan, T.; Karavelioğlu, Y. Effectiveness of High-Intensity Interval Training vs Moderate-Intensity Continuous Training in Patients with Fibromyalgia: A Pilot Randomized Controlled Trial. *Arch. Phys. Med. Rehabil.* **2020**, *101*, 1865–1876. [CrossRef]
16. Sveaas, S.H.; Bilberg, A.; Berg, I.J.; Provan, S.A.; Rollefstad, S.; Semb, A.G.; Hagen, K.B.; Johansen, M.W.; Pedersen, E.; Dagfinrud, H. High intensity exercise for 3 months reduces disease activity in axial spondyloarthritis (axSpA): A multicentre randomised trial of 100 patients. *Br. J. Sports Med.* **2019**, *54*, 292–297. [CrossRef]
17. Verbrugghe, J.; Agten, A.; Stevens, S.; Hansen, D.; Demoulin, C.; Eijnde, B.O.; Vandenabeele, F.; Timmermans, A. Exercise Intensity Matters in Chronic Nonspecific Low Back Pain Rehabilitation. *Med. Sci. Sports Exerc.* **2019**, *51*, 2434–2442. [CrossRef]
18. Batacan, R.B.; Duncan, M.J.; Dalbo, V.J.; Tucker, P.S.; Fenning, A.S. Effects of high-intensity interval training on cardiometabolic health: A systematic review and meta-analysis of intervention studies. *Br. J. Sports Med.* **2017**, *51*, 494–503. [CrossRef]

19. Mugele, H.; Freitag, N.; Wilhelmi, J.; Yang, Y.; Cheng, S.; Bloch, W.; Schumann, M. High-intensity interval training in the therapy and aftercare of cancer patients: A systematic review with meta-analysis. *J. Cancer Surviv.* **2019**, *13*, 205–223. [CrossRef]
20. Weston, K.S.; Wisløff, U.; Coombes, J.S. High-intensity interval training in patients with lifestyle-induced cardiometabolic disease: A systematic review and meta-analysis. *Br. J. Sports Med.* **2014**, *48*, 1227–1234. [CrossRef]
21. Doury-Panchout, F.; Métivier, J.C.; Fouquet, B. VO2max in patients with chronic pain: The effect of a 4-week rehabilitation program. *Ann. Phys. Rehabil. Med.* **2014**, *57*, 1–10. [CrossRef] [PubMed]
22. Moher, D.; Liberati, A.; Tetzlaff, J.; Altman, D.G. Preferred reporting items for systematic reviews and meta-analyses: The PRISMA statement. *Int. J. Surg.* **2009**, *8*, 6.
23. Stone, P.W. Popping the (PICO) question in research and evidence-based practice. *Appl. Nurs. Res.* **2002**, *15*, 197–198. [CrossRef] [PubMed]
24. Terwee, C.B.; Jansma, E.P.; Riphagen, I.I.; de Vet, H.C.W. Development of a methodological PubMed search filter for finding studies on measurement properties of measurement instruments. *Qual. Life Res.* **2009**, *18*, 1115–1123. [CrossRef]
25. Shariff, S.Z.; Bejaimal, S.A.; Sontrop, J.M.; Iansavichus, A.V.; Haynes, R.B.; Weir, M.A.; Garg, A.X. Retrieving clinical evidence: A comparison of PubMed and Google Scholar for quick clinical searches. *J. Med. Internet Res.* **2013**, *15*, e164. [CrossRef]
26. Haddaway, N.R.; Collins, A.M.; Coughlin, D.; Kirk, S. The Role of Google Scholar in Evidence Reviews and Its Applicability to Grey Literature Searching. *PLoS ONE* **2015**, *10*, e0138237. [CrossRef]
27. Moher, D.; Pham, B.; Jones, A.; Cook, D.J.; Jadad, A.R.; Moher, M.; Tugwell, P.; Klassen, T.P. Does quality of reports of randomised trials affect estimates of intervention efficacy reported in meta-analyses? *Lancet* **1998**, *352*, 609–613. [CrossRef]
28. Kwon, Y.; Lemieux, M.; McTavish, J.; Wathen, N. Identifying and removing duplicate records from systematic review searches. *J. Med. Libr. Assoc.* **2015**, *103*, 184–188. [CrossRef]
29. Furlan, A.D.; Pennick, V.; Bombardier, C.; van Tulder, M. 2009 updated method guidelines for systematic reviews in the Cochrane Back Review Group. *Spine* **2009**, *34*, 1929–1941. [CrossRef]
30. Higgins, J.; Green, S. *Cochrane Handbook for Systematic Reviews of Interventions*; Version 5.1.0[M]; Wiley-Blackwell: Hoboken, NJ, USA, 2008.
31. de Morton, N.A. The PEDro scale is a valid measure of the methodological quality of clinical trials: A demographic study. *Aust. J. Physiother.* **2009**, *55*, 129–133. [CrossRef]
32. Hariohm, K.; Prakash, V.; Saravankumar, J. Quantity and quality of randomized controlled trials published by Indian physiotherapists. *Perspect. Clin. Res.* **2015**, *6*, 91. [CrossRef] [PubMed]
33. Landis, J.R.; Koch, G.G. An Application of Hierarchical Kappa-type Statistics in the Assessment of Majority Agreement among Multiple Observers. *Biometrics* **1977**, *33*, 363. [CrossRef] [PubMed]
34. Guyatt, G.H.; Oxman, A.D.; Vist, G.E.; Kunz, R.; Falck-Ytter, Y.; Alonso-Coello, P.; Schünemann, H.J. GRADE Working Group GRADE: An emerging consensus on rating quality of evidence and strength of recommendations. *BMJ* **2008**, *336*, 924–926. [CrossRef] [PubMed]
35. Andrews, J.; Guyatt, G.; Oxman, A.D.; Alderson, P.; Dahm, P.; Falck-Ytter, Y.; Nasser, M.; Meerpohl, J.; Post, P.N.; Kunz, R.; et al. GRADE guidelines: 14. Going from evidence to recommendations: The significance and presentation of recommendations. *J. Clin. Epidemiol.* **2013**, *66*, 719–725. [CrossRef]
36. Balshem, H.; Helfand, M.; Schünemann, H.J.; Oxman, A.D.; Kunz, R.; Brozek, J.; Vist, G.E.; Falck-Ytter, Y.; Meerpohl, J.; Norris, S.; et al. GRADE guidelines: 3. Rating the quality of evidence. *J. Clin. Epidemiol.* **2011**, *64*, 401–406. [CrossRef]
37. Sanabria, A.J.; Rigau, D.; Rotaeche, R.; Selva, A.; Marzo-Castillejo, M.; Alonso-Coello, P. GRADE: Methodology for formulating and grading recommendations in clinical practice. *Aten. Primaria* **2015**, *47*, 48–55. [CrossRef] [PubMed]
38. Barendregt, J.J.; Doi, S.A. *MetaXL User Guide Version 5.3*; EpiGear International Pty Ltd.: Brisbane, Australia, 2016.
39. Hedges, L. Estimation of effect size from a series of independent experiments. *Psychol. Bull.* **1982**, *92*, 490–499. [CrossRef]
40. Hopkins, W.G.; Marshall, S.W.; Batterham, A.M.; Hanin, J. Progressive statistics for studies in sports medicine and exercise science. *Med. Sci. Sports Exerc.* **2009**, *41*, 3–13. [CrossRef]
41. Huedo-Medina, T.B.; Sánchez-Meca, J.; Marín-Martínez, F.; Botella, J. Assessing heterogeneity in meta-analysis: Q statistic or I^2 index? *Psychol. Methods* **2006**, *11*, 193–206. [CrossRef]
42. Doi, S.A. Rendering the Doi plot properly in meta-analysis. *Int. J. Evid. Based. Healthc.* **2018**, *16*, 242–243. [CrossRef]
43. Furuya-Kanamori, L.; Barendregt, J.J.; Doi, S.A.R. A new improved graphical and quantitative method for detecting bias in meta-analysis. *Int. J. Evid. Based. Healthc.* **2018**, *16*, 195–203. [CrossRef] [PubMed]
44. Suurmond, R.; van Rhee, H.; Hak, T. Introduction, comparison, and validation of Meta-Essentials: A free and simple tool for meta-analysis. *Res. Synth. Methods* **2017**, *8*, 537–553. [CrossRef] [PubMed]
45. Bressel, E.; Wing, J.E.; Miller, A.I.; Dolny, D.G. High-intensity interval training on an aquatic treadmill in adults with osteoarthritis: Effect on pain, balance, function, and mobility. *J. Strength Cond. Res.* **2014**, *28*, 2088–2096. [CrossRef] [PubMed]
46. Keogh, J.W.; Grigg, J.; Vertullo, C.J. Is high-intensity interval cycling feasible and more beneficial than continuous cycling for knee osteoarthritic patients? Results of a randomised control feasibility trial. *PeerJ* **2018**, *6*, e4738. [CrossRef] [PubMed]
47. Sveaas, S.H.; Berg, I.J.; Provan, S.A.; Semb, A.G.; Hagen, K.B.; Vøllestad, N.; Fongen, C.; Olsen, I.C.; Michelsen, A.; Ueland, T.; et al. Efficacy of high intensity exercise on disease activity and cardiovascular risk in active axial spondyloarthritis: A randomized controlled pilot study. *PLoS ONE* **2014**, *9*, e108688. [CrossRef] [PubMed]

48. Verbrugghe, J.; Agten, A.; Eijnde, B.O.; Olivieri, E.; Huybrechts, X.; Seelen, H.; Vandenabeele, F.; Timmermans, A. Feasibility of high intensity training in nonspecific chronic low back pain: A clinical trial. *J. Back Musculoskelet. Rehabil.* **2018**, *31*, 657–666. [CrossRef] [PubMed]
49. Verbrugghe, J.; Agten, A.; Stevens, S.; Hansen, D.; Demoulin, C.; Eijnde, B.O.; Vandenabeele, F.; Timmermans, A. High Intensity Training to Treat Chronic Nonspecific Low Back Pain: Effectiveness of Various Exercise Modes. *J. Clin. Med.* **2020**, *9*, 2401. [CrossRef]
50. Hanssen, H.; Minghetti, A.; Magon, S.; Rossmeissl, A.; Rasenack, M.; Papadopoulou, A.; Klenk, C.; Faude, O.; Zahner, L.; Sprenger, T.; et al. Effects of different endurance exercise modalities on migraine days and cerebrovascular health in episodic migraineurs: A randomized controlled trial. *Scand. J. Med. Sci. Sports* **2018**, *28*, 1103–1112. [CrossRef]
51. Berg, O.K.; Paulsberg, F.; Brabant, C.; Arabsolghar, K.; Ronglan, S.; BjØrnsen, N.; TØrhaug, T.; Granviken, F.; Gismervik, S.; Hoff, J. High-Intensity Shoulder Abduction Exercise in Subacromial Pain Syndrome. *Med. Sci. Sports Exerc.* **2020**, *53*, 1–9. [CrossRef]
52. Sandstad, J.; Stensvold, D.; Hoff, M.; Nes, B.M.; Arbo, I.; Bye, A. The effects of high intensity interval training in women with rheumatic disease: A pilot study. *Eur. J. Appl. Physiol.* **2015**, *115*, 2081–2089. [CrossRef]
53. Flehr, A.; Barton, C.; Coles, J.; Gibson, S.J.; Lambert, G.W.; Lambert, E.A.; Dhar, A.K.; Dixon, J.B. #MindinBody—Feasibility of vigorous exercise (Bikram yoga versus high intensity interval training) to improve persistent pain in women with a history of trauma: A pilot randomized control trial. *BMC Complement. Altern. Med.* **2019**, *19*, 234.
54. Thomsen, R.S.; Nilsen, T.I.L.; Haugeberg, G.; Bye, A.; Kavanaugh, A.; Hoff, M. Impact of High Intensity Interval Training on Disease Activity and Disease in Patients with Psoriatic Arthritis: A Randomized Controlled Trial. *Arthritis Care Res.* **2019**, *71*, 530–537. [CrossRef] [PubMed]
55. Palma, S.; Hasenoehrl, T.; Jordakieva, G.; Ramazanova, D.; Crevenna, R. High-intensity interval training in the prehabilitation of cancer patients—A systematic review and meta-analysis. *Support. Care Cancer* **2021**, *29*, 1781–1794. [CrossRef]
56. Milanović, Z.; Sporiš, G.; Weston, M. Effectiveness of High-Intensity Interval Training (HIT) and Continuous Endurance Training for VO2max Improvements: A Systematic Review and Meta-Analysis of Controlled Trials. *Sports Med.* **2015**, *45*, 1469–1481. [CrossRef]
57. Ramos, J.S.; Dalleck, L.C.; Tjonna, A.E.; Beetham, K.S.; Coombes, J.S. The impact of high-intensity interval training versus moderate-intensity continuous training on vascular function: A systematic review and meta-analysis. *Sports Med.* **2015**, *45*, 679–692. [CrossRef] [PubMed]
58. Gibala, M. Molecular responses to high-intensity interval exercise. *Appl. Physiol. Nutr. Metab.* **2009**, *34*, 428–432. [CrossRef] [PubMed]
59. MacInnis, M.J.; Gibala, M.J. Physiological adaptations to interval training and the role of exercise intensity. *J. Physiol.* **2017**, *595*, 2915–2930. [CrossRef] [PubMed]
60. Belviranli, M.; Okudan, N.; Kabak, B. The Effects of Acute High-Intensity Interval Training on Hematological Parameters in Sedentary Subjects. *Med. Sci.* **2017**, *5*, 15. [CrossRef]
61. Huang, Y.-C.; Tsai, H.-H.; Fu, T.-C.; Hsu, C.-C.; Wang, J.-S. High-Intensity Interval Training Improves Left Ventricular Contractile Function. *Med. Sci. Sports Exerc.* **2019**, *51*, 1420–1428. [CrossRef]
62. Lundby, C.; Montero, D.; Joyner, M. Biology of VO(2) max: Looking under the physiology lamp. *Acta Physiol.* **2017**, *220*, 218–228. [CrossRef]
63. Kaminsky, L.A.; Arena, R.; Ellingsen, Ø.; Harber, M.P.; Myers, J.; Ozemek, C.; Ross, R. Cardiorespiratory fitness and cardiovascular disease—The past, present, and future. *Prog. Cardiovasc. Dis.* **2019**, *62*, 86–93. [CrossRef] [PubMed]
64. Kodama, S.; Saito, K.; Tanaka, S.; Maki, M.; Yachi, Y.; Asumi, M.; Sugawara, A.; Totsuka, K.; Shimano, H.; Ohashi, Y.; et al. Cardiorespiratory fitness as a quantitative predictor of all-cause mortality and cardiovascular events in healthy men and women: A meta-analysis. *JAMA* **2009**, *301*, 2024–2035. [CrossRef] [PubMed]
65. Williams, A.; Kamper, S.J.; Wiggers, J.H.; O'Brien, K.M.; Lee, H.; Wolfenden, L.; Yoong, S.L.; Robson, E.; McAuley, J.H.; Hartvigsen, J.; et al. Musculoskeletal conditions may increase the risk of chronic disease: A systematic review and meta-analysis of cohort studies. *BMC Med.* **2018**, *16*, 167. [CrossRef] [PubMed]
66. Fayaz, A.; Ayis, S.; Panesar, S.S.; Langford, R.M.; Donaldson, L.J. Assessing the relationship between chronic pain and cardiovascular disease: A systematic review and meta-analysis. *Scand. J. pain* **2016**, *13*, 76–90. [CrossRef]
67. Imboden, M.T.; Harber, M.P.; Whaley, M.H.; Finch, W.H.; Bishop, D.L.; Fleenor, B.S.; Kaminsky, L.A. The Association between the Change in Directly Measured Cardiorespiratory Fitness across Time and Mortality Risk. *Prog. Cardiovasc. Dis.* **2019**, *62*, 157–162. [CrossRef]
68. Laukkanen, J.A.; Zaccardi, F.; Khan, H.; Kurl, S.; Jae, S.Y.; Rauramaa, R. Long-term Change in Cardiorespiratory Fitness and All-Cause Mortality: A Population-Based Follow-up Study. *Mayo Clin. Proc.* **2016**, *91*, 1183–1188. [CrossRef]
69. Geneen, L.J.; Moore, R.A.; Clarke, C.; Martin, D.; Colvin, L.A.; Smith, B.H. Physical activity and exercise for chronic pain in adults: An overview of Cochrane Reviews. In *Cochrane Database of Systematic Reviews*; Geneen, L.J., Ed.; John Wiley & Sons, Ltd: Chichester, UK, 2017; Volume 4, p. CD011279.
70. Rice, D.; Nijs, J.; Kosek, E.; Wideman, T.; Hasenbring, M.I.; Koltyn, K.; Graven-Nielsen, T.; Polli, A. Exercise-Induced Hypoalgesia in Pain-Free and Chronic Pain Populations: State of the Art and Future Directions. *J. Pain* **2019**, *20*, 1249–1266. [CrossRef]
71. Sluka, K.A.; Frey-Law, L.; Hoeger Bement, M. Exercise-induced pain and analgesia? Underlying mechanisms and clinical translation. *Pain* **2018**, *159* (Suppl. S1), S91–S97. [CrossRef]

72. Nijs, J.; George, S.Z.; Clauw, D.J.; Fernández-de-las-Peñas, C.; Kosek, E.; Ickmans, K.; Fernández-Carnero, J.; Polli, A.; Kapreli, E.; Huysmans, E.; et al. Central sensitisation in chronic pain conditions: Latest discoveries and their potential for precision medicine. *Lancet Rheumatol.* **2021**, *3*, e383–e392. [CrossRef]
73. Mijwel, S.; Backman, M.; Bolam, K.A.; Olofsson, E.; Norrbom, J.; Bergh, J.; Sundberg, C.J.; Wengström, Y.; Rundqvist, H. Highly favorable physiological responses to concurrent resistance and high-intensity interval training during chemotherapy: The OptiTrain breast cancer trial. *Breast Cancer Res. Treat.* **2018**, *169*, 93–103. [CrossRef]
74. van den Berg, R.; Jongbloed, E.M.; de Schepper, E.I.T.; Bierma-Zeinstra, S.M.A.; Koes, B.W.; Luijsterburg, P.A.J. The association between pro-inflammatory biomarkers and nonspecific low back pain: A systematic review. *Spine J.* **2018**, *18*, 2140–2151. [CrossRef] [PubMed]
75. Farrell, S.F.; de Zoete, R.M.J.; Cabot, P.J.; Sterling, M. Systemic inflammatory markers in neck pain: A systematic review with meta-analysis. *Eur. J. Pain* **2020**, *24*, 1666–1686. [CrossRef] [PubMed]
76. DeVon, H.A.; Piano, M.R.; Rosenfeld, A.G.; Hoppensteadt, D.A. The Association of Pain with Protein Inflammatory Biomarkers: A Review of the Literature. *Nurs. Res.* **2014**, *63*, 51–62. [CrossRef]
77. Adams, S.C.; DeLorey, D.S.; Davenport, M.H.; Stickland, M.K.; Fairey, A.S.; North, S.; Szczotka, A.; Courneya, K.S. Effects of high-intensity aerobic interval training on cardiovascular disease risk in testicular cancer survivors: A phase 2 randomized controlled trial. *Cancer* **2017**, *123*, 4057–4065. [CrossRef] [PubMed]
78. Khalafi, M.; Symonds, M.E. The impact of high-intensity interval training on inflammatory markers in metabolic disorders: A meta-analysis. *Scand. J. Med. Sci. Sports* **2020**, *30*, 2020–2036. [CrossRef] [PubMed]
79. Steckling, F.M.; Farinha, J.B.; da Cunha Figueiredo, F.; Dos Santos, D.L.; Bresciani, G.; Kretzmann, N.A.; Stefanello, S.T.; Courtes, A.A.; de Oliveira Beck, M.; Sangoi Cardoso, M.; et al. High-intensity interval training improves inflammatory and adipokine profiles in postmenopausal women with metabolic syndrome. *Arch. Physiol. Biochem.* **2019**, *125*, 85–91. [CrossRef]
80. Nunes, P.R.P.; Martins, F.M.; Souza, A.P.; Carneiro, M.A.S.; Orsatti, C.L.; Michelin, M.A.; Murta, E.F.C.; de Oliveira, E.P.; Orsatti, F.L. Effect of high-intensity interval training on body composition and inflammatory markers in obese postmenopausal women: A randomized controlled trial. *Menopause* **2019**, *26*, 256–264. [CrossRef]
81. Zwetsloot, K.A.; John, C.S.; Lawrence, M.M.; Battista, R.A.; Shanely, R.A. High-intensity interval training induces a modest systemic inflammatory response in active, young men. *J. Inflamm. Res.* **2014**, *7*, 9–17. [CrossRef]
82. Pedersen, B.K. Anti-inflammatory effects of exercise: Role in diabetes and cardiovascular disease. *Eur. J. Clin. Investig.* **2017**, *47*, 600–611. [CrossRef]
83. Shanaki, M.; Khosravi, M.; Khoshdooni-Farahani, A.; Dadashi, A.; Heydari, M.F.; Delfan, M.; Jafary, H.; Gorgani-Firuzjaee, S. High-Intensity Interval Training Reversed High-Fat Diet-Induced M1-Macrophage Polarization in Rat Adipose Tissue via Inhibition of NOTCH Signaling. *J. Inflamm. Res.* **2020**, *13*, 165–174. [CrossRef]
84. Eslami, R.; Parnow, A.; Pairo, Z.; Nikolaidis, P.; Knechtle, B. The effects of two different intensities of aerobic training protocols on pain and serum neuro-biomarkers in women migraineurs: A randomized controlled trail. *Eur. J. Appl. Physiol.* **2021**, *121*, 609–620. [CrossRef] [PubMed]
85. Lamé, I.E.; Peters, M.L.; Vlaeyen, J.W.S.; Kleef, M.v.; Patijn, J. Quality of life in chronic pain is more associated with beliefs about pain, than with pain intensity. *Eur. J. Pain* **2005**, *9*, 15–24. [CrossRef] [PubMed]
86. Monticone, M.; Ferrante, S.; Rocca, B.; Baiardi, P.; Farra, F.D.; Foti, C. Effect of a long-lasting multidisciplinary program on disability and fear-avoidance behaviors in patients with chronic low back pain: Results of a randomized controlled trial. *Clin. J. Pain* **2013**, *29*, 929–938. [CrossRef] [PubMed]
87. Kamper, S.J.; Apeldoorn, A.T.; Chiarotto, A.; Smeets, R.J.E.M.; Ostelo, R.W.J.G.; Guzman, J.; van Tulder, M.W. Multidisciplinary biopsychosocial rehabilitation for chronic low back pain: Cochrane systematic review and meta-analysis. *BMJ* **2015**, *350*, h444. [CrossRef]
88. Veldhuijzen van Zanten, J.J.C.S.; Rouse, P.C.; Hale, E.D.; Ntoumanis, N.; Metsios, G.S.; Duda, J.L.; Kitas, G.D. Perceived Barriers, Facilitators and Benefits for Regular Physical Activity and Exercise in Patients with Rheumatoid Arthritis: A Review of the Literature. *Sports Med.* **2015**, *45*, 1401–1412. [CrossRef]
89. Boutevillain, L.; Dupeyron, A.; Rouch, C.; Richard, E.; Coudeyre, E. Facilitators and barriers to physical activity in people with chronic low back pain: A qualitative study. *PLoS ONE* **2017**, *12*, e0179826. [CrossRef]
90. McPhail, S.M.; Schippers, M.; Marshall, A.L.; Waite, M.; Kuipers, P. Perceived barriers and facilitators to increasing physical activity among people with musculoskeletal disorders: A qualitative investigation to inform intervention development. *Clin. Interv. Aging* **2014**, *9*, 2113–2122. [CrossRef]
91. Wewege, M.A.; Ahn, D.; Yu, J.; Liou, K.; Keech, A. High-Intensity Interval Training for Patients with Cardiovascular Disease-Is It Safe? A Systematic Review. *J. Am. Heart Assoc.* **2018**, *7*, e009305. [CrossRef]
92. Heisz, J.J.; Tejada, M.G.M.; Paolucci, E.M.; Muir, C. Enjoyment for High-Intensity Interval Exercise Increases during the First Six Weeks of Training: Implications for Promoting Exercise Adherence in Sedentary Adults. *PLoS ONE* **2016**, *11*, e0168534. [CrossRef]
93. American Thoracic Society; American College of Chest Physicians. ATS/ACCP Statement on cardiopulmonary exercise testing. *Am. J. Respir. Crit. Care Med.* **2003**, *167*, 211–277. [CrossRef]

MDPI AG
Grosspeteranlage 5
4052 Basel
Switzerland
Tel.: +41 61 683 77 34

Diagnostics Editorial Office
E-mail: diagnostics@mdpi.com
www.mdpi.com/journal/diagnostics

www.ingramcontent.com/pod-product-compliance
Lightning Source LLC
Chambersburg PA
CBHW061609210926
51850CB00009B/2268
9783725863020